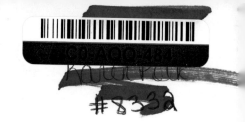

# HANDBOOK OF
## COMMUNITY HEALTH NURSING

**Dorothy D. Petrowski, R.N., Ph.D.,** is a community health nurse who received her diploma in nursing from Swedish Hospital in Minneapolis, B.S. in nursing cum laude from Loyola University in Chicago, M.P.H. from the University of Michigan, and Ph.D. in education from the University of Maryland. She completed theory and practice courses at West Virginia University to prepare herself as a family nurse practitioner. Since 1978, she has been an associate professor at the University of Wisconsin-Milwaukee, where she teaches in a community-based masters and the undergraduate program. Earlier she became the chairperson of the Masters Program in Community Health Nursing at the Catholic University of America, and assisted in the development of and taught in a community masters program that prepared family nurse practitioners at West Virginia University. She had also been a supervisor at the county health department in Ann Arbor, Michigan and at the outpatient department in Chicago Lying-In Hospital. While pursuing doctoral studies in the 1970s, she served as a part-time staff nurse at the Visiting Nurse Association in the District of Columbia. She has done research in curriculum evaluation, widowhood, and alcoholism.

# HANDBOOK OF
# COMMUNITY HEALTH NURSING

## Essentials for Clinical Practice

Dorothy D. Petrowski, R.N., Ph.D.

with contributors

*Foreword by Ruth B. Freeman, R.N., Ed.D.*

## Springer Publishing Company
New York

Springer Publishing Company, Inc.
200 Park Avenue South
New York, New York 10003

84  85  86  87  88  /  10  9  8  7  6  5  4  3  2  1

---

*Library of Congress Cataloging in Publication Data*

Petrowski, Dorothy D.
  Handbook of community health nursing.
  Includes bibliographies and index.
   1. Community health nursing—Handbooks, manuals, etc.   I. Title.   [DNLM: 1. Com-
munity health nursing—Handbooks.   2. Family—Nursing texts.   3. Family health. WY
106 P497h]
RT98.P47   1983        610.73′43        83-16767
ISBN 0-8261-4210-9

---

Printed in the United States of America

This book is affectionately dedicated to my sister,
Mabel Margeret Erion, who devotedly reared
our large family after Mother's early death.

# Contents

# Foreword

Public health nursing and health care generally interact in the effort to serve the community, but as health services expand, the many facets of care need extended and more detailed identification.

This book on community health nursing focuses on clinical nursing care. It covers many of the situations that community health nurses and nurse practitioners face daily, and, as such, complements other community health nursing textbooks. It should well serve students and practicing nurses in the field of community health both in the United States and the rest of the world.

The author, a family nurse practitioner with long and varied experience in providing nursing care and supervision to staff nurses, instructing students, and administering an educational program in community health, combines a scientific and a practical approach. Her additional preparation in education enhances the health education aspects of the book, particularly in the areas of teaching clients and families prevention and wellness, self-care strategies, nursing care, and rehabilitation.

Ruth B. Freeman, R.N., Ed.D.
Professor Emerita
School of Hygiene and Preventive Medicine
Johns Hopkins University
December 5, 1906–December 2, 1982

# Preface

This book was initially conceived when I worked with students in clinical settings in community health. Often my students and I perceived the need for a general reference for nursing care in nonacute settings as we organized our assignments. This volume treats clinical nursing care by the age groups of clients, from conception to death, and includes both wellness and illness. Treatment in home and clinic settings is discussed in each chapter. Additional settings are discussed as appropriate for the various age groups, such as the nursery school for the preschooler, public school for the child and adolescent, the place of work for the young through the middle-aged, and the nursing home for the elderly.

The first chapter outlines the development, definition, and scope of community health nursing practice and the need for community health nursing services. Chapters 2 through 9, following the age continuum, discuss representative clinical nursing care for each age group, with a description of clinical manifestations or characteristics of an illness or health problem and the appropriate nursing care. The last chapter is devoted to terminal illness and death in both the home and hospice settings.

Much emphasis is placed on including wellness and the family in nursing care for maximum benefit to both client and family. Discussions of such topics as nursing care in occupational settings, university health services, and hospices, and current research on specific illnesses, remind the reader that nursing is an ever-changing arena of practice. While recognizing that not all nurses are female, I have simplified the language in this volume by usually using the feminine pronouns in referring to them; similarly, masculine pronouns are used to refer to clients (except in cases that could apply only to women, such as maternity or breast cancer). Suggestions from readers would help to make future editions even more useful.

DOROTHY D. PETROWSKI

# Acknowledgments

I gratefully acknowledge the assistance and support of several friends, colleagues, and relatives who greatly facilitated the preparation of this book. First, I am deeply indebted to Bob Dreher, a friend, for comprehensive editorial assistance throughout the preparation of the manuscript. Nancy Evans, a professional editor and writer, provided valued inspiration at the beginning of the undertaking.

Art Jacknowitz, Associate Professor of Clinical Pharmacy and Director of Drug Information at the West Virginia Medical Center, advised on drug therapies for coronary heart disease and diabetes mellitus. Mary Gainer, graphic artist at the University of Wisconsin–Milwaukee, did most of the original line drawings. Ronald Titkofsky, Professor of Speech Pathology and Audiology at the University of Wisconsin–Milwaukee, critiqued the section on speech therapy for the client with a cerebral vascular accident (CVA). Still another faculty member from the University of Wisconsin–Milwaukee—Kathleen Cowles, Assistant Professor of Nursing—gave assistance by supplying information about dying and death. Margaret Christianson, a public health nutritionist with the Milwaukee school system, provided information about nutrition for infants and clients with diabetes and hypertension. Two community health nurses, Caroline Charonko and Ann Riojas, contributed to Chapter 6.

I also wish to thank Kathleen Gordon of Milwaukee, who ably typed many versions of the manuscript (sometimes at late hours), and my editor at Springer, Barbara Watkins, for her suggestions on content and editing skill. And, lastly, I thank my family—especially my brother, the Reverend Lester Dumer, and my sister, Vivian Ninke, who encouraged me many times and in various ways. To these persons, as well as to others who helped in the preparation of the manuscript, I express my gratitude.

# Contributors

**Marion Mendelsohn Coleman, R.N., M.S.N.,** pediatric nurse practitioner; formerly with the Pediatric Clinic, University of Massachusetts Medical Center, Worcester, Massachusetts

**Patricia Kachelmeyer, R.N., M.S.N.,** Assistant Professor, School of Nursing, University of Wisconsin–Milwaukee, Milwaukee, Wisconsin

**Karen E. Miles, R.N., M.S.N.,** Assistant Professor and Family Nurse Practitioner, School of Nursing, West Virginia University, Morgantown, West Virginia; doctoral candidate, School of Education, Department of Educational Psychology, West Virginia University

**Charlene C. Ossler, R.N.C., M.S.N., M.P.H.,** Assistant Professor, School of Public Health, University of North Carolina, Chapel Hill, North Carolina; doctoral candidate, School of Public Health and Hygiene, Johns Hopkins University, Baltimore, Maryland

**Helen L. Swain, R.N., Ph.D.,** Professor, School of Nursing, University of Wisconsin–Milwaukee, Milwaukee, Wisconsin

**Charlene Tosi, R.N., M.S.,** school nurse consultant; Assistant Professor, School of Nursing, University of Wisconsin–Milwaukee, Milwaukee, Wisconsin

**Phyllis Tyzenhouse, R.N., D.P.H.,** epidemiologist and geriatric nurse practitioner; Associate Professor and Chairperson, Department of Community Health Nursing, Virginia Commonwealth University, Medical College of Virginia, Richmond, Virginia

# HANDBOOK OF
## COMMUNITY HEALTH NURSING

# 1

# Introduction to Clinical Nursing for Community Health Practice

*Dorothy D. Petrowski*

## Introduction

Most clinical nursing textbooks have traditionally focused on hospital care and acute care interventions; the duties and problems of the community health nurse (CHN) are discussed in a few paragraphs at the end of a chapter, if at all. Such a text is inadequate for a nurse practicing outside of a hospital because of the wide range of concerns and responsibilities in community health nursing.

The past two decades have brought a merging of public health science and nursing under the common title of "community health nursing." In some schools, it has been further integrated into nursing theory and practice courses in the baccalaureate curriculum. The textbooks offered thus far for CHNs contain much of the original public health science and treat nursing care with a general focus. Such books are needed, but the specifics of clinical nursing must be addressed also. This textbook, specifically designed for the CHN, is intended to help fill the void of clinical nursing content and to be useful in both traditional and integrated nursing curricula. The book focuses on clinical nursing assessment and intervention along the age continuum in nonacute settings—private homes, clinics, public schools, colleges, nursing homes, and industrial establishments; both wellness and illness are discussed in relation to each age and setting.

This chapter reviews briefly the development of community health nursing during the past century, providing a perspective for a better understanding of modern nursing practiced outside the hospital. "Clinical nursing" and "community health nursing" are defined. The advent of the nurse practitioner (NP) and the expansion of nursing skills are discussed, because these movements began in community health nursing practice and caused significant changes.

## The Development of Community Health Nursing and Its Influence on Today's Practice

The advent of modern nursing is usually traced to the establishment of the Nightingale Training School for Nurses in 1860 at St. Thomas Hospital in London, but visiting nursing actually began a year earlier in Liverpool, England, when William Rathbone founded the first visiting nurse association. These nurses cared for patients of all socioeconomic levels in their homes as well as in the Royal Liverpool Infirmary (Dolan, 1973). Florence Nightingale, who also trained visiting nurses, coined the phrase "health nursing" (as distinguished from "sick" nursing or hospital nursing) to emphasize health promotion (Brainard, 1922).

In the United States, visiting nursing started in 1886 with the Instructive District Nurse Association of Boston, which gave as much emphasis to health education as to bedside care (Brainard, 1922; Wald, 1915). In the early 1920s, the Town and Country Nursing Service of the American Red Cross developed rural and small-town public health nursing. In this same year, county and state health departments became active in public health nursing and, with the passage of the Sheppard-Towner Act in 1921, used allotted federal funds to reduce maternal and infant mortality (Gardner, 1948; Griffin & Griffin, 1973).

Although the terms "visiting nursing," "public health nursing," and "community health nursing" are used interchangeably, "visiting nursing" is the oldest and usually refers to nursing done by voluntary agencies such as visiting nurse associations (Wald originated the term "public health nursing" to distinguish it from private duty nursing). "Community health nursing" is a newer title, encompassing both visiting nursing and public health nursing, and including the addition of the new independent NPs.

The concept of an expanded role for nurses took concrete form in 1966 when public health nurses were prepared at the University of Colorado in physical assessment skills that heretofore had been done by pediatricians, this marking the beginning of the NP movement ("Colorado Studies Upgrading Public Health Nurse Skills," 1966).

## Definitions of Nursing, Clinical Nursing, and Community Health Nursing: Scope of Practice

Virginia Henderson's time-honored definition of "nursing" still provides an important part of nursing's theoretical framework. As she puts it, the unique function of the nurse is

> To assist the individual, sick or well, in the performance of those activities contributing to health, or its recovery (or to a peaceful death) that he would perform unaided if he had the necessary strength, will, or knowledge. It is likewise her function to help the individual gain independence as rapidly as possible. (Harmer & Henderson, 1960, p. 4)

"Clinical nursing" is defined as direct intervention with a client by a professional nurse in any setting. All interventions performed by practical nurses and nursing assistants under the supervision of a professional nurse are included. Observing, assessing or evaluating, diagnosing, treating, teaching, counseling, and serving as a client advocate are all part of clinical nursing and the nursing process.

Changes in the nurse practice acts in the past decade have officially recognized the role of the nurse in diagnosing and treating health problems. New York State was the first to reflect this expanded role with the 1972 revision of its Nurse Practice Act:

> The practice of the profession of nursing as a registered professional nurse is defined as diagnosing and treating human responses to actual or potential health problems, through such services as casefinding, health teaching, health counseling, and provision of care supportive to or restorative of life and well-being and executing medical regimes prescribed by a licensed or otherwise legally authorized physician or dentist. A nursing regimen shall be consistent with and shall not vary any existing medical regimen. (State of New York, 1972)

Community health nursing is defined as follows by the American Nurses' Association and the American Public Health Association (APHA):

> Community health nursing is a synthesis of nursing practice and public health practice applied to the promotion and preservation of the health

of the population. The nature of this practice is general and comprehensive, includes all ages and diagnostic groups, and is directed to individual clients, families and other groups and communities, thereby contributing to the nation's health. (American Public Health Association, 1980)

The major focuses of community health nursing are on the prevention of illness and the promotion and maintenance of health. Therefore, the scope of community health nursing practice includes the provision of needed therapeutic services, counseling, education, management, and advocacy activities. Another significant function is the provision of primary health care. "Primary health care" is defined as the client's first contact for a health problem, plus the needed follow-up, regardless of the presence or absence of organic disease. It includes the well, the "worried well," the presymptomatic patient, and the patient with a disease in the early symptomatic stage (Reynolds, 1975). It further includes the management of chronically ill clients with uncomplicated diseases. The CHN, therefore, has responsibility for the following:

1. Assessing the health status of the client.
2. Diagnosing on the basis of health status data.
3. Implementing health planning in accord with the diagnosis.
4. Involving the client in his care to maximize health potential.
5. Reassessing health practices.

It is important to note that much of this care is given in collaboration with other disciplines and the public (American Public Health Association, 1980).

## Inclusion of Nurse Practitioner Skills in Clinical Nursing

A nurse practitioner (NP) is defined as a professional nurse who usually works in association with a physician to provide primary health care to clients. Her main functions include physical assessment and exercising collaborative and independent judgment in health care management of clients (Chen, Barkauskas, Ohlson, & Chen, 1982). A certain degree of ambiguity presently exists in the definition of the NP's role and functions. Clinical nursing done by the baccalaureate graduate may include some nurse practitioner skills (primarily health assessment), while not requiring the American Nurses' Association's NP certification. Guidelines for health histories and physical assessment are included at the end of this textbook (Appendixes A and B), because the baccalaureate graduates who practice in community health settings perform them. Some of the activities listed may be too complex for the undergraduate student or beginning graduate, and she may require assistance from an NP. Although assessment skills are taught in most baccalaureate programs, there may be wide variation in the degree of expertise.

The development of the NP concept seemed to legitimize the role of CHNs, who had been functioning in an expanded role from necessity. In rural areas, where shortages of physicians were most acute, CHNs had been the primary care providers for entire population groups. Evidence that these nurses have been effective and acceptable to the people they treat has been documented by the success of the Frontier Nursing Service in Kentucky, which has a long history of serving communities at a level beyond the traditional scope of nursing.

A variety of NPs in a community setting serve as invaluable assets to the health care delivery system. The community NP may collaborate with a physician to staff a public health or rural health clinic. They may share clients for whom the nurse provides the majority of the primary care: health assessments, guidance and education. As a primary care provider in a less well-staffed area, the NP may be the *only* source for all levels of health care. The work of the pediatric NP is discussed in reference to the toddler in Chapter 4, and the contributions of the school and the gerontological NPs are outlined in Chapters 6 and 9, respectively.

## The Need for Community Health Nursing Services Today

Community health nursing services are essential today because of several factors:

1. Almost all categories of hospitalized patients are discharged earlier and often require CHN follow-up at home.
2. The maintenance of chronically or terminally ill clients at home necessitates supportive nursing services for both the clients and their significant others. Morbidity and mortality rates have changed significantly in the United States, since many of the

communicable diseases have been conquered. The three leading causes of death—heart disease, cancer, and stroke, accounting for 66% of all deaths—are especially prevalent among the ill at home.
3. The continuing high infant mortality rate in the United States (11.7 per 1000 live births in 1981), which gives this country the poor ranking of 14th among all nations in infant mortality, demands CHN intervention (National Center for Health Statistics, 1982a, 1982b).
4. Prevention occupies a more prominent place in community health than ever before. Since more people are living longer, it is imperative that they learn healthy ways to cope with life. Consumers have become more vocal and are demanding information about health and disease processes in order to prevent or minimize effects of disease.

This textbook specifically discusses the care of the following groups in nonacute care settings: (1) antepartum and postpartum mothers and their infants; (2) toddlers; (3) preschoolers; (4) school-age clients; (5) young adults; (6) the middle-aged; (7) the elderly; and (8) the dying. The nursing interventions include current practices in clinical and primary care where indicated.

## References

American Public Health Association. *The definition and role of public health nursing in the delivery of health care.* Washington, D.C.: Author, 1980.

Brainard, A. *The evolution of public health nursing.* Philadelphia: W. B. Saunders, 1922.

Chen, S. C., Barkauskas, V. H., Ohlson, V. M., & Chen, E. H. Health problems encountered by nurse practitioners and physicians. *Nursing Research,* 1982, *31,* 163–168.

Colorado studies upgrading public health nurse skills. *American Journal of Nursing,* 1966, *66,* 1480.

Dolan, J. A. *Nursing in society: A historical perspective* (13th ed.). Philadelphia: W. B. Saunders, 1973.

Gardner, M. S. *Public health nursing.* New York: Macmillan, 1948.

Griffin, J. G., & Griffin, J. K. *History and trends of professional nursing* (7th ed.). St. Louis: C. V. Mosby, 1973.

Harmer, B., & Henderson, V. *Textbook of the principles and practice of nursing.* New York: Macmillan, 1960.

National Center for Health Statistics. *Infant mortality rates: Selected countries from the 1978 yearbook of the United Nations.* Washington, D.C.: U.S. Department of Health and Human Services, 1982. (a)

National Center for Health Statistics. *Monthly vital statistics report* (Vol. 30, No. 12). Washington, D.C.: U.S. Department of Health and Human Services, 1982. (b)

Reynolds, R. J. Communications—primary care, ambulatory care, and family medicine: Overlapping but not synonymous. *Journal of Medical Education,* 1975, *50,* 893–895.

State of New York. The Nurse Practice Act of New York (Education Law, Article 139, Section 69021). Albany: Author, 1972.

Wald, L. D. *The house on Henry Street.* New York: Holt, 1915.

# 2

# The Prenatal and Postnatal Client

*Dorothy D. Petrowski*

## The Prenatal Client in the Clinic or the Physician's Office

### Introduction

When a woman suspects she is pregnant, she will usually make an appointment in a clinic, a neighborhood health center, or a doctor's office. Occasionally, a woman may seek the services of a certified nurse midwife (CNM), although this service is not now utilized in the United States as often as it is in many other countries. At the time of the appointment, the client is probably more than 2 months pregnant. The clinic nurse, who may or may not be a community health nurse (CHN), performs a variety of services for the client.

During the first clinic visit, a comprehensive health assessment of the client is accomplished. This assessment includes not only the obvious physical aspects, such as vital signs and general appearance, but factors related to the client's patterns of self-care, including nutrition, provision of exercise and rest, and personal hygiene. Of equal importance are the history and assessment of the client as a unique psychosocial being. An assessment of her ability to understand and comply with prescribed regimens and a review of her personal network of support are essential during this initial contact.

Establishment of rapport between the clinic nurse and the client promotes the client's ability and willingness to carry out prescribed health practices during her pregnancy. This is accomplished in a variety of ways, most important of which is the establishment of open communication. A willingness to listen to the client's concerns about her pregnancy and its possible impact on her and/or her family, and an ability to respond to even the simplest questions with a genuine regard for the integrity of the client, are necessary to the beginning of rapport.

If the clinic nurse is a CNM or a nurse practitioner (NP), she will frequently complete the entire health and physical assessments and review the findings with the clinic physician and the client. In a few clinics in the United States, it is the nurse, rather than the physician, who manages a major portion of the prenatal client's primary care. Medical consultation, however, is available and is utilized as necessary.

## Clinic Care

### Comprehensive prenatal assessment

The initial assessment should include a health history; physical and laboratory examinations; nutrition assessment; and social, psychological, and client education assessments. The CHN in the clinic is most likely to be involved with all aspects of this assessment, but more so with the prenatal health history and the nutrition, social, psychological, and client education assessments. If, however, she has NP skills, she also performs the physical examination. She should be acquainted with all aspects of prenatal clinic care in order to implement and evaluate the care. All assessments must include a provision that encourages the client, if she desires, to add to her information on any clinic visits. Guidelines for a comprehensive initial prenatal health assessment follow:

A. Health history (subjective data)
  1. Client profile
     a. Age, marital status, and family composition.
     b. Significant others and how they adjust to pregnancy and parenting.
     c. Smoking, alcohol consumption, and drug-taking habits.
  2. Prenatal history
     a. Progress of present pregnancy, listing gravid and parous status, last normal menstrual period, and any complaints such as spotting.
     b. Menstrual and contraceptive history, age at menarche, previous pregnancies and deliveries, and complications (if any).
     c. Previous illnesses—a checklist format that serves to help the

client remember past illnesses may be utilized.

    d. Review of body systems, noting any problems.

    e. Family history of health problems, particularly multiple pregnancies, cardiovascular problems, diabetes, epilepsy, congenital anomalies, hereditary diseases, and mental problems.

B. Physical and laboratory examination

An initial physical examination is done by an NP, a CNM, or a physician.

  1. Blood pressure examination.

  2. Weight check.

  3. Vaginal examination to check for discharges, and bimanual examination to estimate weeks of gestation.

  4. Pelvimetry done by physician or CNM.

  5. Abdominal examination for two purposes:

    a. Auscultation for fetal heart tones (FHTs) if the client is 18–22 weeks pregnant, using a fetoscope. The Doppler principle (Dopptone) can detect them earlier (at 11–16 weeks).

    b. Measurement of height of fundus from symphysis pubis to over top of the fundus to assist in determination of the gestational age. Then calculate using McDonald's rule: Height of fundus (in centimeters) $\times 8/7 =$ weeks of gestation (Jensen, Benson & Bobak, 1981).

  6. Laboratory analyses, including a complete examination of the urine and blood.

    a. Urine is examined for glucose, protein, and identification of significant bacteria.

    b. Blood is taken for hemoglobin, hematocrit, red cell index, and blood type tests; tests for abnormal antibodies, such as the Rh titer and rubella antibody titer; and a serologic test for syphilis, such as the Venereal Disease Research Laboratory (VDRL) blood test (Pritchard & MacDonald, 1976).

C. Nutrition assessment

This assessment is done to establish past and present deficiencies in the diet and to allow the client to inquire about the dietary changes required in pregnancy to her eating habits.

  1. Assessment of dietary intake.

  2. Identification of need for nutrition education.

  3. Identification of need for financial assistance.

D. Social assessment

The positive outcome of any pregnancy is related to the social network that each client has established before her pregnancy. The following should be assessed:

  1. Economic situation.

2. Occupation of pregnant woman and her partner.
3. Relationship with father of the baby.
4. Feelings about effect on avocation and vocation.
E. Psychological history and current status
   These should be assessed in terms of the following:
   1. Desirability of pregnancy by client and her partner.
   2. Feelings associated with pregnancy.
   3. Feelings about body image and sexuality.
   4. Patterns of self-care, both physical and emotional.

The client is instructed to return to the clinic on a predetermined schedule, unless there are complications or the client elects to come at other times for any reason. The client is usually seen monthly from the initial visit through the seventh month. Then she attends bimonthly during her eighth month and weekly thereafter until delivery. On subsequent clinic visits, specific observations and interventions are made about the client's health by the clinic nurse and/or physician. These should be altered to suit the individual client's unique problems. For example, she may be tearful, and the nurse may want to explore this further with her. Guidelines for subsequent clinic visits should include the following:

1. Investigate complaints and answer questions. Some unusual questions relate to such items as the stages of fetal development, counseling about sexual intercourse, and the validity of such old wives' tales as "lifting the arms above the head causes the umbilical cord to become wrapped around the baby's neck."
2. Weigh the client. She can safely gain 10–12 kg (22–27 pounds) if her weight at conception is normal. The American College of Obstetrics and Gynecology recommends a minimal weight gain in the first trimester and approximately 1 pound a week in the last two trimesters (International Childbirth Education Association, 1978). An average, steady weight gain would be approximately 2 to 3 pounds in the first trimester and a pound a week during the remainder of the pregnancy.
3. Record temperature, pulse, and respirations (TPR) to detect bladder and other infections.
4. Check blood pressure to detect signs of toxemia and hypertension.
5. Examine abdomen as recommended for the initial visit, with these three additions:
   a. Determination of fetal presentation utilizing abdominal palpation after the 24th week.

   b. Identification of fetal presentation, position, and station (en-
      gagement) at the 32nd week and following, utilizing ab-
      dominal palpations. The fundal height is measured and
      compared with the reported estimated date of confinement
      (EDC).
   c. Determination of FHTs; these can be heard by Doppler
      method at approximately the 10th week and with a feto-
      scope after the 18th.
6. Examine the mucosa via a vaginal examination in later weeks
   to confirm presenting part, station, and cervical effacement and
   dilatation. Leukorrhea caused by *Trichomonas vaginalis* and *Candida albicans* is investigated and treated. *Trichomonas vaginalis*,
   which thrives in an alkaline medium, is common in pregnancy. In pregnancy, the pH of the vagina changes from the nonpregnant acid range of 3.5 to 4.5 to about 7.
7. Test for glucose or albumen, neither of which should be present. Blood work is ordered as needed. A cervical culture for
   gonorrhea is done near term if this disease is prevalent in the
   population. Gonorrhea is treated to prevent Gonorrheal oph-
   thalmia (neonatorum).
8. Update history and physical, psychological, and social assessments as required.

*Implementation of clinic care*

Before leaving any clinic appointment, the client should be counseled in areas relative to the comprehensive prenatal assessment. Any
specific questions should be answered to her satisfaction. Some examples of anticipated problems relative to the clinic assessment are detailed here. Only one aspect has been selected from each clinical assessment area, because the implementation of health care is further
developed under the "Nursing Care at Home" section (see p. 15).
There is necessarily some overlap among assessment, implementation,
and evaluation of care in the clinic, home, and work settings. However,
this overlap may also be reinforcing for the client.
   *Health history—progressing with pregnancy.* If there is a problem
in coping with the pregnancy or if the pregnancy is unwanted, the CHN
should discuss this further with the client. The client may need additional time to discuss this with the obstetrician or NP. It may necessitate
referral to a mental health nurse clinician, psychiatric social worker,
psychologist, psychiatrist, or clergyman. The CHN may want to urge
the husband or significant other to spend more time with the client.
   *Physical and laboratory examinations—explanations about tests and pre-*

*scriptions.* All aspects of the physical and laboratory evaluations should be discussed with the client. The client should be told her blood pressure, her prospects for a normal pregnancy and delivery, outcomes of laboratory tests, and the beginning of FHTs. The reasons for prescribing medication should be explained. Prescriptions often include multiple vitamins, although many physicians feel these can be gotten through an adequate diet. There is some evidence that folic acid should be supplemented. Iron requirements are increased in pregnancy, so iron supplements are usually ordered in the least expensive form of ferrous sulfate (Pritchard & MacDonald, 1976). The client should be told to take no drug (prescription or nonprescription) that is not prescribed.

*Nutrition assessment.* This material is discussed in the "Nursing Care at Home" section (see pp. 15–22).

*Social assessment—financial counseling.* Clinics are usually located in hospitals where the fee is adjusted according to the client's ability to pay, ranging from no payment to full payment. A hospital-based social worker assists if the patient needs financial help. However, the CHN should be alert to the client's needs in this area and refer her to the county department of welfare and the state's Medicaid regulations in her locale if necessary. Costs of clinic, hospital, and CHN home visits should be reviewed. Usually the CHN visits are at no direct cost to the client because they are subsidized by government or United Way funding.

*Psychological assessment and promotion of psychological well-being.* The psychological care of the mother, newborn, father, and siblings is as important as the physical care the CHN provides. Much of the joy and satisfaction in planning a pregnancy, the pregnancy itself, labor, delivery, and the postpartal period are greater if the client is mentally healthy prior to conception. Past good physical health and present good hygienic measures are in great measure responsible for a noncrisis pregnancy. The significant male's positive role in the pregnancy plays a tremendous role in reducing stress. A woman's perception of herself influences the childbirth experience and depends to an extent upon her husband's perceptions of the event. When a mother's needs are met, she can better reach out to her baby, the rest of her family, and others.

The nurse provides psychological counseling adapted to what the client or her partner expresses, what the nurse thinks the client will accept, or what the physician recommends. Occasionally a client will not accept necessary protective or preventive measures. Then the CHN attempts to ascertain why and includes this in her nursing diagnosis. The client may lack motivation because of low self-esteem or some undetermined reason. Psychological well-being plays a considerable part in the client's acceptance of her pregnancy. The CHN can assess this by the client's mood, her willingness to cooperate with clinic routines, and her questions. If problems with pregnancy are recognized early, counseling by the CHN is usually sufficient, and referral to a psychologist, a mental health nurse clinician, or a psychiatrist is not needed. Examples of clients who may require counseling are those with unplanned pregnancies and those with many domestic problems.

*Client health education assessment.* The CHN should approach health education in terms of the client's perceptions of needed health care information and should mention alternatives. The CHN in the clinic can supply much of the health education—for instance, information about the importance of the prenatal clinic visits, normal fetal development, and crisis situations that may arise between clinic visits. Regular clinic visits are necessary to promote the health of mother and baby and to detect problems that may arise. Fetal development can be described with visual aids; allowing the mother to listen to the FHTs is also helpful. If the client contacts the clinic by telephone and describes a possible medical problem, the CHN usually asks the client to make an emergency clinic appointment. To enhance interaction with clinic personnel, informational tapes and literature can be placed in the waiting area.

## Referrals to Classes

### Childbirth Education Classes

The CHN may refer a client and her partner to childbirth education classes, which teach physical exercise, breathing, and relaxation. Childbirth education classes are taught to parents by nurses or childbirth educators who are usually employed by hospitals, community health agencies, or the Red Cross. The usual class content includes reproductive physiology, conception and fetal development, changes in the maternal body, preparation for labor and delivery through breathing and physical exercises, normal labor and delivery, contraception, infant feeding, and care of a newborn. The CHN should encourage clients and their partners to attend these classes. The CHN can reinforce and clarify class content during home visits.

### Physical Exercises, Breathing, and Relaxation Classes

The expectant mother may consult the CHN about physical activities that are allowed or encouraged during pregnancy. Teaching in this area can be done on a one-to-one basis or in a formal class. Walking, swimming, and dancing are beneficial for any pregnant client, unless there are obstetric complications such as vaginal bleeding. Physical activities that include the risk of falls, such as skiing and horseback riding, should be avoided. The main purpose of exercises is to strengthen the abdominal, lower back, and pelvic muscles. Examples of specific abdominal and lower-back exercises are pelvic rocking and the pelvic tilt. Kegel exercises—the relaxing and contracting of the pelvic floor by interrupting the urine flow—improve pelvic muscles (Noble, 1978). A client should seek a physician's approval for extra physical exercises during pregnancy.

Prenatal exercises should ideally begin in the first trimester, coordinated with breathing and relaxation preparation, and should continue throughout pregnancy. These exercise classes may be taught by a nurse or physical therapist, usually with a physician's approval. Prepared childbirth methods, such as the Dick-Read and Lamaze methods, teach correct breathing exercises and relaxation for labor and delivery. Physical exercises accompany these as well. The ultimate purpose of these exercises is to enable the client to maintain control during labor, thereby decreasing or obviating the need for medication during labor and delivery. I recall two women who were in superb physical condition; one was an avid sportswoman, and the other a physical education teacher. They were admitted directly to the delivery room when they entered the hospital, bypassing the labor area. They had short labors with very little medication.

## Nursing Care at Home

### Responding to the Referral

There are many reasons for prenatal follow-up in the client's home by a CHN. First, the client has much to learn about her own health and that of her unborn child, so teaching may conveniently be shared by inpatient care providers and community health agencies. Second, a number of clients do not keep prenatal clinic appointments and must be encouraged to do so. Teaching these clients is doubly important. They may not go to the clinic because they do not understand the importance of regular health supervision. Reinforcement of clinic teaching in the home increases such clients' retention of content. This is especially important for clients with primigravidas, high-risk pregnancies, and complicated pregnancies. Finally, clients are usually more comfortable discussing concerns with a nurse at home.

After the initial clinic visit, the clinic sends a brief referral to the

CHN in the community health agency. It includes identifying information, such as the name, address, and assessment data such as EDC, parous and gravid status, prescriptions, vital signs, urinalysis, and abnormal findings such as vaginal bleeding or plans for Caesarean birth. The CHN plans visits in accordance with this information. For example, an immediate visit by the CHN is warranted by a complication such as vaginal bleeding, especially during the last trimester.

A CHN visits a client approximately once a month, attempting to space her visits between the prenatal clinic visits in order to allow the client optimal contact with health professionals. The nurse may visit more often if this is indicated by a client's needs, especially during the last trimester. The total number of prenatal home visits would normally vary from five to eight. The basic purposes are ongoing assessment and implementation of planned care through teaching and counseling.

### Teaching and Counseling

The content described below is designed primarily for a primipara and for use when a CHN makes a home visit. It can be supplemented by additional advice for high-risk or complicated pregnancies. Preparation for childbirth can come through various media, primarily clinic visits, group parents' classes, and home visits by the CHN. Other channels may include literature, television, and listening to tapes while waiting in the clinic or a physician's office. A CHN may be asked to prepare the content for literature or tapes. Although the medium for disseminating information varies, the content should not, except that some clients require more information and repetition than others. A guide for teaching prenatal care is outlined in Table 2-1.

> *Discussion of prenatal care between client and community health nurse*

The information provided in Table 2-1 can also be divided by trimester. This division corresponds with clients' interest and need for essential information at certain time periods. For example, sections A through C fit nicely in the "Early Bird" lessons or discussions during the first trimester and the beginning of the second. During the second trimester, section D can be reviewed, leaving sections E and F to the last trimester. The client and her partner, if he is present, should be involved in the decision as to what content will be discussed during the visits. The CHN should also anticipate what a prenatal client wants to discuss (Sumner, 1976). This anticipation is facilitated by the CHN's

## Table 2-1
## Guide for Teaching Prenatal Care

A. Body Changes

   1. Physical
      a. Average weight gain
         about 25 pounds
      b. Fetal development
      c. Reproductive biology
      d. Morning sickness

   2. Psychological
      a. Adjustment to pregnancy
      b. Hormonal
      c. Role changes

B. Special Intake Requirements

   1. Nutritive
      a. Based on the "four
         foods" plan
      b. Additional supplements
         for pregnancy

   2. Medicinal
      a. Iron
      b. A and D
      c. Take nothing not pre-
         scribed

C. Supervision and Support
   Systems

   1. Medical-Nursing Providers
   2. Partner
   3. Significant others such as
      boy friend or mother
   4. Extended family
   5. Friends and neighbors
   6. Parents' class participants
   7. Clergy
   8. Mental health nurse clini-
      cian

D. External Bodily Adjustment

   1. Physical Exercises
   2. Work - home or outside
   3. Rest and Sleep
   4. Clothing
   5. Sexual intercourse
   6. Cleansing body
   7. Preparation of breasts
      for breastfeeding
   8. Recreation

E. Labor and Delivery

   1. What to take to the hos-
      pital
   2. When to go to the hospital
   3. Labor
      a. Anesthesia and analgesia
      b. Contractions
      c. Other preparations, such
         as the prep and enema
   4. Delivery

F. Postpartum and Newborn Period

   1. Acute phase or hospital
      phase
      a. Mother
      b. Newborn
 *2. From hospital discharge to
      4-6 weeks postpartum
      a. Mother
      b. Newborn
      c. Partner

*This phase is discussed in further detail in the "Postpartum Care at Home and in the Clinic" section of this chapter (see pp. 27–44).

being mindful of the tasks of pregnancy by trimester. During the first trimester the client may experience ambivalence and may need to discuss the fact that she is pregnant. This need usually results in the woman's seeking care. During the second trimester, the fetus is beginning "to show"; the woman wears maternity clothes and views herself as pregnant. During the last trimester she needs to prepare for separation and so may be identifying concerns about labor, delivery, and the postpartum period.

The CHN has a background in maternal-infant care that she must adapt to the client at home in a particular culture and class in society, using literature and audiovisual aids as conditions indicate. The client learns more if she is motivated, and motivation can be increased by addressing specific client concerns and needs and by presenting information attractively. For example, if the client is Spanish-speaking, literature in that language should be provided. Several of the government pamphlets such as *Prenatal Care* are printed in Spanish.

One example from each of the six categories in Table 2-1 is expanded here to demonstrate how material can be accommodated to the client in her own environment.

*Fetal development (section A, no. 1b).* Ordinarily the pregnant woman is fascinated with the development of a human embryo inside her uterus. In discussing fetal development, the CHN can use the *Birth Atlas* published by the Maternity Center in New York City, an excellent aid to use in the home. Or she can review a commercial pamphlet with the client, such as the *Expectant Mother's Guide* by Gerber (see Appendix 2A for addresses for these materials). At the initial medical checkup, about 2 months into the pregnancy, the client may be surprised to learn that the embryo is about an inch long and weighs 2/3 of an ounce, and that the main characteristics of human form have taken shape already. The CHN can go through the development month by month with the client, answering her questions as they review the fetal progress.

*Nutritive requirements (section B, no. 1).* The CHN is one of the main sources of nutrition information for the client. Most health agencies employ a nutritionist, who can be an invaluable consultative resource to the CHN. Diet counseling for pregnancy should not just begin in pregnancy; ideally, it should begin with teenagers at the time of the menarche or earlier. When the CHN visits a pregnant client in a home to counsel about diet, the cardboard food models from the National Dairy Council are an excellent resource because they show portion sizes. *You and Your Contented Baby*, by the Carnation Company, is a high-quality pamphlet on the subject. (See Appendix 2A for address.)

It is a good idea to show a pregnant woman the differences in her requirements from those of the nonpregnant woman. This can be done by referring to the recommended daily dietary allowances advised by the National Research Council (National Research Council, 1980).

The CHN must translate this information into an understandable diet; a daily food plan for pregnancy and lactation is shown in Table 2-2. Most clients will have had some teaching by the clinic dietitian. In

Table 2-2
Daily Food Plan for Pregnancy and Lactation

| Food | Nonpregnant woman | Pregnancy | Lactation |
|---|---|---|---|
| Dairy Products: Milk (whole, 2%, skim, non-fat dry milk, buttermilk) & foods prepared with milk; cheese, yogurt, & ice cream. | 2 cups | 3-4 cups | 4-5 cups |
| Meat (lean meat, fish, poultry, cheese, dried beans or peas)--skip occasionally. | 1 serving (3-4 oz) | 2 servings (6-8 oz); include liver frequently | 2 1/2 servings (8 oz) |
| Eggs--skip occasionally | 1 | 1-2 | 1-2 |
| Vegetable (dark green or deep yellow) | 1 serving | 1 serving | 1-2 servings |
| Vitamin C-rich foods* Good source--citrus fruit, berries, cantaloupe Fair source--tomatoes, cabbage, greens, potatoes in skin | 1 good source or 2 fair sources | 1 good source & 1 fair source or 2 good sources | 1 good source & 1 fair source or 2 good sources |
| Other vegetables and fruits | 1 serving | 2 servings | 2 servings |
| Bread** and cereals (whole grain or enriched) | 3 servings** | 4-5 servings | 5 servings |
| Butter or fortified margarine | As desired or needed for calories | As desired or needed for calories | As desired or needed for calories |

*Note.* Adapted from S. R. Williams, *Nutrition and diet therapy* (4th ed.). St. Louis: C. V. Mosby, 1981. Copyright 1981 by S. R. Williams. Reprinted by permission.
*Use some raw daily.
**One slice of bread equals 1 serving.

any event, the CHN should understand the nutritional requirements of pregnancy and should tailor them to the client's needs in a manner the client can understand. Explaining the reasons for increased nutrient requirements, such as the need for four glasses of milk, will increase the likelihood of the client's adherence to such a recommendation.

*Fathers and significant others (section C, nos. 2–3).* Fathers are very special, but they are often treated as bystanders in our society during pregnancy, delivery, and the immediate postpartum period. During the client's visits to a clinic, the father is often at work. For this reason, the nurse must be his advocate by involving him in discussions with the mother about parents' classes and ways he can assist his partner, such as preparing her breasts for breast feeding (discussed below), and also by emphasizing joys and stresses of the changes in her body and their life style. If the CHN sees the father, it is usually during a home visit. It is all the more crucial to involve the father, because the extended family is no longer available in most cases for support, as in some cultures.

Some expectant mothers do not have partners. If this is the case, the nurse should ask whether a client's mother or other special person is at home and would like to take part in the home visit. Such a significant other often is very supportive and may have additional concerns, ranging from the type of anesthesia during delivery to the cost of the hospital stay.

*Preparation of breasts for breast feeding (section D, no. 7).* The nurse should discuss with the client her plans for feeding the infant. Information on both breast and bottle feeding should be presented. Whichever method is chosen, the CHN should support the decision. Formula preparation is discussed in Chapter 3. Breast feeding is enjoying a renewed popularity. Before going to the client's home, the nurse could review the movie *Breast Feeding: Prenatal and Postpartal Preparation* (Case Western Reserve University, Health Sciences Communications Center, 1974), prepared for nurses and physicians to help them instruct new mothers, or a literature source such as the handbook from the American Academy of Pediatrics, which describes the steps required for a client to prepare her breasts and the advantages of breast feeding (American Academy of Pediatrics, 1979).

The CHN should assess a pregnant woman for inverted nipples. All women who are going to breast-feed should practice some techniques to thoughen the nipple's skin. These techniques are best practiced in the third trimester. Nipple rolling—gently rolling each nipple for two minutes twice daily, using the thumb and first finger while applying gentle traction to the nipple as well—is one technique. A second suggested technique is rubbing each nipple with a terry cloth for about 15 seconds once daily. A woman can be assisted in these techniques by her partner (Atkinson, 1979).

*What to take to the hospital (section E, no. 1).*   The nurse will probably discuss items to take to the hospital with the client in the last trimester. The items basically include a layette; slippers, robe, and the like; clothes for the mother to return home in if she does not want to wear her maternity dress; and personal items (such as deodorant) that will be used during hospitalization. The CHN can remind the client to take reading material, important telephone numbers, birth announcements, and stamps; she should also remind her to pack her suitcase a couple of weeks ahead of her EDC. It is a good idea to have the mother make a written list and then go over it with her. This suggested list for mother and baby is as follows:

*For the Mother:*

1. Two or three washable nightgowns
2. A washable robe
3. A pair of slippers
4. A bed jacket
5. Two or three bras (nursing type if nursing; regular if not)
6. Sanitary belt
7. Hair brush and comb
8. Toothbrush and toothpaste
9. Cosmetics and deodorant
10. Shower cap
11. Reading material
12. Birth announcements and stamps
13. Hospital insurance card
14. _____
15. _____

*For the Baby:*

1. Two cloth diapers with pins, or disposable diapers
2. A nightgown, kimono, or sleeper
3. A shirt
4. Cotton receiving blanket
5. Plastic pants or quilted pad
6. If warm weather, a lightweight blanket; if cold weather, a warm blanket, sweater, and cap

*Newborn (section F, no. 1b).*  During pregnancy, women are usually more interested in the prenatal period than they are in the postpartum. It is, however, a good idea to discuss the postpartal period with
her, so she can anticipate her baby with joy. This approach aids in
bonding during the days she is in the hospital. Bonding is discussed
in more detail in Chapter 3. The client will undoubtedly initiate a discussion of problems that can occur with a newborn, such as prematurity, deformities, infections, and so on. Each problem should be discussed by addressing the client's concerns and providing relevant facts.
She should be reminded that the hospital will usually notify the CHN
of her discharge and that the CHN can make home visits to a new
mother and baby in the first few days and weeks at home. The mother
can also be instructed to request a CHN home visit.

### Encouragement of self-care

The traditional health care system in the United States has not fostered self-responsibility for health. This results in the pregnant woman's relying too much on medical support to maintain her state of wellness during pregnancy. Objectives need to be refocused on what the
woman and her partner can do for themselves. Conception, pregnancy, and childbirth are normal processes for which a woman and her
partner need knowledge, support, and preparation from health professionals. The CHN should motivate and encourage the client in self-
care in areas where it is practical, such as diet, exercise, rest, nipple
preparation for breast feeding, comfortable maternity clothes, and so
on. Self-care should be coordinated appropriately with medical care for
maximum adaptation to the physiological and psychological changes
in pregnancy.

## High-Risk Pregnancies

High-risk pregnancies are a concern of the federal government as well
as of health providers. Congress passed the Maternal Child Health and
Mental Retardation Planning Amendments of 1963 to develop and support mother and infant care programs. The primary purpose of this legislation, which is part of the Social Security Act, was to provide comprehensive care for high-risk pregnant women and infants. This law
defines a ''high-risk pregnancy'' as one in which the prospective

mother has or is likely to have conditions associated with childbearing which indicate hazards to the health of the mother or infant.

The "high-risk infant" has been defined by the U.S. Children's Bureau as one who has or is likely to develop a physical, intellectual, personality, or social handicap capable of interfering with his normal growth, development and capacity to learn. This disability may originate in the prenatal or postnatal period and may be the result of unfavorable hereditary or environmental influences (Wallace, Gold, & Lis, 1973).

The usual examples of clients at high risk in pregnancy are teenagers under 16, older primiparas (i.e., women 35 years or over), unmarried women, multiple-child pregnancies, women with a 10-year lapse since their last pregnancy, grand multiparas (those with seven or more pregnancies), women with one or more previous Caesarean births, and those from seriously disadvantaged families. Other examples of high-risk clients are women with a history of miscarriages, premature births, or stillbirths, and women with diabetes, hypertension, or heart disease.

### The Unmarried Pregnant Adolescent

The largest and most rapidly growing category of high-risk pregnancies is that of teenage pregnancies. Usually teenagers are not mature enough physically to produce full-term infants and to develop the necessary bonding and continued psychological support babies need to grow to their potential fullness. Some obstetricians suggest that a female is not developed enough to conceive and deliver a full-term infant until about 5 years after the menarche. A CHN should plan to expand and reinforce every aspect of teaching and counseling for an unmarried pregnant teenager. The immature mother needs much more teaching about the physiological changes in her body, her diet, and the plan for regular clinic follow-up. She is adjusting to two crises at this time, adolescence and the unplanned pregnancy. A prudent course for the CHN is to discuss frankly with the teenager what she needs to know to make her pregnancy as normal as possible. The CHN should inquire about the father of the baby, his interest in the pregnancy, and his ability to offer psychological and financial support. This section is expanded in Chapter 6, "Health during the School-Age Years," in which teenage pregnancy is discussed.

Other types of problem pregnancies are those with complications related to the mother's health. Examples are clients with diabetes, hypertension (blood pressure over 140/90), and a postterm pregnancy. Only the diabetic is discussed in this chapter.

## The Pregnant Woman Who Is Diabetic

The addition of pregnancy to diabetes adds stress. Recent studies have, however, demonstrated that excellent diabetic control can be achieved through education, proper diet, twice-daily insulin injections, and close medical and nursing supervision. A very new trend in care for the prenatal client with diabetes is the provision of frequent, comprehensive ambulatory care, decreasing hospitalizations. This keeps the family unit intact and aids in the emotional and social well-being of the client. Because more and more pregnant women with diabetes will be at home, the CHN will play a bigger role in their nursing care (Kreitzer, 1980; Schneider, Curet, Olson, & Shay, 1980).

Diagnostic screening for diabetes is an important aspect of prenatal care. A family history of diabetes, obesity, a history of infants weighing over 4500 grams (10 pounds), and unexplained stillbirths are danger signals. During the first trimester, there is an improvement in the diabetic condition because of fetal drain on glucose. Therefore, there is a tendency toward hypoglycemia (Schuler, 1979). Because the duration of insulin effectiveness decreases in pregnancy, the client is often placed on split dosages of short-acting (regular) and intermediate-acting (NPH or Lente) insulins in the morning and evening (Kreitzer, 1980).

As the pregnancy advances, the circulating levels of human placental lactogen (HPL), estrogen, progesterone, and cortisone increase and intensify the diabetes. An insulin-dependent client may need her insulin dosage increased. In the last two trimesters, there is a tendency toward acidosis, necessitating a further increase in insulin. Uncontrolled maternal acidosis can harm the neuropsychological development of the fetus (Schuler, 1979).

The CHN should counsel the diabetic who becomes pregnant about diet, weight control, exercise, insulin, monitoring glucose levels in the urine or blood, and prevention of infections. A pregnant client who is diabetic should have an individual diet plan adjusted periodically to her caloric needs. A daily intake of about 2300 calories (or 20–40 calories/kg of body weight) is required for a client who is of average body size. The diet composition is usually 40–50% carbohydrate, 30–40% fat, and 20% protein (Guthrie & Guthrie, 1977). The CHN will probably want to consult the health agency nutritionist to insure that the prenatal diet is adequate and that weight is being controlled. Early in the pregnancy, the CHN should request that the client write down her food intake for a 3-day period and then compare it to the diet prescription. See Chapter 8 for instructions on analyzing a 3-day diet study.

The client should test her urine regularly, as determined by the severity of her disease. Very recent literature indicates that a blood test may be devised for the woman to test blood glucose levels at home, thus enabling her to control her diabetes more effectively ("Diabetic Mothers-to-Be Get Aid," 1982). She must be taught to recognize signs of ketoacidosis and hypoglycemic reactions. The balance between rest and activity is critical in adjusting insulin. Oral hypoglycemics are not recommended because of cardiovascular problems they may cause in the mother. She is more prone to urinary infections because of the added glucose and the threat of hyperglycemia and ketoacidosis.

At present, most physicians prefer to deliver prenatals who are diabetic 2 weeks before the EDC to decrease risks associated with placental dysfunction. Very current research indicates that women may be delivered closer to term as the control measures such as monitoring blood glucose at home are improved (Schneider et al., 1980). Therefore, tests, ultrasonography, and amniocentesis are used to establish the EDC. Ultrasonography is almost always used to measure the fetal biparietal diameter, which indicates growth rate. An amniocentesis may be performed to evaluate fetal lung maturity in order to establish a delivery date, thereby decreasing the chance of a stillbirth or an extremely large baby. Throughout the pregnancy, the CHN evaluates the client's understanding of the diabetic controls required and assists her to adjust to them. She is seen in the prenatal clinic as often as every 1 to 2 weeks in the first two trimesters and weekly in the last month (Guthrie & Guthrie, 1977; Jensen et al., 1981; Schuler, 1979).

Two types of high-risk pregnancies have been discussed here, the unmarried teenager and the diabetic. The CHN should set these and all other high-risk and complicated pregnancies as priorities and make certain she visits such clients regularly. For each type of high-risk case, she will have to supplement the information given to a normal primigravida or multigravida.

## The Prenatal Client in High School

There is a definite need for parenting and homemaking classes in the junior and senior high schools, not only because of the increase in adolescent pregnancies, but also because many young people get married shortly after high school. (This topic is expanded in Chapter 6.)

## The Pregnant Client
## in the Occupational Setting

About 40% of pregnant women work outside the home during their pregnancy; this means that there are a little over 1.25 million pregnant females in the work force at any given time (Health Resources Administration, 1977). If a pregnant working woman is having obstetric complications such as vaginal bleeding or premature labor, she should stop work and seek the advice of her physician about resuming employment. She should be aware of the hazards of inhalation or ingestion of, or skin contact with, toxic chemicals.

In 1977, the American College of Obstetricians and Gynecologists published guidelines for pregnant workers; these essentially state that the pregnant worker (1) can continue to perform the same type of work she did before pregnancy, and (2) can work as long as her physician says she can. The burden of the responsibility for her condition now rests with her and her doctor. However, the nurse in an occupational health setting is responsible for assessing the safety of the work setting.

True disabilities of pregnancy fall into three basic categories: (1) disabilities of pregnancy per se (labor and delivery), (2) disabilities related to complications (eclampsia, cardiac involvement, and excessive fatigue), and (3) disabilities related to job exposures (toxic substances and abnormal fatigue). Pregnancy itself is now considered as any other temporary disability, so the client *cannot* refuse to do her job or aspects of it because of fatigue or other complaints. There are no longer "resting" rooms, because this would discriminate against male employees. The pregnant employee must follow company policies as for any other temporary disability.

There are, however, a few problems with the new freedom of the pregnant woman at work, if she works in the last trimester. She is awkward because of her weight redistribution and a new center of gravity, so she may trip and fall more often. She also can work right up to term if she wishes, so the nurse in the work setting must be able to recognize symptoms of early labor and should keep supplies on hand for a spontaneous delivery.

## Alternate Approaches to Prenatal
## Health Care Management

A couple who are expecting a baby should be made aware of the choices they have for health care during pregnancy and later. In the health supervision during pregnancy, the client should feel that clinic appoint-

ments are for her convenience and care. She should have the freedom
to discuss her concerns frankly. In addition, the clinic nurse should describe labor, delivery, and postpartal procedures, including aspects
such as enemas, fetal monitoring, and rooming-in. There is controversy at present as to the need for shaving the perineum and the excessive
use of fetal monitoring, because of the discomfort involved in the first
practice and the expense in the second. Rooming-in (i.e., having the
newborn in a nursery adjacent to the mother's room or directly in the
mother's room) allows the father to be present and allows bonding to
begin with his child.

The pros and cons of hospital deliveries should be available to the
expectant couple. Although most American births occur in hospitals,
where the latest equipment is available, there is an interest in home deliveries and midwife care because they are both less expensive and more
personal. Hospitals are beginning to permit fathers in the delivery room,
and even in the operating room for Caesarean births (Feldman, 1978).

Birthing centers, out-of-hospital delivery sites, are another innovation founded on the premise that normal persons can and should be
treated differently from high-risk ones, as well as on consumers' demand for homelike births. The client receives prenatal clinic, labor/de-
livery, and postnatal services from a CNM, a nutritionist, and physicians who take referrals and provide consultations. The client and her
partner are considered the leaders of their own health team, with the
health personnel serving as consultants to them for their individual experiences (Nielsen, 1978).

## Postpartum Care at Home and in the Clinic

### The Postpartum Client at Home

#### *Definitions and implications of the postpartum period*

The immediate postpartum period encompasses two phases,.the
concerns of which are different. The first phase consists of the 3 to 5
days following delivery when the client is hospitalized and when the
client and her newborn require careful observation and physical care
by health personnel. The new mother and father also need emotional
support and have numerous questions as they begin adjusting to parenthood.

The second phase continues from hospital discharge through 4
to 6 weeks after delivery; this is a time when the CHN makes home
visits. In the case of a birth at home, the CHN's role is similar. This

second phase is a period of physical restoration of body tissue for the mother and adjustment of the family to new roles and responsibilities. At the end of this phase, the mother is considered physically healed. Her breasts are no longer engorged; the lochia has ceased, signaling a healing at the placental site of the uterus; and the episiotomy is healed. Bonding with her newborn should be established, and the family should have adjusted to the requirements of a newborn.

### The client's vulnerability after hospital discharge

The second phase of the immediate postpartum period is the phase most often neglected by health personnel. The acute medical and nursing care received in the hospital is no longer available, and the clinic is not really considered the place to handle the physical and psychological difficulties the family experiences during this time. Even in the best circumstances, it is a time of extreme vulnerability for the mother and her newborn and the mother-father relationship (Rubin, 1975). During this period in the maternity cycle, the CHN can be very valuable, because she comes to the home to care for the client and offers needed information and emotional support. She supports the integration of the infant into the family. She monitors the baby's progress and supports the mother-father relationship. The CHN praises the new mother's accomplishments in infant care and reassures her that the fatigue will disappear; alleviates tension by pointing out that quirks in the newborn such as the startle reflex are normal; and encourages the father when he is fearful of handling the neonate.

### The father's involvement

A CHN may not encounter the pregnant or postpartum client's partner as often as the hospital nurse may encounter him. The father frequently takes time off to take his wife to the hospital and generally sets evenings aside to visit her and the new baby in the hospital. When the CHN comes to the home or sees the mother and baby in the clinic, the father is usually at work. A great effort should be made to include the father in discussions with the CHN whenever possible. The CHN can try to schedule times convenient for the father. It is a good idea for him to assist in the feeding, diapering, and rocking of the infant to relieve the mother and to allow him to get to know his baby. Frequently, new mothers may also need to be encouraged to accept help from fathers.

Nursing Care of the Mother

After discharge from the hospital, the mother should receive nursing care until about 6 weeks after delivery. Anticipatory guidance related to potential problems is usually very helpful. Some mothers may need extra guidance until they are 3 months postpartum (the "fourth trimester" concept). The bonding between the mother and baby that has started in the hospital should be guided and nurtured to insure a stable family group in society (Barnes, 1978).

The CHN is in a unique position, because she sees the mother in the mother's environment. Hospital nurses provide care and teach each client, but the postpartum stay in the hospital is too brief to enable them to guide and support the client over the long-term adjustment to parenthood. In the home, nursing care and teaching can be adapted to the home environment and life style. The CHN can examine the mother and infant and discuss issues in the place where the mother is most comfortable.

The hospital refers postpartal clients to the CHN by telephone or written referral. The first two or three visits to the postpartum client should receive high priority in the CHN's client load.

A CHN visit immediately after hospital discharge greatly enhances postpartum care. The nurse reinforces the hospital's teaching in such subjects as proper perineal care and adapts it to home care. The nurse should make her first visit on the day the mother returns home or the next, and an additional visit or two may be necessary during the first week. The suggested frequency of visits during the first 6 weeks postpartum is as follows: one to three visits the first week, one to two the second and third weeks, and every other week (unless oftener seems appropriate) for the next 3 weeks. The total suggested number of visits is from two to seven. This provides the family members with support when they are alone with the newborn and may be slightly apprehensive. In fact, the family is often helped just to know there is support in case of need!

The schedule of home visits should be adjusted for clients who have had a Caesarean birth or a complication such as an infection. If a CHN has visited a mother prenatally, rapport and teaching have already been accomplished. One or two visits may be sufficient because such a client feels comfortable about telephoning the CHN for additional information or visits. The frequency of visits is dictated by the client's self-assessment, the CHN's assessment, and agency policy.

Health concerns during the postpartum period can be conveniently divided into those for the mother and the baby. They can be further divided into physical, psychological, and social concerns during the first 6 weeks and from the sixth week to the third month postpartum. Infant care is discussed in the last portion of this chapter.

On the initial visit, the CHN examines the client, answers her questions, and offers supportive guidance as necessary. The CHN takes the TPR and blood pressure and examines the breasts, fundus, perineum, and legs, asking the mother to undress as necessary and to lie on the bed or couch, insuring privacy. There should be adequate light to ensure a sound assessment.

### Physical care

*Breast care and lactation.* Breast care after the third day postpartum differs between clients who do breast-feed and those who do not. By the second day postpartum, a modest amount of colostrum can be expressed from the nipples or may even leak. Colostrum secretion continues for about 1 week, with a gradual change to mature breast milk. Colostrum contains more minerals and protein than breast milk, but less sugar and fat, providing nourishment and protection for the newborn. It is rich in antibodies such as IgA, which protects against enteric infections (Pritchard & MacDonald, 1976).

Lactation has been described as a very intimate experience, and for the mother who is prepared and supported in her decision to breast-feed, the experience can be very satisfying. Lactation begins abruptly when the placenta is delivered, at which time progesterone and estrogen levels are profoundly decreased; prolactin from the pituitary and the stimulus of newborn sucking control lactation. "Letting down," or the release of milk, is initiated especially by the baby's sucking or crying. It can be suppressed by fright, stress, or a physical illness.

Lactation continues unless it is interrupted by medication or the absence of infant sucking. Medications are given to suppress engorgement and lactation in those mothers choosing to bottle-feed. Medications for this are estradiol valerate (Delestrogen) and testosterone enanthate (Deladumone) given intramuscularly (Willson, Beecham, & Carrington, 1979). At present there is some controversy about suppressing lactation with medication.

By the second day in multiparas and the third day in primiparas, the breasts become engorged, firm, and tender, with prominent veins. This vascular stasis usually disappears spontaneously in 36 to 48 hours, but may still be present when the client is discharged to her home. If the new mother is not planning to nurse her infant, the CHN should establish whether she has had medication to suppress lactation. Cold packs, such as ice in a hot water bottle, can be applied twice daily to relieve the congestion, swelling, and pain of engorgement. Nonprescription analgesics such as Tylenol and aspirin can be suggested, and a prescription for codeine could be requested from the client's physician. Her temperature should be taken to check for a possible beginning breast infection, and nipples should be examined for cracks and irritation.

Nursing an infant accelerates uterine involution. Repeated nipple stimulation causes a release of oxytocin, which increases contractions of the uterine muscles.

As with the nursing mother, the CHN should pay attention to providing necessary information and emotional support for the mother who chooses to bottle-feed her infant. In some cases a mother may want to breast-feed, but cannot because of problems she is having such as an illness or a premature baby. Both breast-fed and bottle-fed babies experience some of the same problems, such as "fussy" feeding times when nothing seems to satisfy a baby, sleepiness, and absence of the mother and/or need for someone else to do the feeding. The CHN should help the mother to anticipate these irregularities, so that they do not become crisis situations.

*Uterine-perineal care.* A good example of utilizing the client's equipment and home environment to provide nursing care and teach self-care is perineal care. As the client leaves the hospital, she is probably told to continue perineal care; however, at home she may not have the equipment or sterile supplies used in the hospital. It is suggested that she wash her perineum, including the episiotomy, gently with soap and water once daily and after each bowel movement, using a clean washcloth and towel or clean (not sterile) cotton balls. After urination, she can pour some warm water over the perineum to promote healing. If the client has not brought home the equipment she used in the hospital, the CHN can suggest that she use one of her small kitchen pitchers, a measuring cup, or some other container with a lip. The CHN should impress upon the client that the purpose of the cleansing is to promote healing of the episiotomy and to prevent infection.

EPISIOTOMY. If the episiotomy is swollen and painful, the client can take a sitz bath in warm water for about 20 to 30 minutes once or twice daily in her own tub. If the episiotomy is especially sore, air drying of the perineum for 20 minutes twice daily is effective. Also, a light can be applied to the area for about 20 minutes once or twice daily to supply dry heat and to promote healing. A variety of home lamps can be adapted for this use by removing the shades. Safety should be stressed by instructing the client to place the lamp at least 3 feet away from her to avoid burning her thighs or perineum. Topical anesthetics can be obtained from the physician or over the counter for relief of pain. The cream, spray, or ointment should be applied to the pad rather than directly to the stitches.

FUNDUS.   After the second postpartum day, the fundus goes down a finger's breadth daily (1 cm) until the 10th day, when it is non-palpable. The CHN determines the height and firmness of the fundus at each home visit in the first couple of weeks by placing the edge of her left hand (little finger side) at the level of the umbilicus and moving down (or up if necessary) slowly until it rests on the top of the uterus. She then palpates the fundus with her right hand, using finger breadths to determine location below the umbilicus. Before the maneuver the client should empty her bladder, because a full bladder may raise the level of the fundus, making palpation difficult or inaccurate. Establishing the correct level of the fundus and its firmness confirms that the uterus is returning to the correct size and that the placental site is healing. It is important to explain to the mother what is being assessed and why. She or her husband may want to check the height and firmness of the fundus themselves.

LOCHIA.   The healing of the placental site is also indicated by assessing the three stages of lochia. "Lochia rubra" (bright red) lasts about 3 days postpartum, and "lochia serosa" (pinkish) is usually present when the CHN makes her first visit. Lochia serosa lasts from the fourth to the ninth day, after which time "lochia alba" (yellowish-white) begins and continues to approximately the 21st day postpartum. The CHN should check for any infectious process, which is evidenced by foul-smelling lochia, excoriated perineum, an unusually small or large amount of flow, fever, and complaints of general discomfort.

*Elimination.*   The CHN should inquire about elimination. Constipation can be a problem for the first 2 to 3 weeks. If so, the mother should be instructed to take adequate fluids, roughage in her diet, warm prune juice, and/or a mild laxative. If cystitis is a problem, the client should telephone the physician for medication such as Gantrisin. The CHN should suggest an adequate fluid intake and careful perineal care as outlined above.

*Showering and bathing.*   Most physicians recommend showering 2 days postpartum and tub bathing or showering about a week postpartum. The procedure depends upon the facilities in the client's home and the way she feels.

*Rest, activity, and exercises.*   A discussion of exercises, activity, and rest for the client is beneficial. Some doctors prescribe a set of exercises for the mother a few days after delivery; these may be started while the client is still in the hospital. If so, the four exercises included here would be appropriate for her to begin on the eighth day after delivery. (See Figure 2-1.) They represent a good variety, even though they may be different from those recommended in the hospital. These exercises are intended to tighten the abdominal, lower-back, and pelvic muscles. More exercises can be done if desired. If the client has had a Caesarean birth, these exercises could be started gradually 2 to 4 weeks later. It has been my own experience that a postpartum client feels better and regains her strength and shape much faster if she does exercises daily for 3 months. The CHN can help the new mother select appropriate and enjoyable prepregnancy activities such as walking or bicycling as she feels able. Exercises help both physically and emotionally (Noble, 1978).

Some other activities are permitted and others are not after the client returns home. Activities too strenuous may interfere with the return of the uterus to normal and with the healing of the perineal stitches. The client should not go up and down stairs more than a very few times a day for the first 2 to 3 weeks after delivery. She may ride or drive in a car for short distances at any time. The amount of activity should be gradually increased, letting the feeling of fatigue be the guide. If the client feels tired, she should sit down or lie down. She certainly may do some of the minor household activities, but no heavy work or lifting until 6 weeks after delivery. A good rule of thumb is not to lift anything heavier than the baby for the first 6 weeks.

Fatigue is a common postpartum problem and should not be treated lightly. The new mother often suffers interruption of sleep in addition to the physiological effects of labor and delivery. The mother and father may be surprised at the fatigue and may need to be reassured that it is normal and that it is all right to rest frequently. The father often becomes fatigued as well because he is awakened at night, and the stress of worrying about his new family is tiring. Both parents require rest to keep fit. At home, the mother should lie down at least an hour or two every forenoon and afternoon until the baby is about a month old.

It is strongly advised that the mother have help at home for a few weeks following the birth of the baby, so that she can devote time to infant care and can rest adequately. It may also be necessary to restrict visitors during the first few days at home to insure rest periods. Although giving birth is a normal event, the mother goes through a great deal of physical exertion with the labor, blood loss, and minor surgery (the episiotomy). If she has had a Caesarean birth, she may need even more help and rest during the early postpartal period.

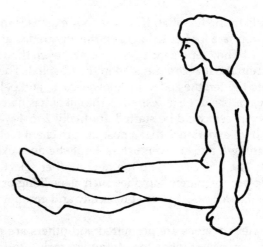

A. Tightening Pelvic Muscles: Sit with legs outstretched and crossed. Tighten inside thigh muscles, buttocks, and pelvic muscles. Hold for a count of 5, then relax. Do five times. This feels the same as trying to prevent urination. You can practice this exercise by stopping the flow of urine in midstream.

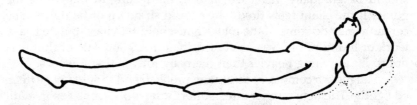

B. Head Raising: On your back, with arms at your sides and legs straight, raise your head. Attempt to put your chin on your chest without moving any other part of your body. Repeat 10 times.

Figure 2-1.   Postpartum Exercises. (Drawings by Mary Gainer,

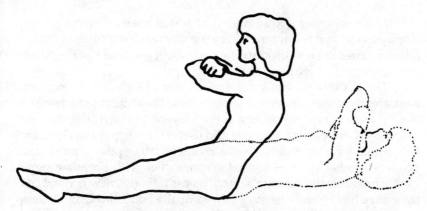

C. Shoulder Raising and Sitting Up: On your back with arms across chest and feet braced against the wall, raise your head and shoulders slowly to a half-sitting position, then slowly lower them back to the floor. Repeat several times, and as you improve, raise yourself to a full sitting position.

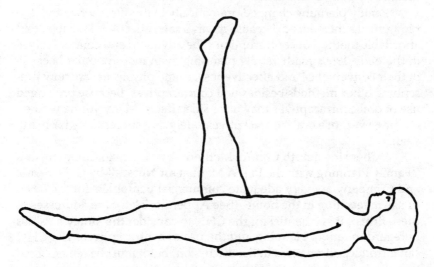

D. Leg Raising: On your back with arms flat at your side, raise one leg (with knee straight) halfway to the horizontal position, then lower slowly. Do the same with the other leg. Then raise and lower both legs together. As you feel stronger, repeat several times and gradually increase the height to which you raise your legs.

University of Wisconsin–Milwaukee, Milwaukee, Wisconsin.)

*Family planning.*   Resumption of sexual intercourse can usually begin as soon as it is comfortable for the woman. Most couples resume relations after the episiotomy is healed, about 4 to 6 weeks after delivery, or after the first postpartum checkup.

The diaphragm and intrauterine device (IUD) are the non-oral contraceptives that are currently prescribed. The diaphragm reportedly has no known side effects, but it is awkward to insert, remove, and maintain. Condoms are effective and useful if a postpartum client and her partner have intercourse before another contraceptive is prescribed. Foam or another spermicide used in conjunction with a condom significantly increases the condom's effectiveness rating. A new nonoral contraceptive has recently been approved by the Food and Drug Administration. It is a soft, disposable polyurethane sponge permeated with a spermicide, which does not require fitting by a physician. It is reportedly 85% effective in preventing pregnancies (The Sponge . . . , 1983). Some couples practice sexual abstinence in such forms as the rhythm method to plan their families.

Family planning changed dramatically in the 1930s when the diaphragm was introduced, because it was a safe, effective, available, and affordable method of contraception. The advent of oral contraceptives in the early 1960s made family planning even more popular because of their convenience and effectiveness. Some physicians are now prescribing other methods besides oral contraceptives, because prolonged use of oral contraceptives may have side effects. Many young women do, however, use oral contraceptives safely and successfully for many years.

"Choosing a Birth Control Method" by the Emko Company and "Family Planning with the Pill: A Manual for Nurses" by G. D. Searle and Company are very adequate commercial pamphlets for the CHN to use in teaching in the home. (See Appendix 2A for the addresses of these firms.) It is essential for the CHN to consider the family's values in regard to family planning and the use of contraceptives. The CHN can introduce alternatives in the discussion, but it must be remembered that the family selects the alternative that is most agreeable to them. Fathers should be invited to enter the discussion about family planning.

*Psychological care*

As noted earlier in this chapter, the psychological care of the mother, newborn, father, and siblings is as important as the physical care the CHN provides. The emotional support that the CHN should offer takes a number of forms.

*The mother's relationship with the father.* The relationship of the mother with the father of the infant has a great influence on the support she will receive from him after she returns home. The CHN should provide every opportunity to foster a good relationship by including him in discussions and decisions. If the client is unmarried, her mate may still play a crucial role in helping her care for herself and the baby. The nurse should respect whatever relationship exists, but be cognizant that some fathers may not be as involved as others or may not be involved at all.

*The parenting role and bonding.* Parenting is an exciting adventure, but new parents often need guidance in making it a satisfying experience. They should learn that because the baby is growing and developing and the feeding and crying times change, they may not always be able to maintain a planned schedule. Some undesirable situations have to be accepted. The mother and father should be encouraged to enjoy their infant and should be assisted in establishing touch and verbal communications with the baby, so that bonding can continue. Attachment to a newborn and bonding between the baby and his parents begins with pregnancy, continues at birth, and goes on into the caretaking phases of the postpartal period and later.

*Primiparas and other special cases.* A client usually requires more assistance from the CHN if this is her first baby, if it has been 10 years or more since the last baby, or if she has a multiple birth. Many of these mothers require much psychological support to reassure them that they are progressing in their role development as mothers. The CHN should assist them in expressing their feelings of anger and inadequacy, as well as the joyous and satisfying emotions. A mother faced with the care of her first offspring, in particular, has many moments when she is discouraged and not at all sure she is providing care as she should be doing. Mothers with other children appreciate assistance from the CHN in the first few weeks, but usually do not require as much nursing care or for as long a period as does a primiparous client.

*Time with other siblings.* Any sibling(s) must be included in the care and satisfactions of the new baby in order to feel a part of the total family. Many hospitals permit sibling visitations, so the relationship between siblings can begin early. A CHN can encourage family togetherness by involving a sibling when she gives a bath demonstration for a new mother. She can also focus attention on siblings as individuals, assuring them that they, too, are valued. Anticipatory guidance in regard to the inevitability of sibling rivalry and its various symptoms, such as regressive behavior or acting out of anger, is helpful to the parents. The CHN should suggest that special time for the siblings be provided by each parent.

### Social concerns

*Support systems.*   Because of our nuclear family pattern, the new mother may be alone after hospital discharge, unless she invites someone to assist for a short period. Quite often a relative, the mother or mother-in-law of the client, moves in to help out for a few days or weeks. Relatives, friends, and neighbors mainly come to see the mother and her newborn during this period and congratulate her. Members of such support systems often bring food to celebrate the birth, perform household chores on a limited basis, and run errands for the family during the first few weeks. The CHN should encourage such activities.

*Resuming household and career tasks.*   Most women resume their usual household tasks, especially light housework, gradually during the first month postpartum. Very few new mothers return to a job outside the home prior to the 6-week checkup by a physician, CNM, or NP, unless prior arrangements have been made. Then the working mother returns to her job at 6 weeks if she is considered well, she desires to return, the family needs her income, and/or the employer applies pressure. Many women stay at home with their new babies for 3 to 6 months or longer. Others change positions, often moving to part-time employment. A goodly number do not return to the work force until their children start school or complete it. Industries have different monetary policies relative to maternity leave, but they must follow the federal government's guidelines about returning to work, discussed earlier (see p. 26). The decision to return to work is often difficult for the mother, and whatever she decides should be supported by the CHN and her family.

*Recreation.*   Recreation helps fill physical, emotional, and social human needs. The types of recreation that new postpartum clients engage in, and when, vary. For example, if a client is an artist, she might begin painting very soon after hospital discharge, but another client might not resume cross-country skiing until the next season. Her partner's wishes play a great part in her decisions and activities regarding her avocations. The importance of outside interests should be discussed with each client, because they fill so many personal needs for happiness and well-being for her and her family.

### Research needed on the postpartum period after hospital discharge

Little research has been done on the postpartum period after hospital discharge, because nursing has only recently become involved in research. Research involving CHNs traveling to various homes in the community is costly and time-consuming. Given further study, the incidence of "postpartum blues" may be found to be significantly related to fatigue after hospital discharge, as well as to role change stresses associated with childbirth.

### Health assessment guide

Because a great part of primary or ambulatory care of the postpartum client is done by the CHN, Table 2-3 presents a guide for the CHN to use in assessing the mother in the home.

## Clinic Care

When the client is discharged from the hospital, an appointment for a postpartum examination will be made for her in a clinic, or she is requested to make one with her private physician. When the CHN visits the home, she should confirm whether this is the case. Usually the client has only one postpartum checkup by a physician, unless there are complications. The postpartum history and physical and psychological assessments should include the following aspects:

1. Checking of weight and blood pressure
2. Examination of breasts and nipples (including axilla check for lumps)
3. Pelvic examination, including checks of the following:
   a. Episiotomy for indications of healing
   b. Uterine size for involution
   c. Cervix for evidence of tears
   d. Absence of lochia and if menses have been established
   e. Cervicovaginal cytology (if none within last 12 months)
   f. Presence of hemorrhoids
4. Examination of legs for varicosities
5. Examination of any other body areas if client has complaints
6. Laboratory work, including:
   a. Hematocrit or hemoglobin test
   b. Rubella vaccination if prenatal titer negative
7. Assessment of exercises, activity, and rest
8. Family planning, counseling, and initiation of client's choice of contraceptive method
9. Assessment of self-directed health care behavior
10. Assessment of infant care plan
    a. Reinforcement of lactation diet if necessary
    b. Determination of whether mother enjoys caring for the infant

## Table 2-3
## Postpartum Assessment Guide after Client is at Home

|  | Baseline Initial Visit | 2nd Visit | 3rd Visit | 4th Visit |
|---|---|---|---|---|
| Date of Home Visit | | | | |
| **Physical Examination** | | | | |
| Vital signs | | | | |
| Breast/Nipples | | | | |
| Uterus – Fundus | | | | |
| Perineum | | | | |
| Lochia/Episiotomy | | | | |
| Bladder/Bowels | | | | |
| Pretibial areas/calves | | | | |
| Ambulation | | | | |
| Other areas | | | | |
| **History** | | | | |
| Nutrition (diet, appetite, fluid intake) | | | | |
| Rest, activity/exercises | | | | |
| Other areas | | | | |
| **Psychological/Social** | | | | |
| Enjoys infant | | | | |
| Has outside help | | | | |
| Assistance from husband or significant other person | | | | |
| Other areas | | | | |

*Note.* Adapted from S. Campbell and J. Smith, "Postpartum: Assessment Guide," *American Journal of Nursing,* 1977, 77(7), 1179. Copyright © 1977, American Journal of Nursing Company. Adapted by permission.

The counseling and teaching can be in large measure accomplished by the professional nurse. If the client returns to a health department clinic for her checkup, a CHN will be on the staff. Otherwise the clinic nurse is usually not a CHN.

*The client's return to usual activities,
including employment*

After a 4- or 6-week checkup, the client is usually able to resume her normal activities at home or return to employment. The CHN should insure that she feels comfortable discussing any concerns she has about her future activities. She usually makes an appointment to see the physician or NP in 3 to 6 months (or sooner) for another gynecological checkup, in order to have her oral contraceptives refilled or to determine whether a problem such as a vaginal infection exists.

## Care from the Sixth Week to the Third Month after Delivery

Postpartum care from the sixth week to the third month focuses on a few special aspects. If the client returns to work, the CHN will no longer be visiting her. And if she remains at home, the CHN will visit only for special concerns, such as assistance in parenting to increase her confidence, instruction in a weight reduction diet if this need has been determined earlier, and infant feeding. A few clients continue in parenting groups for support, sharing of experiences, and information. Concerns during this portion of the postpartum period focus on being a good parent and looking for new sources of support in this area. Special physical concerns during this period might be attention to anything abnormal found in the clinic visit, such as a vaginal discharge, obesity, or fatigue. The client should be psychologically ready to terminate relationships with the CHN and physician, and should possibly locate a support group or supportive neighbors.

From 6 weeks to 3 months postpartum, many women are still adjusting socially, physically, and psychologically to the outcome of their pregnancy and delivery. The client may not yet have attained her prepregnancy weight and muscle tone and may never do so, unless she continues the exercises begun a few days after delivery. Society assumes that by now the adjustment has been made, but the new mother may not feel this way when her infant awakens her each night to be fed. If she has a career, her employer and colleagues expect her to return, and she herself may feel that she is falling behind. This period is sometimes referred to as the "fourth trimester" to emphasize that the mother still needs attention, particularly support and praise.

Three months after delivery the mother is no longer considered a postpartum case, and the baby is referred to as an infant, not a neonate. (He is actually a neonate for only 28 days.) The work of raising a child has been launched. The requirements of both mother and child for support and care begin to change. In addition to focusing on the infant, the mother can now begin to reinvest energy in other aspects of her life—other family members, job, and hobbies.

## Classes

### Parenting classes

Parenting groups can begin at any time after birth and can be started by a variety of individuals or groups, including mothers, nurses, nursing students, and psychologists. Groups in mothering, parenting, and child care for babies and toddlers exist in many communities to assist parents in their new role and responsibilities. Some parenting groups continue with discussions focusing on older children and adolescence.

The University of Minnesota provides an example of a parenting group that parents can join very early in the postpartum period. It was begun to fill a void between hospital discharge and the first clinic visits 4 to 6 weeks later. Groups of four to eight couples attend four weekly discussions, beginning when their babies are about 1 week old. Crying, feeding, safety needs, and minor illnesses as rashes and colds are examples of baby-related topics. Other areas of concern are parental fatigue, changing roles, and decreased time with one's spouse. This group experience is part of the family-centered maternity care at that university (Stanik & Hogberg, 1979). The Nursing Center at the University of Wisconsin–Milwaukee offers parenting classes for parents of children from birth–2 years, focusing on communication skills, discipline, values clarification, and growth and development (Riesch, 1982). It should be noted that these types of experiences may not be for every new mother and father. A group or class may not be available in their community; the mother may not feel physically well enough to attend; or the father may not be able to take time off from his work. A CHN who sees such a need in her community may wish to start such a group herself.

*Postpartum exercises*

Exercise classes do exist in some locales, in such places as the YWCA, to assist mothers in regaining abdominal and pelvic muscle control and losing weight. These are also places to socialize. Mothers need to be reminded that focusing on themselves and their problems is normal and necessary. Many mothers are also eager to regain their prepregnancy weight and shape and feel better about themselves when they do.

## Community Resources

*La Leche League*

The La Leche League is the largest and most successful self-help group of mothers in the world. It was started in 1956 by seven breast-feeding mothers in Franklin Park, Illinois, to provide mutual support for breast-feeding women when bottle feeding was the predominant method. Their basic philosophy is good mothering through breast feeding and good comradeship among women. Chapters of La Leche are available in most cities, so the CHN can refer a mother to this group. The address is in Appendix 2A.

*The International Childbirth*
*Education Association*

The International Childbirth Education Association was formed in 1960 by both parents and professionals to promote family-centered maternity care. It promotes better childbirth and pediatric care by professionals, trains teachers for childbirth education, and publishes literature on maternity and childbirth, among other activities. This organization can be contacted for individual or group membership at the address given in Appendix 2A.

*American Society for Psycho-Prophylaxis*
*in Obstetrics*

The major goal of the American Society for Psycho-Prophylaxis in Obstetrics is to promote natural childbirth (the Lamaze method). The Society's address is in Appendix 2A.

Interconception Period

Health care of women during interconception, the period between pregnancies, is a new concept receiving some attention. It is felt that this is necessary for women to be concerned about their health between pregnancies in order to insure future normal conception (Barnes, 1978). Spermatozoa should also be healthy. This concept of positive health during the interconception period should in essence apply to the entire potential family.

## Appendix 2A

1. Maternity Center Association (publisher of the *Birth Atlas*)
   48 East 92nd Street
   New York, NY 10028
   (212) EN9-7300

2. Gerber Products Company (publisher of the pamphlet, *Expectant Mother's Guide*)
   Fremont, MI 49412

3. The Carnation Company (publisher of the pamphlet, *You and Your Contented Baby*)
   Medical Department
   5045 Wilshire Boulevard
   Los Angeles, CA 90036

4. Schering Corporation (publisher of the pamphlet, *Choosing a Birth Control Method*)
   The Emko Products Div.
   Kenilworth, NJ 07003

5. G. D. Searle and Company (publisher of the pamphlet, *Family Planning with the Pill: A Manual for Nurses*)
   Special Services Dept.
   P.O. Box 5110
   Chicago, IL 60680

6. La Leche League International
   9616 Minneapolis Avenue
   Franklin Park, IL 50131

7. International Childbirth Education Association
   P.O. Box 20084
   Minneapolis, MN 55420
   (612) 854-8660

8. American Society for Psycho-Prophylaxis in Obstetrics
1523 L Street, N.W.
Washington, DC 20025
(202) 783-7050

# References

American Academy of Pediatrics. *Pediatric nutrition handbook.* Evanston, Ill.: Author, 1979.

American College of Obstetricians and Gynecologists. *Guidelines on pregnancy and work* (NIOSH Research Report). Chicago: Author, 1977.

Atkinson, L. D. Prenatal nipple conditioning for breastfeeding. *Nursing Research,* 1979, 23, 267–271.

Barnes, F. E. F. (Ed.). *Ambulatory maternal health care and family planning services, policies, principles, practices.* Washington, D.C.: American Public Health Association, Committee on Maternal Health Care and Family Planning, 1978.

Case Western Reserve University, Health Sciences Communication Center (Producer). *Breast feeding: Prenatal and postpartal preparation.* Cleveland: Producer, 1974. (Film)

Diabetic mothers-to-be get aid. *Milwaukee Journal,* January 1, 1982, Part 6, p. 2.

Feldman, S. *Choices in childbirth.* New York: Grosset & Dunlap, 1978.

Guthrie, D. W., & Guthrie, R. A. *Nursing management of diabetes mellitus.* St. Louis: C. V. Mosby, 1977.

Health Resources Administration. *Advancedata: Vital and health statistics of the National Center for Health Statistics* (No. 11). Washington, D.C.: U.S. Department of Health, Education and Welfare, 1977.

International Childbirth Education Association. *ICEA News,* 1978, 65, 10.

Jensen, M. D., Benson, R. C., & Bobak, I. M. *Maternity care* (2nd ed.). St. Louis: C. V. Mosby, 1981.

Kreitzer, M. S. *Pregnancy and diabetes.* Hackensack, N.J.: American Diabetes Association, New Jersey Affiliate, 1980.

National Research Council (Food and Nutrition Board, Committee on Dietary Allowances). *Recommended dietary allowances* (9th ed.). Washington, D.C.: Author, 1980.

Nielsen, I. Anatomy of a birth center. In C. Reinke & P. Simkin (Eds.), *Kaleidoscope of childbearing: Preparation, birth, and nurturing* (highlights of the Tenth Biennial Convention of the International Childbirth Education Association). Seattle: International Childbirth Education Association, 1978.

Noble, E. Rationale for prenatal and postpartum exercises. In C. Reinke & P. Simkin (Eds.), *Kaleidoscope of childbearing: Preparation, birth, and nurturing* (highlights of the Tenth Biennial Convention of the International Childbirth Education Association). Seattle: International Childbirth Education Association, 1978.

Pritchard, J. A., & MacDonald, P. C. *Obstetrics* (15th ed.). New York: Appleton-Century-Crofts, 1976.

Riesch, S. Personal communication, January 4, 1982.

Rubin, R. Maternity nursing stops too soon. *American Journal of Nursing*, 1975, 75, 1634.

Schneider, J. M., Curet, L. B., Olson, R. W., & Shay, G. Ambulatory care of the diabetic. *Obstetrics and Gynecology*, 1980, 56, 144–149.

Schuler, K. When a pregnant woman is diabetic: Antepartal care. *American Journal of Nursing*, 1979, 79, 448–450.

The sponge: New contraceptive ok'd. *Milwaukee Journal*, April 8, 1983, p. 1.

Stanik, M. K., & Hogberg, B. L. L. Transition into parenthood. *American Journal of Nursing*, 1979, 79, 90–93.

Sumner, G. Giving expectant parents the help they need: The ABC's of prenatal education. *The American Journal of Maternal-Child Nursing*, 1976, 1, 220–225.

Wallace, H. M., Gold, E. M., & Lis, E. F. *Maternal and child health practices*. Springfield, Ill.: Charles C Thomas, 1973.

Willson, J. R., Beecham, C. T., & Carrington, E. R. *Obstetrics and Gynecology* (6th ed.). St. Louis: C. V. Mosby, 1979.

# 3

# Infant Care at Home
# and in the Clinic

*Dorothy D. Petrowski*

Because newborn and infant care logically follow maternity care, they are included in this chapter. The growth and development periods of infancy described are (1) the neonatal period (up to 4–6 weeks of life), and (2) the period from 6 weeks to 1 year. For both periods, the discussion focuses on physical, psychological, and social health care domains during wellness and illness. The nursing care encompasses the "traditional" type given by a community health nurse (CHN), with incorporation of in-depth health assessment skills.

## The Newborn at Home

The newborn whose life has begun in the hospital usually arrives home at 3 days of age. The CHN plans a home visit upon notification of the mother's release from the hospital. Although most mothers experience fatigue and soreness, they all too often are left alone to care for themselves and their babies. I have visited many such mothers and must stress the importance of encouraging mothers to arrange for some help at home during the first 2 or 3 weeks after birth, even if it is only for a few hours daily. A few women deliver at home; a CHN should visit these mothers even sooner in the newborn period.

### Characteristics, Growth, and Development of the Neonate

A newborn is a tiny being whose body is out of proportion to an adult's. The head, 13 to 14 inches in circumference, is about one-fourth of the body size. The body is about 1/20th the size of an adult's, with rela-

47

tively short extremities. The average length is 20 inches. Most newborns weigh between 6 and 9 pounds, with 7½ pounds the average weight.

The neonate loses weight at first. This loss of weight is less than 10% of the birth weight and is usually regained by the tenth day of life. Subsequently, the newborn gains an average of 1 ounce daily (six to 8 ounces weekly) and doubles birth weight in five to six months. During the first weeks of life, a baby lies on his back or abdomen with the head to one side. When on his stomach, he can raise his head slightly. He can focus his eyes on objects in his line of vision and can follow the object to a limited extent. His hands are usually clenched into fists. For about a month, sudden noises or movements of his crib make him cry and move his arms. Crying is his predominant language, though he "speaks" through smiling, touching, and cuddling. He eats, sleeps, cries, and thrusts his extremities much of the time (Kaluger & Kaluger, 1974; Ross Laboratories, 1977).

Examination of the Neonate by the Nurse

Health assessment of the newborn has traditionally been done by a CHN on her first home visit to a newborn. Portions of it are repeated as necessary on subsequent visits. After the CHN obtains a health history related to present complaints, sleeping and eating patterns, and so forth, she performs a physical examination. The newborn is placed on a pad or folded blanket that has been spread on a firm surface such as the kitchen table, is undressed, and is covered with a small blanket. The CHN observes and inspects him carefully in an organized sequence from head to toe, reviewing various body systems in the process. The size, position, and symmetry of body parts are always checked to determine their normality. If the CHN has nurse practitioner (NP) skills, she can use the fourfold method—inspection, percussion, palpation, and auscultation (IPPA) of the body systems—for the examination. She should utilize IPPA or a portion of it only as appropriate. For example, she can inspect the face while palpating the lacrimal sac and duct system, and she should auscultate the four quadrants of the abdomen before palpating and percussing in order to be able to hear undisturbed bowel sounds. Sections appropriate for a nurse with NP skills are marked with an asterisk on the guidelines for physical examination and health assessment of a neonate that follow. Pieces of equipment needed for the examination include a tape measure marked in centimeters and inches, a penlight, a tongue blade, and a stethoscope. An ophthalmoscope may also be used. The physical examination described here is adapted for a home visit. It includes all body systems and should take no longer than 30 minutes.

A. Head (eyes, nose, ears, and mouth) and neck
   1. Head
      a. Note whether scalp and skin are pinkish and clear of "cradle cap" and rashes. Milia are present during neonatal period.
      b. Check if fontanels are flat (not bulging), smooth, and taut. Anterior fontanel is diamond-shaped and 2.5–4.0 cm (1–1.75 in.) in size. Posterior fontanel is triangular-shaped, 0.5–1 cm (0.2–0.4 in.). The posterior one closes by 2 months of age, and the anterior one closes in 18 months to 2 years.
      c. Measure largest circumference of head.
      d. Head should flex and rotate within normal limits (WNL).
   2. Eyes
      a. Note whether eyes blink at light (use penlight). Neonate can fix on an object only momentarily.
      b. Check to see whether tearing is present. Palpate lacrimal gland and sac for swelling. Tearing should be present. If not, the lacrimal ducts may be plugged and might need massage (from medial canthus of eyes across the lacrimal ducts and downward on the nasolacrimal duct) a few times daily.
      *c. Check to see whether sclera are clear and conjunctiva are WNL.
      *d. Check for red or orange reflex and for any opacities interrupting it. (If mother holds baby over her shoulder, the newborn will keep eyes open.) Set the opthalmoscope at "0" diopter.
   3. Nose
      a. Nasal patency, thin mucus, and sneezing should be present. Check for discharges and mouth breathing.
      b. Note whether septum is at midline.
   4. Ears
      a. Check position, size, and symmetry of ears.
      b. Hearing can be checked by ringing bell or clapping hands close to baby's head, and he will respond with generalized random movements.
      *c. Pull ear down and back to examine canal, tympanic membrane, and the pars tensa with the triangular cone of light reflected on it to check for otitis media. Remember to use the smallest speculum on the otoscope; remember also that crying distorts the membrane.
   5. Mouth and pharynx
      a. Examine mouth for pinkish mucous membrane, intact soft and hard palates, and freely moveable tongue. Note whether there is a monilia or thrush infection (flat white spots that do not rub off).

      b. Check closure of both soft and hard palates (this is usually done at birth).

   6. Neck

      a. Neck should be short, thick, with skin folds.

      b. Check for cleanliness, because regurgitated milk and blanket fuzz can collect in the folds and cause irritation.

B. Chest (lungs and heart)

Chest should be narrow and abdomen should be prominent and cylindrical in shape.

   1. Lungs

      a. Respirations should range between 30 to 50 in the neonate for the first 6 months of life and be irregular and abdominal. Cough reflex should be present.

      b. Note if lungs are resonant anterior and posterior, with breath sounds WNL (use bell of stethoscope or child adapter).

   2. Heart

      a. Check rate. Apical pulse should be about 130 for the first 6 months of life (use bell of stethoscope).

C. Abdomen, back, and buttocks

  *1. Check bowel sounds (do first).

  *2. Palpate for abdominal masses.

   3. Check for rashes.

   4. Spine should be straight.

   5. Scapulae, gluteal, and knee folds should be symmetrical.

D. External genitalia

   1. Check to see whether diaper is wet.

   2. Make sure circumcision is healing on males.

E. Extremities

   1. Check both lower and upper extremities for equal length and symmetry.

   2. Do exercises to check range of motion (ROM) on selected joints, such as the ball-and-socket ones (shoulder and hip) and hinge ones (elbow and knee). See Appendix 3A, "Passive Range of Motion Adapted for Nursing," if examiner wishes to do other ROM exercises on the baby (or an adult).

   3. Check the hip joint for a congenitally dislocated hip by abducting hip joint (Ortolani test). Perform the Ortolani test to ascertain whether femur rotates properly in the acetabulum. The sign is negative if the examiner cannot touch abducted hips to examining table and hears no click (ball of femur slipping out of joint).

   4. Check to see whether longitudinal arches of feet are obscured by fat pads, giving the appearance of flat feet.

F. Neurological data
  1. The infant should be able to turn head from side to side when prone.
  2. He should be able to hold head in horizontal line with back when held prone.
  3. During breast feeding, the infant should suck vigorously.
  4. He should have a keen tactile sense (should respond even to the gentlest touch).
  5. Reflexes should be checked (these can be elicited when specific body parts are examined). Select two or more as representative, such as rooting, palmar grip, Moro, and Babinski. Check to see whether these are present and equal. These reflexes disappear in 2–4 months.
     a. Moro reflex (the infant flings both arms out and brings them toward center of body)—observe for symmetry, presence of response, and symmetrical movement.
     b. Babinski reflex (when sole of the infant's foot is stroked from heel forward, toes turn down)—examine for same qualities.
G. Miscellaneous
  1. Measure the infant's length.
  2. Weigh him.
  3. Take his temperature. (Jensen, Benson, & Bobak, 1981; Whaley & Wong, 1979).

The infant should be referred to a clinic or physician if questionable pathology is noted. The CHN discusses this with the parent(s). The nurse may assist the parent in making the medical appointment. For example, if conjunctivitis is suspected, referral is necessary for confirmation and antibiotic treatment. During and after a physical examination, the CHN should teach and give counsel related to the mother's questions and her own findings.

Newborn Care, Counseling, and Teaching

Goals for newborn care are organized as physical, psychological, and social. They encompass the main topics the CHN would discuss with the parents in the first home visits.

Physical Care

Physical care focuses on three main aspects: (1) intake and output requirements; (2) skin care; and (3) environmental or external influences. Intake and output concerns center on food, including vitamins and minerals, and normal elimination and circumcision. Bathing and umbilical cord care are the skin care measures addressed. Environmental or external influences include warmth (clothing and room temperature), safety, and equipment required for a newborn.

*Intake and output requirements:*
*food, including vitamins and minerals*

One of the mother's main concerns is feeding her newborn by breast or bottle. Burping, holding, and cuddling are similar with both.

*Nutritional requirements.* The infant's first year is the time of most rapid growth, development, and maturation. He doubles his birth weight between 4 and 6 months of age and triples it at 1 year. This growth depends upon adequate nutrition. The CHN should review the nutritional requirements, including calories, protein, fat, and carbohydrates, with the parents. The average calorie requirement is about 100 to 110 kcal/kg/day throughout the first year. This is derived from approximately 2.2 gm of protein per kg of body weight, fats in the range of 3.3 to 6.0 gm/100 kcal (30 to 45% of calories from fat), and about 500 to 1000 gm of carbohydrate daily (Woodruff, 1978; Christianson, 1982).

*Vitamins and minerals.* Both breast milk and prepared formulas contain adequate vitamins and minerals for infants, with the exception of Vitamins C and D and iron and fluoride. An infant has an adequate iron supply from his mother until about 4 months of age, if the mother had an adequate diet prenatally. Vitamin D is low in breast milk, but is added to commercial formulas. See Table 3-1 for a breakdown of supplementary vitamins and minerals for infants.

*Breast feeding.*

SCIENTIFIC BASIS FOR BREAST FEEDING. Current scientific research suggests that human milk is superior to cow's milk. Most commercial formulas, based on cow's milk for protein and lactose and using polyunsaturated vegetable oils instead of butterfat, meet the same nutritional requirements as human breast milk. For years evaporated milk was the standard formula. It meets most requirements if it is diluted (13 ounces or one can of evaporated milk and 18 ounces of water) and if 5% carbohydrate (2 tablespoons of dark Karo syrup) is added. Vitamin C in the past was supplied by orange juice, but the lack of fatty acids and Vitamin E in this formula may affect brain development. Fresh cow's milk is the same as evaporated milk if it is diluted and heated (Woodruff, 1978). All lowfat milks, such as skim milk and 1% or 2% milk, are unsatisfactory for infants.

Table 3-1

Supplementary Vitamins and Minerals for Infants

| | | Vitamins | | | | Minerals | |
|---|---|---|---|---|---|---|---|
| | | A | B | C | D | Iron | Fluoride |
| Full-term | Breast-fed | none | none | at 2* wks. | at 2 wks. | at 4 mos. | at 2 wks. if not in water supply |
| | Bottle-fed | not if in formula; otherwise at 2 wks. | not if in formula; otherwise at 2 wks. | at 2 wks. | not if in formula; otherwise at 2 wks. | " | " |
| Prematures | | └──at birth──┘ | | | | 2 mos. or before | |

*Note.* From M. Christianson, Nutritionist, Milwaukee Public Schools. Personal communication, February 1982.

*Necessary if infant becomes conditioned by mother's taking a high dosage (1 gm daily) prenatally.

It should also be noted that the protein content of cow's milk is about two times greater than that of human milk (1.5 gm/100 ml and 3.3 gm/100 ml, respectively), and that the calcium and sodium content of cow's milk is four times that of human milk. These excess protein and minerals can inhibit utilization of essential nutrients, such as magnesium, zinc, and iron; they can also significantly increase the renal solute load, which can damage the kidneys. The high calcium content also interferes with fat absorption and fat-soluble vitamins. Thus, cow's milk must be diluted. The fat in cow's milk is of limited value to an infant because it is poorly absorbed (Mead Johnson and Company, 1978; Pipes, 1977). Only the tip of the iceberg has been uncovered in reference to the values of breast milk for an infant.

TECHNIQUES OF BREASTFEEDING. When the breast-fed baby arrives home, a pattern has begun to be established. The new breast-feeding mother requires assistance and encouragement at home; she needs to know about caring for her nipples, scheduling feedings, positioning and placing the baby at the breast, burping the baby, and insuring that the baby is receiving enough milk. The mother may also seek advice about exposure of her breast when visitors come to her home and in public, in which case the CHN could suggest that she use her bedroom and a ladies' lounge when in public.

A full "demand" schedule is appropriate—if it does not become *too* demanding. A "semi-demand" schedule is probably more ideal, whereby the baby nurses on demand, but not oftener than every 2 to 3 hours. A newborn of normal birth weight will nurse on the average of every 2 to 3 hours. The following guidelines for breast feeding should be helpful during the first few weeks at home:

1. The mother should wash the breasts with a mild soap and water (or just water) daily, and wipe nipples with a warm, damp cloth before each feeding.
2. The mother should sit or lie down. Lying down affords her an extra chance to rest, and sitting up promotes complete empty-ing of the breasts. One breast-feeding session should take only about 30 to 45 minutes or less (feeding of 10–30 minutes and burping or bubbling time of about 10–15 minutes). If it is longer, the mother gets tired and frustrated, and the baby learns a pattern of procrastination. An infant receives nearly 90% of the milk requirements in the first 5 to 10 minutes of good, strong nursing, so the remainder of the time fulfills a sucking need (Chinn, 1974).
3. The mother should feed the baby from 5 to 15 minutes on one breast. This should satisfy the baby's immediate hunger if sucking is done actively. Before going to the other breast, the mother should gently but firmly break the suction between the baby and the nipple/areola.
4. The mother should take a brief break (if the infant allows this) before switching to the other breast. This allows time to burp the baby, change a diaper, and play with him a moment or two.
5. The mother should then put the baby to the second breast and allow him to nurse another 5 to 10 minutes or within reason. He may take longer to empty the second breast as the hunger was satisfied on the first breast, and now he is fulfilling a suck-ing need as well.
6. At the next feeding, the mother should alternate breasts. At-taching a safety pin to the bra as a reminder of which breast was used last is a good idea. (Most mothers use a nursing bra; the breast can be exposed without removing the bra.)
7. Alternatives to the above guidelines include starting with the breast that fills up the most, or using only one breast at a feed-ing (Warner, 1975).

*Bottle feeding.* A mother usually requires assistance with her decision to bottle-feed. Decisions must be made concerning (1) the type of formula (powder or liquid), (2) the kind of equipment to use (bottles, nipples, and sterilizer), (3) the scheduling, and (4) the method of sterilization (terminal or aseptic). After these decisions have been made, the CHN can assist the new mother by demonstrating formula making and bottle warming, as well as by discussing the amount of formula the baby should take, reuse of unconsumed formula one time, and methods of burping or bubbling.

Liquids are more popular than powders because producers have calculated them, so the mother merely adds a can of water, as in preparing a commercial soup for a meal. Glass or Pyrex bottles can be sterilized. Although sterilization is not routinely recommended, it may be necessary for a premature infant. Glass or Pyrex bottles are more economical than plastic bottles with disposable inserts. Many mothers do use plastic bottles or plastic bottles with disposable inserts very successfully. The mother should be instructed to wash the plastic bottles with warm, soapy water and rinse; boiling would melt them. The inserts are sterilized by the manufacturer. The feeding schedule is similar to that recommended for breast feeding.

Various sterilizers are appropriate. In fact, a large kettle with a cover can be used by placing a washcloth in the bottom. Sterilization of infant formula is not true sterilization of the type that is done in surgery. It is a step beyond pasteurization (a partial sterilization), and its purposes are to kill enough bacteria in the milk to make it safe for the infant and to reduce curds.

Terminal sterilization is preferred over aseptic because it is safer. The aseptic method is usually recommended as a last resort when a mother does not have a sterilizer or if she is preparing only one bottle. In some metropolitan areas, sterilization of formula after the newborn phase is no longer recommended because of improved water quality. Directions for the terminal and aseptic methods follow:

*Terminal Heat Method**

1. Wash all equipment—bottles, nipples and caps—in the dishwasher or in hot, soapy water, using a bottle brush on bottles and nipples to remove milk residue.
2. For commercial formula, follow label directions.
3. Pour required amount of formula into bottles, and cover with nipples and caps loosely.

*Sterilized water can be prepared in the same manner. Water can be kept about 10 days and does not require refrigeration.

4. Place bottles on rack in sterilizer. Add tap water to a depth of 2 inches and boil 20 minutes.
5. When cool enough to touch (about 30 minutes), tighten bottle covers, rotate bottles gently (prevents scum on surface), and store formula in refrigerator. (Modern refrigerators can accommodate the introduction of very warm foods.)

*Aseptic Method**

1. Wash all equipment as above, plus a 32-ounce measuring cup, a measuring spoon, and tongs to handle equipment.
2. Place all equipment that is to be used in making formula in the sterilizer, *cover* with water, and boil 10 minutes. Pour off the water. (Do not boil plastic equipment.)
3. At the same time that the equipment is being boiled, boil water 10 minutes in a *second* kettle. Measure required amount in the 32-ounce measuring cup, and add necessary amount of commercial formula.
4. Divide the formula among the six to eight bottles, put on nipples and caps, and store in refrigerator.

If the mother feels unsure about the method of sterilization, the CHN can set up a home visit to demonstrate this. At this time, she can also discuss warming of the bottle, the amount of formula the infant takes, and one-time reuse of the formula. Bottles are warmed by placing them in a kettle with 2 or 3 inches of water and boiling the water for about 10 minutes or in a microwave oven by following directions. The mother should test the temperature of the milk on the inner part of the wrist or a similarly sensitive body part before offering it to the baby. A baby who is bottle-fed should be held when fed.

Most mothers ask the CHN how much formula a baby should take. The usual weight gain per week for the normal infant during his first 6 months of life is 3 to 5 ounces (90 to 150 gm) (Whaley & Wong, 1979). To gain at this rate, a newborn eats between 18–24 ounces of formula in 24 hours during his first month, gradually increasing this until he approaches 28–32 ounces at 6–9 months. A percentage of infants may consume considerably more than a quart (1 liter) at an age when they are too young for solids; this is an acceptable practice. The amount of formula is naturally reduced as solids are added. Most nutritionists recommend that most infants should not exceed 32 ounces

*Recommended for making one bottle of formula; the procedure can be adapted for filling plastic bottles and plastic bag inserts for plastic bottles.

of formula daily, in order to insure that other needed nutrients are supplied from solids.

Bacteria begin to grow in milk after about 2 hours' exposure at room temperature. On this scientific basis, only one reuse of unconsumed formula can be recommended. The used bottle, however, must be placed in the refrigerator immediately after use (i.e., after the feeding and burping), or at least within 1½ to 2 hours. This recommendation considers the facts that formula is expensive; that it is difficult for the mother to prepare; and that each day a newborn is home he can tolerate less sterile conditions.

Burping (or bubbling) the baby should be discussed with the mother to relieve her anxiety and to inform her about different methods of bubbling. Burping is necessary because an infant swallows air as he sucks, and because most of his first 6 months are spent in a horizontal position. Unless a baby is bubbled, the air will be forced up on its own and milk will accompany it, resulting in regurgitation. Holding a baby during his feeding instead of propping a bottle also insures that less air is swallowed and furthers the bonding between mother and infant. Attention to psychological needs enhances the manner in which physical needs are met.

One feeding should take about 30–45 minutes, including the burping time. It is reasonable that a mother would burp the baby once or twice during the feeding and once or twice after. Only a very few minutes should be spent at burping time, or the baby will fall asleep. These bubbling moments can be good times just to enjoy the baby, feel his soft skin, and cuddle him.

There are several different methods of burping a baby: (1) lifting him to the shoulder; (2) laying him across the knee with stomach down; or (3) keeping him in the lap in a sitting position with head and chest supported. The mother should place a diaper under the baby's face because milk often comes up with the air. Because the stomach is on the left, the mother should pat the left side of the baby's back when bubbling him with the palm of her hand. It is often necessary to pat quite vigorously. The mother can softly rub the infant's back from the thoracic area up to the neck. If a baby does not burp after the feeding, it is a good idea to place him on his stomach (not his back) with the head to either side, or to place him on the right side. These positions permit any air to rise easily and come out without carrying milk with it.

*Weaning.* A mother can begin weaning the infant from the breast by gradually replacing one breast-feeding session with solids. Using a bottle or cup is a preferred method of weaning. After the infant is adjusted to losing the nursing session, a second replacement can be made at the other end of the day. This schedule should be continued until only two breast-feeding sessions remain—preferably morning and evening, but whatever is most convenient for mother and baby is the ideal. These two feedings may be continued throughout infancy or longer. In some countries, a baby is breast-fed until he is 2 years of age or older (Lawrence, 1980).

Weaning from the bottle is similar, in that a baby usually continues to have a bottle in the forenoon and at bedtime. Most babies cut teeth between 6 and 9 months of age; this readies them for foods they can chew, so weaning during these months is natural and logical. Many mothers allow their infants to use pacifiers to take care of their sucking need. Most children who use pacifiers or thumbs give up regular use of these comfort devices by the end of the preschool years.

It should be emphasized that infants ought to be breast-fed or kept on formula for the first year of life.

*Extra water and orange juice.*   Water and orange juice need not be given routinely. Extra water may be offered, but is not required except during very warm weather, and/or if the child has an infection. (Orange juice was introduced into the neonate's diet about 1900, because pasteurization destroyed the Vitamin C in cow's milk.) Ascorbic acid requirements for an infant are based on levels in human milk, so breast-fed infants and those receiving fortified formula do not require extra ascorbic acid. Consequently, diluted apple or orange juice is now considered a liquid food to be added when the child is developmentally ready to drink from a cup or when fruits are added, somewhere past the sixth month of life (Christianson, 1982).

*Solids.*   From a nutritional point of view, human milk or commercially prepared formula meets the infant's recommended requirements for the first 6 months. During the second half-year of life, these substances meet only between one-half and two-thirds of the child's caloric needs. Therefore, semisolid foods should be started when the child is developmentally ready to swallow solids, such as when the tongue protrusion reflex disappears. At this stage he is about 4 to 6 months of age and has reached 6 to 7 kg (13 to 15 pounds) or somewhat less, depending upon his birthweight. Early introduction of solids (at 3 months of age or sooner) can lead to gastrointestinal irritation and/or overfeeding. Solids are well tolerated at 6 months of age, and at 9 months a baby can swallow lumpy foods (American Academy of Pediatrics, 1979; Christianson, 1983; Pipes, 1977).

The American Academy of Pediatrics (1979) recommends the introduction of semisolids when the infant is at least 3 months old. Cereal is usually introduced first (at 3–6 months of age) because of its high iron content (7 mg/3 tablespoons). Rice cereal is the preferred first choice because of its low allergic reaction. Other cereals may include oatmeal, barley, and mixed. Each should be introduced separately to acquaint the baby with a new taste and consistency and to note any allergic reactions. Hence, mixed cereals should be started last. Cooked rice cereal or farina can be used if cooked longer to break down the complex carbohydrates. Formula is added to cereals to obtain the right consistency.

Vegetables are introduced after cereals, because they have a lower sugar content than fruits. It is easier to introduce vegetables if this is done before the baby gets accustomed to the sweet taste of fruits first. The baby does not need the extra sugar that fruits provide at this point. Fruits are the third solid started, followed by meats (at 6–7 months of age). Meats provide protein and iron. When any new solid is begun, only a few teaspoons of it should be offered, and it should be given for a few days to a week before a new one is introduced in order to observe the baby's ability to tolerate it.

*Anemia and obesity in infancy.* Anemia or obesity are nutritional problems of concern in infancy. Anemia, which is rare in breast-fed infants, is the most common nutritional deficiency in infants. The present recommendation for iron, of 0.15 mg/100 kcal, is based on the amount in human milk. Therefore, fortification of infant formulas at the level of 10–12 mg/l is recommended. Infant cereals are also fortified with iron (Woodruff, 1978).

A 6-month-old infant is often given cow's milk, which is low in iron. In addition, if he drinks more than a quart (1 liter) daily, the protein in fresh cow's milk can cause irritation of the gastric lining and occult blood loss from the intestines, resulting in increased anemia. This can occur despite an earlier adequate iron intake (Mead Johnson and Company, 1978).

An infant's diet should be limited to the number of calories recommended, and should not exceed it. If an infant is fed too much, he develops extra fat cells. Then weight reduction becomes more complicated later in life, because it is not as simple to reduce the body fat when there are extra fat cells. Obesity is the most common nutritional problem in the United States.

*Elimination (stools, urine, and circumcision).* The type of feeding greatly affects the color and consistency of the stools. Observation of the quantity and quality of stools is necessary, because dehydration from diarrhea can be fatal to a newborn. The number of stools ranges from one to eight daily, with the breast-fed infant having more frequent ones at first than the bottle-fed infant. However, it is normal for the baby to miss a daily bowel movement sometimes. Normal stools contain solids, are yellow or brown, and do not smell foul. Stools of breast-fed babies are yellow and liquid, with small particles like cottage cheese. Each formula produces a characteristic stool; however, stools should still be in a normal range.

Urine is clear, has an ammonia odor, and is excreted from at least five to 20 times in 24 hours. The number of wet diapers per day is a good indicator of the hydration status of the infant.

Circumcision care, discussed here because of its close relationship to elimination, includes assessment of healing and cleansing. Healing is usually completed within 10 days. Cleansing with warm water at bath time and when there is a bowel movement is sufficient. The CHN may need to recommend air drying to promote healing. A small amount of Vaseline can be applied to the circumcision site to relieve redness and irritation. Within the first 24 hours after the circumcision, the child should not sleep on the abdomen to avoid pressure to the area. If bleeding from the site occurs, direct pressure should be applied with a firmly (*not tightly*) wrapped gauze dressing. If the bleeding continues, the newborn should be seen on an emergency basis by a physician or an NP.

### Skin care

*Bathing.* Bathing the baby every other day in a baby's bathtub or the kitchen sink is recommended after the umbilical area is healed. If the mother chooses to bathe the baby less often, she should wash his face, neck creases, and perineal area each day with mild soap and water. The perineal area is also cleansed at each diaper change with a damp washcloth or a disposable towelette. The hair should be shampooed and brushed at each bath time or several times weekly to prevent seborrheic dermatitis, commonly called "cradle cap" (crusty, yellowish, adherent lesions of unknown cause). Often mothers are afraid to rub the area of the fontanel vigorously; failure to do so contributes to cradle cap.

*Umbilical cord care.* At delivery, the umbilical cord is cut about 1 inch from the neonate's body and clamped with a plastic or metal clamp or tied with a cord. The clamp may be removed within a few days of the baby's birth, or left until the cord falls off, 7 to 14 days after delivery. The umbilical stump becomes very dry and black or moist and foul-smelling before it drops off, and this discoloration can alarm the mother if she does not anticipate it. After the cord drops off, the area will have a serosanguinous drainage for a few days. It should be gently cleansed daily with 70% alcohol on cotton until it is completely healed. To prevent infection, tub baths are not usually recommended until the umbilical area is completely healed.

The umbilical area heals best when it is exposed to the air. Drying and healing are facilitated by folding the baby's diaper below the umbilicus and the shirt slightly above it. The mother should make certain the room temperature is warm before exposing the baby's midriff in this manner.

The falling off of the cord and the healing of the umbilicus are very normal processes and occur without problems in most newborns. However, if the umbilicus becomes red and develops a purulent discharge, the mother should call the clinic for advice.

### Environmental or external influences

*Warmth.* A normal newborn does not require a room warmer than is comfortable for the rest of the family. A baby usually cries if he experiences an uncomfortable temperature change. Maintenance of an axillary temperature of 36.4°C (97.6°F) is normal. A drop in rectal temperature to 35.8°C (96.6°F) or rise to 38.1°C (100.6°F) should be a signal for action, such as an increase in clothing or fluids.

*Clothing.* The CHN should suggest size 6 to 12 months for shirts and other sized items, because an infant grows rapidly. Clothing should be washable. A basic layette includes the following:

| | |
|---|---|
| Baby clothes | 48 diapers or disposable diapers |
| | 4 shirts—at least size 6 months |
| | 8–10 sleepers or nightgowns |
| | 2 jackets or sweaters |
| | 1 bunting |
| | 2 pairs plastic panties |
| | Dressy suits or dresses and slips as desired |
| Linens | 2 large, soft bath towels |
| | 2 baby washcloths or thin adult ones |
| | 1 plastic mattress protector |
| | 1 mattress cover |
| | 6 contour-bottom crib sheets |
| | 2 crib blankets |
| | 8 small rubberized pads |
| | 6 receiving blankets |

Feeding supplies                        12 bottles—8-ounce size rec-
                                        ommended—and nipples
                                        Bottle brush
                                        Sterilizer

Tray supplies                           2 bars mild soap (Ivory, Cas-
                                        tile, etc.)
                                        Bottle baby oil
                                        Jar Vaseline
                                        Package cotton balls or roll of
                                        cotton (does not need to be
                                        sterile)
                                        Safety pins and diaper pins

Miscellaneous supplies                  Pacifier
                                        Baby hot-water bottle
                                        Rectal thermometer
                                        1- to 2-gallon pail for diapers
                                        1 hamper for soiled linen

*Safety.*   Most serious childhood accidents can be prevented. Studies show that certain types of accidents are more prevalent at one stage
of development than at another. To prevent them, the CHN and the
parents must be alert to a very young child's insatiable need to explore,
feel, touch, and taste.

Choking, suffocation, automobiles, fire, and falls cause the greatest number of infant deaths. An infant should be held when fed, not
propped, to avoid choking. If a mother breast-feeds in bed, she should
be cautioned about the risk of her falling asleep and rolling onto the
baby. The baby's face must be kept free of covers in the crib, so he will
not suffocate. A newborn is safer in a car seat than in a lap. The parents should look for a car seat with a label certifying that it complies
with the Federal Motor Vehicle Standard Number 213. A parent should
keep matches and lighters out of reach, cap electrical outlets, use guards
for hot air registers, and keep the baby away from hot stoves and hot
liquids. An infant should *never* be left unattended in any place where
he might roll and fall. A high-chair harness is advocated.

A CHN should instruct parents to make their house accident-
proof—to buy safe toys, lock up medicines, place poisonous household
substances in a safe place, and remove sharp objects from reach. Toys
for a small child should be larger than his mouth (a good rule of thumb).
Furniture and toys should be checked to insure lead-free paint. Paint
should conform to standards set by the American National Standards
Institute (ANSI) Standard 266.1-1972. Paint on imported toys may not

conform to these standards, and thus such toys should be purchased with caution. Although child-proof covers are required by law on medicine containers, the containers should be placed in a locked medicine cupboard. In addition to storing cleaning fluids, bleaches, hair sprays, and pesticides in out-of-reach places, such substances should be tightly covered. Scissors and knives should not be left on any accessible surface (Metropolitan Life Insurance Company, 1970).

Although infants cannot be responsible for their actions, the CHN should advise parents to begin warning children as young as 6 months of age about hazards, so that they will grow up with increasing awareness of the dangers in their lives. The nurse should explain the functions of a poison control center, assist the parents in locating the nearest one, and instruct them to post the telephone number in a convenient place.

*Equipment needed.* The CHN should ascertain that the crib protects the baby from falling out, and that it has a firm mattress. A firm mattress is required for proper development of vertebrae. The infant may spend more than half the day on this mattress, so it is worthwhile to have a good one! A rocking chair may be a luxury, but it does add to the psychological dimension of caring for a baby.

## Psychological Care

Psychological care involves physical contact and communication with parents (bonding) and acceptance by siblings.

### Physical contact and communication with parents—bonding

"Bonding," or attachment between a mother and her infant or between the parents and the newborn, should ideally begin in the delivery room to insure optimal nurturing of the offspring. When a newborn arrives at home on the third day of life, hospital personnel have already greatly influenced the bond (Klaus & Kennell, 1976). The CHN, in her home visit, should discuss the following relevant bonding issues with the new mother: when the mother first saw and held her infant; whether the father was present at the delivery; and the quantity and quality of subsequent contact between the parents and the infant during the hospital stay. If these contacts were unsatisfactory or inadequate, a CHN should discuss ways to overcome them and to increase contact with the infant.

The CHN should reinforce satisfactory bonding begun in the hospital by encouraging the parents to communicate with their infant through touching, cuddling, smiling, and talking. If an attachment has not been well established (as evidenced by the mother's lack of total attention to the infant's physical care, extreme fear of the infant, or lack of enjoyment of the baby), the CHN should assist the mother in developing psychological caring for her baby. She should encourage the discussion of any ambivalence the mother has, should reinforce positive aspects of the mother's caring, and should help her set realistic goals for herself and the infant. She can demonstrate cuddling and cooing, and can point out its importance as a stimulant to the infant's social interaction and to the flow of breast milk. (See Appendix 3B for audiovisual aids for discussions on parenting.)

### Acceptance by siblings

Integration of the newborn with any siblings is essential for the newborn's and the parents' physical and mental well-being. Siblings should be allowed and encouraged to hold and care for the new baby. This enables them to understand the baby and focuses attention on the siblings as well as on the new baby. The current emphasis on attachment between a newborn and his parents should be supplemented by the attachment between siblings in order that a functional family unit may develop.

## Social Concerns

Important social concerns are space, economics, the mother's tasks, and baby sitters.

### Space

Newborns require space within a home, and the CHN should determine whether the family has maximized existing space before the baby is born. It is ideal for a baby to have his own room to minimize disturbance of other family members with his cries.

### Economics

Besides space, a newborn requires a bedroom with a crib, a chest, bathing supplies and (ideally) a rocker. The purchases necessary for a new baby, especially a first baby or twins, can add up to hundreds of dollars. Baby showers are one way in which society assists parents with some of the financial burdens. Medical expenses may also concern some parents. The financial drain can add psychological stress to a marital relationship, especially if the baby was not planned.

### The mother's tasks

Another social aspect of the newborn's presence is that of the new tasks created for the baby's mother, such as feeding, diapering, doing laundry, and meeting the baby's other needs; all of these consume a lot of time and create stress. Neighbors in an apartment building may complain that the mother spends a disproportionate amount of time in the laundry facilities, for example. Although a new mother wants to take the best possible care of herself and her infant, she needs added rest and encouragement to cope with the new responsibilities, the extra work, and the stress.

### Baby sitters

Baby sitters will be needed from time to time. Even if relatives are asked, the mother still must be concerned for the baby's comfort and safety. A newborn requires the care of a mature person at least 16 years of age. The mother should write down the tasks (such as feeding the baby) that the sitter is to perform in the mother's absence, as well as the telephone number(s) where she can be reached. The mother can also call her home to check that all is going well.

If the mother returns to work, a long-term arrangement must be made for the care of the infant. In this case it is ideal, but not always feasible, to have an adult come to the home.

## Minor Illnesses

Upper respiratory infections (URIs), diarrheas, pain, and rashes (including diaper rashes) are four of the common minor illnesses infants may develop. They can often be prevented or minimized by preventive child care. The mother should be taught how to recognize symptoms of illness, such as general irritability, flushed face, runny nose, husky cry, or vomiting, and how to take a rectal temperature. A rectal temperature over 102.8°F is usually the cutoff point at which the mother should immediately contact a health professional for advice. Only humidifiers that spray a cool mist should be used to loosen secretions during a URI. Clear liquids are more important than food if the baby has a fever or diarrhea. Infants with mild or moderate diarrhea usually respond quickly to simple measures: dietary changes (possibly withholding food for 12 hours), bed rest, and nonprescription medication. If the loose or liquid stools continue and are frequent the second day, the physician should be notified so that dehydration can be prevented. Aspirin or Tylenol in an infant dosage is often recommended for fever and/or pain.

If the pain continues, the physician or CHN should be telephoned.

Nothing that is not prescribed should be applied to a rash. Meticulous diaper and skin care can often prevent diaper rashes. Diaper dermatitis—irritation or excoriation of the skin in the diaper area—is a common annoyance caused by bacteria from the intestinal tract acting on the urea and forming ammonia, or by diarrhea. It can be prevented by prompt and frequent diaper changes and prompt cleansing of the skin. Air drying can be used for a mild rash, and steroid or antibiotic ointments should be prescribed if it progresses to a very uncomfortable state (Scripien, Barnard, Chard, Howe, & Phillips, 1979).

## Clinic Care in the Neonatal Period

The mother takes her baby to the physician or NP for the first well-baby checkup at 1 month to 6 weeks of age. The physician or NP does a physical examination, including measurements of length, weight, and head size. (See the guidelines for physical examination and health assessment of a neonate by a CHN, pp. 48–51.) Questions about feeding, weight, crying periods, minor illnesses, and so forth are discussed with the parents.

During the first year of life, clinic care includes a health history and the following seven activities: (1) developmental assessment; (2) examination for physical and psychological problems; (3) specialized screening, such as vision and hearing assessment; (4) laboratory tests such as a hematocrit or lead level; (5) immunizations, (6) questions about feeding; and (7) health education.

Health education includes a discussion of development, safety, stimulation with talking and play, feeding practices, and anticipatory guidance for accident prevention. Table 3-2 is a chart of anticipatory teaching and counseling guidelines for the CHN. Playing with an infant fosters bonding, increases his sense of belonging, and stimulates him. Peek-a-boo, pat-a-cake, clapping hands to music, and shaking a rattle are fun games to play with infants.

## Remainder of the Infant Period: 6 Weeks to 1 Year of Age

### Characteristics of Growth and Development

At 6 weeks a baby makes cooing noises and holds a rattle, but sleep occupies most of his time. At 3 months he has mastered holding his head upright when on his stomach, and at 6 months he can sit up in his crib and recognize his parents. The period of infancy is one of tremendous growth, especially physical and motor development; by the age of 1, the baby has tripled his weight and is able to walk. His cognitive and effective development have progressed to such an extent that he is now a definite personality. He interacts socially by imitating his mother's speech sounds, has temper tantrums if he does not get his way, and smiles in response to pleasant encounters. Observation (the Denver Developmental Screening Test, or DDST, is one type of observation) and physical examination are ways to assess development.

## Care at Home

The CHN usually visits an older infant much less often than she does a newborn. Again, this depends upon the health assessment of the mother and the neonate/infant, as evaluated by the clinic personnel and the CHN. She often makes a home visit every month or every other month until the baby is 6 months of age; these visits continue longer, if warranted. The purposes for CHN visits during this period might be to assist with instruction in feeding, to assess growth and development, to give anticipatory guidance as detailed in Table 3-2, to advise on safety, and to provide direct nursing care for minor and more serious illnesses.

## Clinic Care

### Purposes

The infant should be taken to a clinic or a private physician at approximately 1, 2, 4, and 6 months of age (or monthly) so that health personnel can follow the baby's growth and development, give immunizations, supervise the feeding schedule, and give counsel about physical, psychological, and social needs. The infant is usually seen every 2 or 3 months in the second 6 months of life.

A history and health assessment are done at periodic intervals during infancy. The age and responses of the child dictate the sequence of performance. For example, if the baby is quiet, the examiner should auscultate the heart, lungs, and abdomen first. Talking to the baby and parents before, during, and after the examination fosters a trusting relationship and provides a chance to offer explanations. The physical examination of the infant after the newborn period is similar to that for the neonate; only a brief general outline for health assessment is included here.

## Table 3-2

### Anticipatory Teaching and Counseling Guidelines for the CHN

| Age | Developmental Milestones | Feeding | Safety | Attachment and Stimulation | Health Teaching | Other |
|---|---|---|---|---|---|---|
| 1 month | Sucking<br>Rooting<br>Responds to noise<br>Follows to midline<br>Regards face<br>Lifts head when prone | Support of choice of feedings<br>Delay of introduction of solids<br>Use of pacifier<br>Burping | Rolling and falling<br>Aspiration, suffocation<br>Bottle propping | Cuddling and talking to baby<br>Eye contact<br>Physical contact and movement | Immunization schedule and importance<br>Rashes<br>Family planning | Effect of baby on family<br>Individual differences in babies<br>Taking baby outside<br>Stools |
| 2 months | Lifts head to 90°<br>Listens<br>Cooing sounds<br>Rolling over<br>Hands to midline<br>Responds with smile | Reinforce delay of solid foods<br>Enjoyable mealtimes | Car seat safety<br>Rolling and falling<br>Safe toys | Mobiles<br>Infant seat<br>Talking to baby<br>Swing | Side effects of immunizations<br>Fever management | Parents' need to be away from baby<br>Family schedules<br>Thumbsucking |
| 4 months | Sits with support<br>Holds head erect<br>Follows to 180°<br>Grasps rattle<br>Teething | No bottles in bed<br>Pattern for introduction to solids | Safe toys for grasping and mouthing<br>Gradual exposure to sun | Play pen<br>Mirrors<br>Crib toys<br>Interaction with siblings | Teething<br>Care for upper respiratory infection, diarrhea | Temperament<br>Sharing child care between parents<br>Consistency of care |

| Age | | | | | | |
|---|---|---|---|---|---|---|
| 6 months | Reaches for object<br>Sits without support<br>Smiles spontaneously<br>Crawling; syllables<br>Stranger anxiety<br>Everything into mouth | Finger foods<br>Need for foods with iron | Discipline<br>Accident proofing home<br>Burns and drowning | High chair<br>Walker<br>Jumper | Nutrition—<br>Decrease milk intake to 24 oz. per day<br>Avoid extra sugar, salt | Separation and Stranger anxiety<br>Differences in childrearing between parents |
| 9 months | Transfers objects<br>Feeds self with fingers<br>Pulls self to standing<br>Babbles<br>Pat-a-cake | Finger foods<br>Cup<br>Weaning | Access to stairs, outdoors<br>Car safety<br>Ipecac<br>Safe play environment | Bath and nesting toys<br>Kitchen utensils<br>Sound imitation | Caries prevention<br>Disadvantages of early toilet training and weaning | Soft, inexpensive shoes<br>Bedtime rituals<br>Normal curiosity |
| 12 months | Peek-a-boo<br>Uses Mama; Dada<br>Thumb-finger grasp<br>Walking/cruising<br>Exploring<br>Begins to indicate wants | Lessened appetite<br>Increases independence with cup and utensils | Pica<br>Lead danger<br>Supervision of climbing, bathing, play activity | Push and pull toys<br>Reading to child<br>Naming and pointing to objects | Symptoms of ear problems<br>Review nutritional needs<br>Decrease milk intake to 16–20 oz. per day | Handling of genitals<br>Limit-setting<br>Discipline<br>Need for dependence-independence |

*Note.* From M. Etu, Instructor, School of Nursing, University of Wisconsin–Milwaukee. Unpublished material, March 1980. Used by permission of the author.

A. Preliminaries
   1. Measurements
      a. Vital signs and blood pressure
      b. Height, weight, and head circumference
   2. General appearance and affect
   3. Responses to the parents' comments and questions
B. Physical assessment
   1. Head and neck
      a. Scalp and fontanels
      b. Eyes, ears, and nose
      c. Mouth, tongue, and throat
   2. Chest (lungs and heart)
   3. Abdomen and back
   4. Genitalia
   5. Extremities
C. Neurological assessment
   1. Intellectual behavior
   2. Motor functioning
   3. Reflexes
D. Developmental screening

The CHN in a clinic should have appropriate literature about infants (feeding, immunization, growth, and development) available for parents to read while they wait for their appointments. Parents may also wish to listen to tapes (with a headset) about infant care.

## Infants at Risk

As early as 1953, newborns at risk were assigned lower Apgar scores* at birth; however, early identification and treatment of the high-risk infant (perinatology) as a new science began about 15 years ago. New technologies, such as amniocentesis, ultrasonography to measure fetal head size and growth, and visualization of the fetus with fetoscopy, have allowed perinatologists to achieve some lowering of the long-standing and unacceptably high perinatal morbidity and mortality in the United States. The new techniques for infants at risk include a varie-

---

*Apgar scores: In 1953, Virginia Apgar, M.D., introduced a simple, semiquantitative method to evaluate neonates clinically 5 minutes after birth. The score is based on observations of heart rate, respiration, effort, muscle tone, reflex irritability, and color. Scores of 0, 1, or 2 are assigned to each of the five observations. Scores of 0 to 3 indicate a depressed neonate, and 7 or more a very health one (Hughes, 1975).

ty of stimulation approaches to help these infants reach their maximum potential.

Some conditions of high-risk infants are correctable, and others exist for life. Prematurity and cleft palates can be corrected medically and surgically, respectively; Down's syndrome cannot. Cleft palates and Down's syndrome may or may not be inherited. The goal in any of these conditions is prevention, early identification and prompt treatment.

Six specific conditions are discussed here: prematurity; an infant's being small for gestational age (SGA); cleft palate; meningomyelocele; Down's syndrome; and child neglect and abuse. Families of high-risk infants are best served through continuous and coordinated care between health care and community services. Hospital nurseries and public health agencies communicate with referral forms for high-risk infants, which describe the infants' conditions in detail.

## The Preterm Infant

### Definition and risk factors

Births that occur before 37 weeks' gestation are defined as "preterm births." Prematurity and small birth weight are usually concomitant. In 1948, the World Health Organization defined the "premature infant" as a newborn who weighed 2500 grams (5 pounds, 8 ounces) or less at birth. Today, however, many infants with birth weights over 1000 grams survive with prolonged intensive care. The incidence of preterm births is about 7% of all live births (National Center for Health Statistics, 1980). The risk factors include multiple births, abnormalities of the placenta (previa and abruptio), incompetency of the cervix, maternal metabolic disorders, hypothyroidism and hyperthyroidism, eclampsia, premature membrane rupture, and maternal urinary tract infections. Adolescent mothers deliver more premature infants than do older women.

### Care at home

When a preterm infant reaches approximately 2500 grams, he is usually discharged from the hospital. The CHN may visit or telephone the hospital's intensive care unit and talk to the hospital nurses about the special needs of the infant. A CHN frequently visits the home before discharge of the baby to ascertain readiness for the infant's arrival and teach parents about caring for the baby. Some points that may need to be emphasized at this time are appropriate infant equipment, such as a firm mattress and a warm room for the baby; formula preparation; and ways to increase attachment. The attitude of the parents should be considered along with their questions.

The goals of nursing care of the preterm infant at home are: (1) insuring adequate nutrition and weight gain, (2) preventing infection, (3) preserving body heat, (4) insuring rest, and (5) making allowance for physical and psychological stimulation. The care is very similar to that outlined for the normal infant; it varies, depending upon the individual requirements of each baby and the environment to which he goes home. For example, preterm infants are usually fed formula on a 3-hour schedule when they come home, and receive multivitamin drops daily prior to the formula. Contact with outsiders should be limited until the mother is certain that the infant is gaining weight and appears alert.

### The Infant Who Is Small for Gestational Age

SGA infants are not necessarily preterm (37 weeks' gestation or less) and fall into two general categories: hypoplastic (implying an internal defect) or malnourished. SGA babies who have congenital anomalies (with or without chromosomal defects) or have suffered a uterine infection best typify the hypoplastic classification; examples include newborns with Down's or rubella syndrome, respectively.

By far the largest number of SGA infants suffer fetal malnutrition as a result of maternal disease or an unnatural condition that affects the oxygen and nutrients supplied. These include toxemia, respiratory or cardiac disease, abnormal placenta, and addictions (cigarette smoking, and chemical dependence). This SGA group has an infinitely better prognosis than the former described, and their care is similar to that for most preterm infants (Clark & Affonso, 1979).

### The Infant with a Cleft Palate

The cleft palate is usually diagnosed during a thorough physical assessment or at the initial feeding in the first 24 hours of life. Cleft lip and cleft palates can occur separately or together. Only the cleft palate, not the cleft lip (harelip), is discussed here, because a cleft lip can be repaired as early as 2 weeks of age, and the cleft palate involves much more care. The cleft palate surgery is done when the baby is about 14 months old, weighs 20 pounds, and has two front teeth. This time is preferred so that the child will not develop faulty speech patterns (Hughes, 1975).

### Incidence and etiology

Cleft lip and/or palate is the most common facial anomaly (Hughes, 1975). The incidence of cleft lip with or without cleft palate is about 1 in 1000 live births, and of cleft palate alone is about 1 in 2500 live births (Vaughan, McKay & Behrman, 1979).

Experts agree that there is no familial tendency for the cleft lip and palate to occur together, and that heredity plays a part in the cleft palate's occurring separately. However, there is lack of agreement as to whether the isolated cleft lips have a genetic basis or not. Thus, parents can be told that future siblings of a child with an isolated cleft palate have an increased risk for this anomaly (Schaffer & Avery, 1977).

### Preoperative nursing care—first 1 to 2 years of life

*Feeding.* Feeding is the main concern, because the cleft reduces the infant's sucking ability by limiting compression of the areola (or the nipple of a bottle). This makes breast feeding impossible and bottle feeding nearly so. The mother should hold the infant in an upright position during feeding to lessen escape of liquid into the nasal cavity. At every feeding, there will be some regurgitation of the feeding into the nose.

Normal nipples are not suitable, because infants with cleft palates cannot generate the suction required. A variety of special nipples or feeding devices are available. Large, soft nipples with big holes, such as those used for feeding baby lambs, can be purchased in a pet shop or farm feeding store. Feeding should be attempted with nipples because they encourage use of the sucking muscles. This muscle development aids in speech development later. Continued gentle pressure on the base of the bottle reduces the chances of choking and coughing. At every feeding, the infant makes a lot of noise sucking. Since he swallows more air than normal, more frequent bubbling may be required (Whaley & Wong, 1979).

If the nipple feeding is unsuccessful, I have found a small asepto syringe fashioned with a rubber tubing tip to work well; a Breck feeder can also be used. These implements can be purchased in a drugstore or hospital supply store. A spoon can also be used. Ross Laboratories markets a special kit for feeding babies with cleft lips and palates.

Rubber nipples can be softened quickly by putting them in a pressure cooker for a *few* minutes. Nipples should be washed with water and detergent and boiled for 3 to 5 minutes, as for any neonate or infant. They can be stored in a covered jar that has been washed and sterilized by boiling for 10 minutes about twice weekly.

*Planning for surgery and counseling for parents.*   Although cleft palates require more extensive surgery, they do not elicit as much initial negative parental emotion as does the more visible cleft lip. Parents will have questions about the cause of the defect, as well as about surgery, cosmetic effects, and blending procedures. They will require continued support of their own feelings, especially if heredity is deemed to have played a part in the causation. They should be comforted and reassured that the plastic surgery will be successful. The CHN should allow them to talk about their feelings and should promote bonding. Most children require only one surgical procedure to complete the repair. (For the few who require several operations, the parents should be prepared for the number of operations that will have to be done.) Speech training, special dentistry, and orthodontia will also be needed. The CHN should reinforce the advice of the hospital nurses and physicians and should continue to supervise feeding on her home visits. The care of these children truly requires a multidisciplinary approach.

Referral to the state or local service for the developmentally disabled should be done to insure that the child with cleft palate problems is cared for as long as necessary (approximately 5 to 6 years), and to obtain financial assistance if needed. The CHN or the mother can telephone the local county or city health department for information.

### Postoperative care

*Feeding.*   A child who has had surgical repair of a cleft palate remains in the hospital for about 5 to 10 days. The suture line is usually healed at the end of 2 weeks. The mother is instructed to give clear liquids and soft foods, but no milk, until the suture line is healed.

*Clinic visits.*   A clinic appointment is made for the child with the plastic surgeon within the first month after surgery and periodically as needed to plan for further surgery, dentistry, orthodontia, and speech therapy over the next 5 years. At 5 or 6 years of age, the condition is usually corrected to the maximum extent possible. A few children wear dental braces beyond this time. Between appointments to the plastic surgeon, the child usually returns to the well-baby clinic, pediatrician, or family doctor for the usual routine follow-up and care. It is not unusual for a child with a cleft palate to be followed by a community health agency for about 5 years or until the condition is completely corrected.

*Continued counseling for the parents.* Parents may receive support through a parents' group for children with cleft lips and palates. They may also wish to talk to the CHN about their feelings and the child's care at periodic intervals on a long-term basis. *Bright Promise for Your Child with Cleft Lip and Cleft Palate,* a pamphlet published by the Easter Seal Society, is an excellent resource to suggest to the parents (McDonald & Berlin, 1980).

Some parents blame each other for the child's condition. This is especially true if there is another child with a cleft palate among the relatives. In some instances, the CHN may refer the parents for psychiatric care, in order to insure that the child's growth and development follow a normal course.

## The Infant with a Meningomyelocele

Another tragedy for parents is the birth of an infant with a meningomyelocele. Like a child with a cleft palate, this defect requires a lengthy course of postoperative care at home. A defect of embryonic development of the central nervous system (CNS) has been established in meningomyelocele, but the etiology and pathogenesis are unclear. The incidence of spina bifida cystica (meningocele, meningomyelocele, and lipomeningocele) is 1 in 2000 to 4000. Meningomyeloceles are 10 to 20 times more frequent than meningoceles and have much more serious consequences.

### Clinical manifestations

The meningomyelocele (a herniated sac covering meninges and neural tissue) can be located anywhere along the spinal column. The most common sites are the thoracolumbar, lumbar, and lumbrosacral regions. The type and degree of neurological deficit are determined by the location and size of the lesion. Regardless of the upper level of the lesion, the baby with a meningomyelocele usually has neurogenic bladder dysfunction. Hydrocephalus infrequently complicates meningoceles, but is present in 85–90% of those with meningomyeloceles (Schaffer & Avery, 1977). Hydrocephaly is discussed in Chapter 4.

*Prenatal detection*

There is no primary prevention for open neural tube defects (meningomyelocele, meningocele, and anencephaly), because their cause has not been established. However, there is a secondary prevention through the use of uterine ultrasonography and amniotic fluid examination for an elevated alpha-feto-protein (AFP) level. The optimal time for these tests is between the 14th and 16th weeks of pregnancy, before the AFP concentration normally diminishes and in sufficient time for an abortion, if elected (Whaley & Wong, 1979).

*Surgical intervention*

There is controversy at present as to the best time for surgery for meningomyeloceles. At Children's Hospital in Milwaukee, virtually all babies so affected have surgical repair on the day they are born or the next day to decrease the chances of infection and trauma to the lesion (Browning, 1981). The purpose of surgical repair is to cover the exposed nerve elements with tissue and skin. Permanent impairment of neuromuscular function below the level of the defect depends upon how much CNS tissue is involved. Shunting for the hydrocephalus, which is generally present and diagnosed in the newborn, is usually done at a later date.

The child with an extensive "open," occipital lesion has a slim chance of survival and very little possibility of eventual reasonable intellectual or motor function. The child with this defect would be a poor candidate for surgery.

*Postoperative care at home*

Since most babies with meningomyeloceles have surgery before they leave the hospital, only postoperative care at home is discussed here. The child is discharged about 10 to 14 days after surgery. The baby with a meningomyelocele is usually referred to the CHN for follow-up. The CHN's attention should be directed to the following immediate care: (1) keeping the surgical site clean, (2) positioning, (3) ROM exercises, (4) incontinence care, (5) social stimulation, (6) acceptance of the child by the family, and (7) discussion of the condition.

The surgical site is usually well healed at discharge time, and a gentle daily cleansing of the wound should be done. A dressing may or may not be worn at home for a week or two. The baby's position should be changed every few hours, so that he does not lie continuously on the affected side. A physical therapy regime should be ordered by the physician for ROM exercises of the lower extremities. The Crede procedure of massage insures emptying of the bladder. Diapers are changed frequently for a few weeks to prevent breakdown of the suture line.

Acceptance of the child by the parents comes through a better understanding of the child's condition and the care involved. Therefore, the CHN should anticipate questions about the anomaly: its cause, the anatomy and physiology involved, the care needed, and the prognosis. Although the parents may have received an explanation of the defect, they may not have absorbed the information due to shock, denial, and angry reactions to the event. The surgeon should apprise the CHN of the expected prognosis. Social stimulation can be provided by touching, fondling, talking, singing, and hanging mobiles above the crib. The mother should be encouraged to hold the baby during feeding time. Feeding is usually not a problem.

*Long-term care*

Long-term care is directed at controlling hydrocephalus, encouraging ambulation, preventing urinary infections, and helping the child to attain his maximum physical and mental potential. Shunting may be required if hydrocephalus progresses. The child is often fitted with leg braces and crutches for later ambulation. Urinary infections pose a continual threat. Referral to the local division for the developmentally disabled, the Easter Seal Society, or the United Association for Mentally Retarded Citizens should be suggested to the parents as possible sources of financial assistance if needed, of follow-up for as long as needed, and of literature and advice about parents' groups. Because many of these children live into their teenage years today, they are often placed in curative workshops to promote their individual and unique development. Most make a satisfactory adjustment to their physical and mental handicap in a protected atmosphere; a substantial number are now being "mainstreamed" in regular classrooms. The CHN may follow the families of these children for several years to provide the necessary support and counseling.

## The Infant with Down's Syndrome (Mongolism)

Normal human somatic cells consist of 44 autosomes and two sex chromosomes. Chromosomes occur in pairs, 22 autosomes and one sex pair, with one member of each pair donated by the germ cell of each parent. Trisomy is a very common chromosomal abnormality; it occurs when there are three chromosomes present in a pair instead of the normal two (disomy). The total number of somatic chromosomes is 47 in these babies instead of the normal 46. Down's syndrome was described by John Down, M.D., in 1866, and the term "mongolism" became attached to this abnormality because the facial characteristics of persons with Down's resemble those of the Mongol race. Since 1959, three autosomal trisomy syndromes have been identified: (1) Down's syndrome, or 21 Trisomy; (2) 18 Trisomy; and (3) 13 Trisomy.

### Etiology and incidence

The incidence of Down's syndrome is 1 in 660 live births. Approximately 80% of these babies are first-born children of mothers aged 35 and over. The occurrence rises with age, and is 1 in 50 (2%) in mothers aged 44 and over. The chance of Down's syndrome in women 15–24 years of age is 1 in 1500 live births; about 20% of children born with Down's syndrome are born to these young mothers. It appears that biological aging of the mothers may be more important than chronological aging. Several researchers reported an increased incidence of Down's syndrome in young mothers who evidenced early biological aging (early onset of menarche and grey hair). No statistics were found on the number born to mothers aged 35 and older who had had normal children. The incidence of 18 Trisomy is 1 in 4500 and of 13 Trisomy is 1 in 7600 live births (Hughes, 1975).

### Prognosis

The life expectancy of babies with Down's syndrome is much lower than that of normal individuals, because they often have other anomalies, such as congenital heart defects, esophageal and duodenal atresia, and imperforate anuses. Most babies with 18 and 13 Trisomies die in early infancy (Hughes, 1975; Schaffer & Avery, 1977).

### Clinical and radiological signs

In Down's syndrome, the following signs occur more frequently than others. Most of the following clinical or radiological signs appear in over 70% of the cases.

General—Pallor; SGA

Head—Round shape; flat facial profile

Nose—Flattened bridge

Eyes—Oblique palpebral fissures (upward, outward slant); blunt inner palpebral angles; Brushfield's spots (speckling) around the periphery of the iris

Tongue—Intermittently protruding; more pointed than thickened

Neck—Excessive neck skin

Joints—Hyperflexibility

Radiological signs—Dysplasia of pelvis and middle phalanx of the little finger (Babson, Pernoll, & Benda, 1980).

There are other signs, such as small ears; small penis; and broad, stubby hands and feet, but they do not occur with the same frequency as those listed above.

*Mental and physical problems*

The most significant feature of Down's syndrome is mental retardation, because the brain is smaller in size, especially the brain stem and cerebellum. These children were once considered only minimally trainable, which is one reason many of them were institutionalized in the past. However, modern methods of special education have allowed many children with Down's syndrome to maximize their potential with proper instruction. Much of the social stigma of Down's syndrome and other mentally retarded conditions has been decreased in the past few decades. Mental retardation came "out of the closet" in the 1960s when President Kennedy, motivated by his own mentally retarded sister, set up comprehensive mental health programs, including programs on mental retardation. Former Senator S. I. Hayakawa kept his mentally retarded son at home and has insisted that families can do more for such children than an institution can. Today a CHN can suggest various treatments such as an infant stimulation program to assist the family with home care.

A large number of physical problems are associated with Down's syndrome. About 40–50% of these children have cardiac defects, especially septal defects. Hypotonicity of the chest and abdominal muscles probably accounts for the high prevalence of respiratory diseases in these babies. When combined with cardiac anomalies, respiratory infections are the chief cause of Down's syndrome mortality in infancy. The incidence of leukemia is about 15% greater in these children; this is attributed to the imbalance of genes on trisomic chromosome 21. Common visual defects include strabismus, nystagmus, myopia, and cataracts. Inflammation of the conjunctiva and lids occurs frequently. Tracheoesophogeal fistulas, duodenal atresia, renal agenesis, and agangionic megacolon (Hirschsprung's disease) are often present as well (Whaley & Wong, 1979).

*Care at home and in the community*

An infant with Down's syndrome may be discharged from the hospital later than his mother because of respiratory problems or another problem. He is usually discharged in the neonatal period, at which time the CHN visits. On her initial visit, she would provide the same nursing care and instruction as for a normal neonate, such as the health assessment and instruction in feeding. The CHN's additional care includes discussing (1) diagnosis and prognosis; (2) immediate and long-range care plans; (3) acceptance of a mentally retarded child with complicated physical problems; (4) a stimulation program; (5) the setting of realistic goals for the child; (6) investigation of outside help such as day care programs; and possibly (7) genetic counseling.

On the first visit the CHN should decide whether the parents understand and accept the diagnosis and prognosis. One mother said this about her retarded daughter: "I will never accept it, but I will make the most of it. We do want to have other normal children." The CHN will encounter a wide range of parental reactions to diagnosis and prognosis. The adjustment to a child with Down's syndrome will be a gradual process. The CHN can assist by providing facts and allowing parents to discuss their feelings.

The immediate care is very time-consuming. On the early visits to the home, the CHN should discuss feeding, because the protruding tongue can present problems. Fluids and solid foods should be placed well back on the tongue. Precautions should be taken to minimize respiratory problems, such as not taking the baby into crowds or very cold weather during his first few months of life. These children are like rag dolls because of their flaccid extremities; they do not sit or walk on schedule, which increases the mother's work. (See Table 3-3.) The CHN should help parents make long-range plans and become acquainted with pertinent programs, institutions, and legislation in their com-

Table 3-3
Comparison of Motor and Speech Development
in Normal and Down's Syndrome Babies

| | Age in Weeks/Months When Baby Performs Behavior | |
| --- | --- | --- |
| | Down's Syndrome | Normal |
| **Motor** | | |
| 1. Holds head up when held vertically | 1–18 weeks | 6–16 weeks |
| 2. Rolls over | 1–60 | 2–5 |
| 3. Sits without support when placed in sitting position | 5–72 | 5–8 |
| 4. Stands up | 7–84 | 10–14 months |
| 5. Walks alone | 7–74 | 11–15 |
| 6. Toilet-trained | 8–108 | 36–48 |
| **Speech** | | |
| 7. Speaks first word | 6–72 | 6–10 |
| 8. Speaks first sentence | 17–132 | 18–36 |

*Note.* The statistics in this table are drawn from M. A. Melyn and D. T. White, "Mental and Developmental Milestones of Noninstitutionalized Down's Syndrome Children," *Pediatrics*, 1973, *52*, 542–545; from U.S. Department of Health, Education and Welfare, Office of Child Development, Children's Bureau, *Infant Care* (Washington, D.C.: U.S. Government Printing Office, 1973); and from U.S. Department of Health, Education and Welfare, Office of Child Development, Children's Bureau, *Child from 1 to 6* (Washington, D.C.: U.S. Government Printing Office, 1975).

munity. Plans may include help at home, day care, or part- or full-time institutionalization.

Federal and state legislation has improved the quality of life for children with Down's syndrome and other mentally retarded persons. Significant federal legislation includes the following:

1. The Maternal and Child Health and Mental Retardation Planning Amendments of 1963 (PL 88-156). This act focused on developing community instead of institutional programs. It was a breakthrough both for the mentally ill and for retarded children.
2. The Mental Retardation Facilities and Community Mental Health Centers Construction Act of 1963 (PL 88-164). This act provided money to house the services that the Planning Act of the same year, described above, authorized.
3. The Developmental Disabilities Services and Facilities Construction Amendments of 1970 (PL 91-517). This act emphasized a change of terminology and programming. "Developmental disabilities" became the umbrella term that included mental retardation. The target group, the "developmentally disabled," was defined to include persons whose disability is attributable to mental retardation, cerebral palsy, epilepsy, or another neurological condition closely related to mental retardation; the disability must exist prior to age 18, must be expected to continue, and must constitute an unusual handicap. The law authorized states to develop and implement comprehensive and continuing programs for the developmentally disabled, train specialized personnel, set up demonstration projects, and design university-affiliated programs for training of personnel and related services.
4. The Education for All Handicapped Children Act of 1975 (PL 94-142). This act mandated that any kind of handicapped child had a right to an education appropriate for him. The impetus for this legislation came from Pennsylvania, where citizens won a court case giving mentally retarded persons the right to special education (Pukaite, 1980). This legislation is currently being implemented in schools across the country.

Acceptance of a child with Down's syndrome is almost "double jeopardy," because the parents must often accept massive physical problems together with mental retardation. The aim for parents of any mentally retarded child is to set realistic goals to enable him to reach his potential. In this way, parents can learn to love a child for what he is and not reject him because they expected more of him before his birth. A child with Down's syndrome can learn to walk, communicate, tap out rhythm, and capture the hearts of family members in the same way as a normal child does.

These parents need the help of relatives, friends, and society, in addition to that of the health care profession. There are many creative ways to give such help. If a mother works, she will need to plan for day care. If she does not work, she will need to plan for mature baby sitters to enable her to carry on a normal life. A grandmother who lived in a town far away from a daughter with a Down's syndrome child paid for a cleaning woman to relieve her daughter's plight.

Genetic counseling is encouraged, if this has not been done, to prevent a second birth of the same type. Mothers who have given birth to one Down's syndrome infant are at high risk for another. Through amniocentesis, chromosomal analysis can detect trisomy or transloca-tion. If a mother learns that she is carrying a fetus with Down's syn-drome, she may not want to abort it if abortion is contrary to her beliefs.This makes an even stronger case for genetic counseling prior to conception. Genetic counseling is arranged through the client's phy-sician and is available usually only in larger metropolitan areas.

## Child Neglect and Abuse

### Definition and prevention

Child neglect and abuse have always existed, but the magnitude of abuse as a major health problem became clear in 1961 when Henry Kempe, M.D., coined the phrase "battered child syndrome" and through the literature brought it to the forefront. The current defini-tions of "child abuse" and "neglect" come from the 1974 law passed by Congress (PL 93-247), which states that neglect and abuse include physical and mental injury, sexual abuse, negligent treatment, or other maltreatment of a child under 18 years of age by an adult responsible for his care.

Prevention of child neglect and abuse can be accomplished through several avenues, including (1) parent effectiveness training, (2) promotion of bonding or attachment, and (3) screening for "at-risk" parents in clinic situations and provision of teaching and counseling for them.

### The community health nurse's role in reporting abuse

An infant is particularly vulnerable because he is very dependent, is unable to express himself, and causes stress by crying and making other necessary demands. The CHN is in a strategic position to uncover potential problems in a home visit and to assist in prevention by discussing the problem with the parents and seeking help as indicated; the CHN may even be able to provide some of the necessary counseling. The clinic personnel where the infant is seen should be alerted to the problem. The CHN should be aware of signs of neglect such as poor hygiene, the mother's indifferent response to a crying baby, and abuse as manifested by bruises, burns, and fractures. Abusers, who often have been abused themselves, have some common characteristics: (1) neglect as a child, (2) difficulty in coping with life, (3) social isolation, and (4) low self-esteem.

All states have laws requiring that health professionals report child abuse. If the CHN thinks there is a problem of child abuse in a family, she should discuss it with her immediate supervisor to verify her impressions. Documentation of observations must be written, objective, and factual, and must cite specific instances of abuse. The problem can be reported confidentially to the protective services branch of the local welfare department. The departments have social workers trained to handle child abuse problems; the parents should be referred to them for counseling. The CHN should continue to follow the family until she is certain the problem is resolved.

## Appendix 3A: Passive Exercises to Develop Range of Motion, Adapted for Nursing

A. Head
   1. Flexion-extension.
   2. Rotation.
B. Upper extremity
   1. Shoulder (on back)
      a. Shoulder flexion and extension. Hyperextension accomplished on back if patient is near edge of bed or done in prone position.
      b. Abduction and adduction.
      c. Horizontal abduction and adduction. (Start with arm at 90° angle.)
      d. Internal (toward feet) and external (toward head) rotation.
   2. Elbow
      a. Flexion and extension.
      b. Supination (palm up) and pronation.
   3. Wrist
      a. Flexion and extension.
      b. Ulnar (toward little finger) and radial deviation.
   4. Fingers and thumb
      a. Flexion and extension.

   b. Abduction and adduction.
   c. Thumb opposition.
C. Lower extremity
   1. Hip (on back)
      a. Flexion and extension.
      b. Abduction and adduction.
      c. Internal and external rotation.
      d. (On stomach) extension or hyperextension continued—raise leg from
         bed 10 degrees.
   2. Knee
      a. Flexion and extension.
   3. Ankle
      a. Dorsi flexion (up) and plantar flexion (down—as in foot drop).
      b. Inversion and eversion.
   4. Toes
      a. Flexion and extension.
      b. Abduction and adduction (difficult to do actively).


# Appendix 3B: Audiovisual Aids
# for Discussions on Parenting

*Are You Ready for the Postpartum Experience?* (Film, 17 min., color) Available
   from Parenting Pictures, R.D. #1, Box 355B, Columbia, NJ 17832.

   Explores the joys and problems of the first weeks at home with a new baby.
   Focuses on parents adjusting to new roles. Includes scenes from a mothers'
   discussion group.

*Adapting to Parenthood* (Film, 20 min., color) Available from Polymorph Films,
   311 Newbury St., Boston, MA 02115.

   The arrival of a first baby produces profound changes in a marriage. Thus,
   a number of new parents speak of their initial problems: sleeplessness and
   crying babies; interfering grandparents; husbands unwilling to change
   soiled diapers; and frustration and guilt in not feeling the serenity they anticipated. Shows a young couple with their first baby, adjusting to the
   changes taking place in their lives, with special attention to the role of the
   father.

*Mothers after Divorce* (Film, 20 min., color) Available from Polymorph Films,
   311 Newbury St., Boston, MA 02115.

   Perspective on the divorced, single parent. Four suburban women, divorced
   mothers, discuss their child-rearing concerns as well as their loneliness,
   careers, economics, and emotional needs.

*Parenting: Growing with Children* (Film, 22 min., color) Available from FilmFair Communications, 10900 Ventura Blvd., P.O. Box 1728, Studio City, CA 91604.

Looks at the realities, responsibilities, and rewards of parenting, as seen in the lives of four very different families: a young couple struggling to adjust to the arrival of a new baby; a large family in which each parent plays a distinct and clearly defined role; a household in which both husband and wife are seeking meaningful careers while sharing the parenting responsibility equally; and a single mother trying to raise her children with dignity and humanity in a difficult urban environment. The film demonstrates that successful parenting involves many years of commitment, love, patience, and skill. It also shows that there is no one "right" way, and that each family must find its own parenting style, consistent with the parents' personalities, values, and life goals.

*Joyce at 34* (Film, 28 min., color) Available from New Day Films, Box 315, Franklin Lakes, NJ 07417.

The concrete reality of a woman's caring for a new baby while pursuing a career as a filmmaker. Follows Joyce, awaiting the arrival of her first child at the age of 34; later she takes 6-week-old Sarah with her on assignment and/or lets her writer-husband care for the child while she is on another assignment. Joyce's thoughts and comments about her work and about being a mother convey the pressures, delights, doubts, conflicts, and compromises she experiences as she fits Sarah into her daily routine and resumes her filmmaking.

*Parenting Concerns: The First Two Years* (Film or videocassette, 21 min., color) Available from Perennial Education, Box 236, Northfield, IL 60093.

Explores many common, but perplexing child-rearing situations. Prospective parents are introduced to the boredom of schedules, formulas, and endless diaper changes; breast versus bottle feeding; and how and when to respond to the needs of a crying infant. For veteran parents, the issues examined include when and how a mother should return to work; how to survive a child's drive for independence; toilet training; guidelines for disciplining a child; and problems of sibling rivalry.

*Friends* (Film, 20 min., color) Available from Linhoff Color Photo Lab, 4402 France Ave. South, Minneapolis, MN 55410. (Rental: Free loan from Health Education Section, Minneapolis Health Dept., 250 S. 4th St., Minneapolis, MN 55415.)

Suggests activities to parents that encourage normal growth and development in the child's first year of life. Introduces concepts of Piaget's work in an understandable manner. Focuses on resources available in a low-socioeconomic-level home.

*Parenthood: Myths and Realities* (Two filmstrips with audiocassettes or records) Available from Guidance Associates, 757 Third Ave., New York, NY 10017.

Examines romantic misconceptions about parental "instincts," responsibilities, and rewards. Emphasizes respect for the individuality of parent and child; discusses child development, marital life and family interaction, and parental health attitudes.

*Newborn* (Film, 28 min., color) Available from Johnson & Johnson Baby Products Company, Consumer & Professional Services, 501 George Street, New Brunswick, NJ 08903. (Rental: free loan.)

Follows the growth and experience of one baby and his parents through the first 3 months of life together. Emphasis is on physical, emotional, and intellectual needs of the baby and the parents. T. Barry Brazelton, Sydney Cohen, and Virginia Pomeranz appear in the film.

# References

American Academy of Pediatrics. *Pediatric nutrition handbook*. Evanston, Ill.: Author, 1979.

Babson, S. G., Pernoll, M. L., & Benda, G. I. (with assistance of K. Simpson). *Diagnosis and management of the fetus and neonate at risk: A guide for team care* (4th ed.). St. Louis: C. V. Mosby, 1980.

Browning, C. Personal communication, January 29, 1981.

Chinn, P. L. *Child health maintenance*. St. Louis: C. V. Mosby, 1974.

Christianson, M. Personal communication, February 14, 1982.

Christianson, M. Personal communication, April 25, 1983.

Clark, A. L., & Affonso, D. D. (with T. R. Harris). *Childbearing: A nursing perspective* (2nd ed.). Philadelphia: F. A. Davis, 1979.

Hughes, J. G. *Synopsis of pediatrics* (4th ed.). St. Louis: C. V. Mosby, 1975.

Jensen, M. D., Benson, R. C., & Bobak, I. M. *Maternity care: The nurse and the family*. St. Louis: C. V. Mosby, 1981.

Kaluger, G., & Kaluger, M. F. *Human development: The span of life*. St. Louis: C. V. Mosby, 1974.

Klaus, M. H., & Kennell, J. H. *Maternal-infant bonding*. St. Louis: C. V. Mosby, 1976.

Lawrence, R. A. *Breastfeeding: A guide for the medical profession*. St. Louis: C. V. Mosby, 1980.

McDonald, E. T., & Berlin, A. J. *Bright promise for your child with cleft lip and cleft palate*. Chicago: National Easter Seal Society for Crippled Children and Adults, 1980.

Mead Johnson and Company. *Infant nutrition* (Pamphlet No. L-B98-3-78). Evansville, Ind.: Author, 1978.

Metropolitan Life Insurance Company. *Your child's safety.* New York: Author, 1970.

National Center for Health Statistics. *Factors associated with low birth weight, United States 1976* (Vital and Health Statistics Series 21, No. 37; DHEW Publ. No. PHS 80-1915). Washington, D.C.: U.S. Department of Health, Education and Welfare, 1980.

Pipes, P. L. *Nutrition in infancy and childhood.* St. Louis: C. V. Mosby, 1977.

Pukaite, C. Personal communication, February 6, 1980.

Ross Laboratories. *The phenomena of early development.* Columbus, Ohio: Author, 1977.

Schaffer, A. J., & Avery, M. E. *Diseases of the newborn.* Philadelphia: W. B. Saunders, 1977.

Scripien, G. M., Barnard, M. U., Chard, M. A., Howe, J., & Phillips, P. J. *Comprehensive pediatric nursing* (2nd ed.). New York: McGraw-Hill, 1979.

Vaughan, V. C. III, McKay, R. J., Jr., & Behrman, R. E. (W. E. Nelson, Sr. Ed.). *Nelson textbook of pediatrics* (11th ed.). Philadelphia: W. B. Saunders, 1979.

Warner, M. P. *A doctor discusses breastfeeding* (pamphlet). Chicago: Budlong Press, 1975.

Whaley, L. F., & Wong, D. L. *Nursing care of infants and children.* St. Louis: C. V. Mosby, 1979.

Woodruff, C. W. The science of infant nutrition, and the art for infant feeding. *Journal of the American Medical Association,* 1978, *240,* 657–661.

# 4

## Care of the Toddler in the Home, Clinic, Physician's Office, and Well-Child Conference

*Marion Mendelsohn Coleman and Dorothy D. Petrowski*

## Introduction

Care of the child between the ages of 1 and 3 years can be a delightful yet frustrating experience. Although development is not as rapid as in the first year of life, the toddler makes significant advances at this age. He goes from a mostly horizontal to a vertical or upright position—first walking, then running in every direction. At the beginning of this stage, he has a vocabulary of few words; at the end, he is speaking in sentences. His thought processes are also more fully developed. Socially, he is developing from a dependent infant to a child, separating from his mother, and striving for independence—not an easy task for the child or the parent.

## Overview of Normal Development

This chapter discusses the toddler's normal growth and development and common illnesses in the context of community health supervision. In order to care for the toddler, the community health nurse (CHN) must be knowledgeable about normal growth and development, and also of the great individual variation within the limits of normality. Many factors contribute to the development of the child—heredity, environment, and the child's and parents' individual characteristics. Parents, too, are individuals and have needs that influence the way they react to the child.

## Motor Development

Most of the factors involved in motor development appear to be a combination of the child's neuromuscular abilities and factors in the environment. A child's ability to progress in motor development depends more upon the readiness of his own system than upon practice (Gesell, Ilg, & Ames, 1974). In other words, teaching a child to walk before he is ready does not enhance his progress. However, once he has developed the ability to walk, he needs the opportunity to explore and practice.

In addition, motor capabilities progress similarly for most children. The majority of children have learned to walk without support by 13–14 months of age. Initially, the toddler's gait is unsteady and arrhythmical. He walks with his feet wide apart and his feet turned out. This position helps him keep his balance. As he practices, he becomes more coordinated, keeping his feet closer together and walking with a more regular gait (Cratty, 1970).

Once the child begins to walk, a whole new environment opens up to him. Exploring his environment from an upright position is new and exciting to the toddler, and can lead him into potentially unsafe situations. He is constantly moving—putting objects into his mouth, investigating closets, drawers, and furniture. Toddlers also enjoy climbing, especially climbing up stairs. Child-proofing the house and yard will be discussed in detail later in the chapter.

Gross motor drive is stronger than fine motor drive from 1 to 2 years of age. However, the child at this age can scribble drawings; he can also build a tower of two cubes by 15 months of age and a tower of four cubes by 18 months of age (Frankenburg & Dodds, 1967). He can feed himself, but not without making a mess. Turning pages of a book or magazine is also of interest to the child of this age; according to White (1975), he is practicing his finger skills. A book with stiff pages is best to use.

From 2 to 3 years of age, the toddler is still geared toward gross motor activity, but he has become better coordinated. He runs and jumps. By age 3, he can ride a tricycle. White (1975) states that by 2 years of age there is more emphasis on mastery behavior than on exploratory behavior. A child enjoys taking things apart and putting them together again and again. By age 3, he can usually dress with supervision.

## Cognitive Development

Piaget studied child behavior and developed a theory of cognitive development (see Richmond, 1970). Toddlers, according to Piaget, are in the preoperational stage; this stage is characterized by the use of symbols, particularly in play and speech. The child may use objects to symbolize other things, such as a wooden block to represent a car or truck. However, his use of symbols does not increase his knowledge of the object. To learn, he needs actual contact or experience with the object and/or situation. Again, exploration of the environment is important in growth and learning. Several other characteristics are typical of the preconceptual child's thought, according to Piaget; one of the most important is egocentrism (Richmond, 1970).

## Language Development

Verbal communication increases vastly during toddlerhood. A child understands language before he is capable of speaking. Both understanding and use of language depend upon the child's intellect, stage of growth, and environment. The child usually says his first word at about 1 year of age. For the next several months, however, motor skills seem to be more important. Acquisition of language is quite slow from infancy to 18 months of age.

Toddlers enjoy the repetition of sounds. Chants and rhymes such as pat-a-cake that involve both the child and parent are stimulating (Helms & Turner, 1976). At 14–15 months, a child can understand simple instructions and warnings. These instructions must pertain to the here and now, however, since the toddler cannot comprehend future events. By 18–24 months of age, the child has achieved the mental development to further his language ability. At 18 months, the child is usually speaking in two-word sentences, such as "Mommy go," "Dog run," "Me eat" (Dale, 1972). These structures also appear in the early development of other languages.

By the age of 24 months, the child has the use of several hundred words, mostly nouns. The 2-year-old child may speak in three-word telegraphic sentences; all of the nonessential words of a sentence are left out. For example, a child might say "Go out" instead of "I am going out." By 3 years of age, the child's understanding and use of language have increased.

Although the child's intellectual structures may be most important in language ability, the child's environment seems to be important in developing vocabulary. The mother is an extremely important factor in the child's development of language. A mother who is more accepting and less directing of what the child should say has the most positive effect on the child's verbal development.

There are other factors that seem to stimulate the child's language development, such as his varied experiences outside the home and with adults. Another factor is the level of language spoken with the child. When communicating with the child, speaking at his level or slightly above his level of understanding is helpful (White, 1975).

Studies have also been done on the language development of twins. In one study, Dales (1969) found that the language development in twins was slower than the average; it was postulated that twins have each other as company and thus may have fewer language needs. Dales also found that only children were usually above average in language development.

Social Development

According to Erikson (1963), the toddler is in the stage of autonomy versus self-doubt or insecurity, struggling with independence. As he begins to develop a sense of autonomy, he should be encouraged to establish trust in himself and his environment. However, if his independence is thwarted, he may become frustrated and, instead, may develop a sense of insecurity about himself and his environment. He also seeks parental approval, and at times is torn between pleasing his parents and being independent.

The toddler's ambivalence produces many common characteristics. First, a child's negativistic attitude is at its peak at this age. The word "no" is the word most commonly used, though the toddler does not always mean "no" when he says it. It is one way of expressing his new sense of identity and autonomy. Giving the child too many "don't's" or commands at one time usually feeds into this negativism, as does offering too many choices (Waechter & Blake, 1976). Instead of asking "Do you want to go to sleep?", the parent might say, "It is time to go to sleep now."

Spurts of negativism can lead to temper tantrums. The child may lie on the floor, screaming, kicking, or holding his breath. First, it is important to protect the child from injury. A child having a temper tantrum is out of control, and this can be a frightening experience for him. Second, it is best not to focus on the tantrum, but to try to understand its cause. It is important to be consistent in handling such outbursts. Learning that such outbursts bring him attention may encourage the child to repeat them. After a tantrum, a child often seeks reassurance and security from the parent.

## Nursing Care at Home

### Anticipatory Guidance to Promote Wellness

Parents can deal more effectively with their toddler if they are aware of toddlers' normal patterns of behavior, growth, and development. The CHN can teach parents about normal behavior by giving anticipatory guidance at home, in order to help the parents avoid problems or at least understand them.

#### Discipline

Discipline is usually an area of concern to parents. As with temper tantrums, consistent limits need to be set. These limits, first of all, should be appropriate to the child's age. It is realistic that a young toddler will touch or handle a breakable object within his grasp. Also, too many rules may frustrate and inhibit the toddler.

By 14–15 months of age, children can understand simple rules or limits, as noted earlier. However, if the child breaks a rule, the disciplinary action must take place right away. Tots do not understand threats of future punishment. Discipline need not be physical punishment; it can include other methods, such as giving a verbal reprimand or separating the child from the cause of the problem (Brazelton, 1976). Parents should talk about their feelings with the child. It is important for the child to know that parents can have angry feelings, but still love him. The child needs to understand this prase: "I love you; but I don't love this naughty behavior."

#### Feeding

Appetite is another major concern at this age. During the second year, the child's appetite tends to decrease. There are several reasons for this. First, the rate of growth has decreased. Also, the toddler has trouble sitting still long enough to eat a full meal; his increased mobility and desire to explore may cause occasional lack of interest in food. Refusing to eat can also become part of his struggle for autonomy.

The CHN can offer parents suggestions that may help avoid a struggle at mealtime, such as not forcing or threatening the child. Forcing him may only strengthen his refusal to eat because of his desire to be independent. Allowing him to feed himself gives him a feeling of control. Giving him appropriate "finger foods," such as a cracker, piece of fruit, or piece of meat, increases his sense of autonomy. He can use a spoon, although not without spilling, at about 15 months of age. Parents do not need to be prepared for a mess at mealtime. Use of a bib, unbreakable dishes, and a small spoon and cup is helpful. The floor should be protected with a plastic tablecloth under the chair.

To insure a more nutritious meal, the parent should give milk and desserts at the end of the meal. If these items are given first, the child may fill up on these and refuse to eat the rest. Also, parents should limit the number and type of snacks between meals. When snacks are appropriate, such items as carrot sticks, apple slices, or cheese should be offered.

### Bowel and bladder control

Bowel and bladder control is a major area of social development, usually begun toward the end of the second year. Bowel training is accomplished first; then daytime bladder control is usually achieved by age 3. Nighttime bladder control is usually accomplished by age 4. However, a child may occasionally wet during the night with decreasing frequency over the next year.

The child usually shows signs that he is ready for toilet training. One sign that the toddler is aware of defecation may be straining or tugging at his diaper. By 2 years of age he can understand directions and can also learn by imitating older siblings. The sphincter reflexes are developed at this age to the point where control is possible.

The parents should avoid punishing the child during toilet training. Positive reinforcement, such as parental approval or other rewards, is helpful when the child "goes" at the right time and place. However, punishing the child when he does not "go" or when he has an accident may lead to an autonomy struggle. The child wants to please his parent, but he also wants control over his own body. Limits must be set here also. The child should not sit on the chair for extended periods of time. If he does not have a bowel movement within a short period of time, the parent should try putting him on the potty chair again later. Training a child in a relaxed, positive atmosphere generally appears to be the most successful method.

### Preventing accidents

Safety and accident prevention around the home are other important areas in which the CHN can provide parents with anticipatory guidance. According to the National Poison Control Center in Pittsburgh, the highest number of accidental poisonings occur in children aged from 1 to 3 years (Barton, 1979). The most frequently ingested poisonous substances in this age group, accounting for 90% of accidental poisonings, are cleaning products, over-the-counter drugs, and plants.

If they recognize the child's intense curiosity and desire to explore, parents can prevent most accidental ingestions by child-proofing the house. It is important to lock up all poisonous substances such as cleaning fluids. Medicines should be in child-proof containers and should also be locked up. Pocketbooks or purses that contain medication should be kept out of the toddler's reach as well. Plants, especially poisonous ones such as diffenbachia or philodendron, must be put out of reach or out of the home of a walking, climbing, curious toddler. When child-proofing the home, parents should also put away valuable or breakable objects. Many of these could be broken or swallowed by the child.

Parents should be prepared, in case the child does swallow a poisonous substance, to telephone the nearest poison control center. The telephone number should be kept near the telephone. The center will want to know, if possible, what the child took, when and how much he swallowed. The parent may then be advised to give the child syrup of ipecac, available in 1-oz bottles for emergency use, to induce vomiting, or to bring the child to the nearest hospital emergency room.

Many accidents occur in the kitchen, which is not only an interesting place for a tot to explore, but also a place where family members spend much time. It is important to keep handles of hot pots and pans turned inward when cooking. Also, the parents should be aware of tablecloths, coffee pots, and iron cords that the toddler can pull from his lower position.

To help satisfy the toddler's sense of autonomy and his curiosity, White (1975) suggests giving him one or two lower cabinets in the kitchen or a special area there in which he is free to explore. Pots and pans, large spoons, and unusual containers fascinate him. Allowing him to explore or play with several of these objects in his special area gives him some control and the opportunity to satisfy curiosity.

Another safety precaution is to have all windows above the first floor screened to prevent the child from falling out. Toddlers enjoy looking out windows and will do so if possible at various times during the day. If there are stairs in the home, a gate should be placed at the top of the stairs to prevent the child from falling. It may also be necessary initially to place a gate at the bottom or at the first three or four stairs, since the young toddler can climb stairs but has difficulty going back down the stairs.

Car safety is another area to discuss with parents. It is not safe for a parent to hold a child in the car, even if the adult is wearing a seat belt. Until the child reaches a weight of 40 poinds, he needs a safety seat with a harness. After he weighs 40 pounds or is 4 years of age, he can use an adult belt.

### Stimulation

It is important to support and encourage a child's awareness of his environment. This enables him to be curious about and enjoy people, objects, experiences, and so on; it increases the likelihood that the toddler will develop self-esteem, a sense of well-being, and independence. Parents can provide such encouragement through such activities as reading books, playing music, and providing human interactions for the child. It is entirely possible that in deprived situations the CHN will have to teach families how to stimulate their children.

### Anticipatory Guidance to Prevent Illness

There are two problems associated with dietary habits that may be prevented: nursing-bottle caries, and iron deficiency due to a low dietary intake of iron.

### Nursing-bottle caries

Nursing-bottle caries, or "nursing-bottle syndrome," occurs in many children who take a bottle of milk or juice to bed with them at naptime and bedtime beyond the age of 12 months. Some of the liquid remains around the teeth after the child falls asleep. Because of this increased exposure of the teeth to the milk and the decreased salivary flow rate during sleep, the teeth are more susceptible to decay. The teeth most affected are the primary maxillary incisors, followed by the primary first molars.

Referral to a pedodontist is recommended if this condition is noted upon examination of the mouth. To help prevent this syndrome, the topic can be discussed as part of a well-child visit; parents should be counseled to discontinue the bottle. The CHN can suggest giving the bottle before the child goes to sleep, then brushing his teeth. If it is necessary that the child go to sleep with a bottle, it should contain only water, no milk or juice (Shelton, 1977).

*Iron deficiency*

Iron deficiency is another problem associated with feeding habits. It usually occurs between 6 months and 24 months of age (Githens & Hathaway, 1976). Analysis of a child's diet during the well-child history is essential. Children with iron deficiency usually have a diet of solid foods low in iron and an intake of milk (a poor source of iron) greater than one quart per day.

If iron deficiency is suspected, a hemoglobin (Hgb) or hematocrit (Het) test may be done. Another simple method of screening for iron deficiency is the blood test for free erythrocyte protoporphyrin (FEP) level. Conditions such as iron deficiency cause the FEP to increase. The FEP will be elevated in mild cases of iron deficiency before there is a change in the Het or Hgb. However, the FEP is also elevated in lead poisoning, so a lead-level test must also be made. If the FEP is elevated and the lead level is normal, the most common cause is iron deficiency.

The most commonly used medication for this iron deficiency is oral ferrous sulfate, 2–3 mg iron/kg/day, for 3–4 months (Dallman, 1977). Although the drug is better absorbed between meals, it can cause gastrointestinal irritation, so it may need to be given with food. Parents should also be told that the iron causes the child's stools to turn black. the child needs to return to the clinic for a repeat Hgb or Het test in 3–4 months. If the child has not responded to the iron, other causes of the deficiency should be investigated, or a home visit may be requested by the clinic in order to check on adherence to the regimen.

The CHN should ask the mother to demonstrate administration of the medication. Petrowski visited a child at home whose Het was not reaching a satisfactory level on return clinic visits. On the first home visit, she discovered that the mother misunderstood the clinic instructions and was giving only one-half of the iron preparation ordered. On the other hand, a parent could administer too much medication, thinking that "more is better."

The nursing approach of dietary instruction should be introduced simultaneously with the prescribed medicine or before. On the same home visit, Petrowski reviewed the child's diet with the mother and found it almost totally lacking in iron-rich foods. A child needs a diet high in iron, including red meats, liver, eggs, and fortified cereals. His milk intake may need to be limited to one quart per day. Using the cardboard food models from the National Dairy Council in the discussion allows the mother to communicate more freely about her concerns regarding the child's diet and the family diet. One of the most important aspects of treatment and prevention of iron deficiency is nutritional education for the parents.

## Common Illnesses

A nurse usually visits a toddler at home for health supervision. There are, however, several acute and chronic illnesses for which the CHN may receive a referral from a clinic, a hospital, or the mother.

### Acute illnesses

A few typical examples of acute illnesses are discussed here: upper respiratory infections (URIs), otitis media, rashes, gastrointestinal disorders, and fractures.

*Upper respiratory infections.* One of the most common URIs is the "common cold." Approximately 200 different types of viruses can cause the cold. The child may present initially with a fever (100.6–102°F rectally). This is followed by nasal congestion and a clear, thin nasal discharge. The discharge may become thick and purulent after several days. There is also an increase in secretions running down the posterior pharynx, which can cause irritation, coughing, and spreading of infection to the lungs. One of the most frequent complications of the cold at this age is otitis media (Vaughan, McKay, & Behrman, 1979).

Although all contributing factors are not clearly understood, the number of colds a child has a year is related to the number of exposures he has received. If a toddler has older siblings in school, or if the child himself goes to nursery school, he will be exposed to many more viruses and has greater chances of getting more colds. There is no proven prevention for the cold. However, good general hygienic measures, such as a balanced diet, enough sleep, and exercise, aid in preventing colds.

Treatment of a cold usually includes increased fluids to help thin the drainage, rest, and baby aspirin or liquid acetaminophen for the fever. (There is a new warning against using aspirin with children who have influenza or chicken pox because it is associated with Reyes syndrome. See Center for Disease Control, 1982.) The parents should be counseled in the use of a thermometer at home. If the body temperature is dangerously high (103°F), the CHN should teach the parent how to do a tepid sponge bath (a bath with lukewarm water) until the temperature decreases. A cool mist vaporizer to increase humidity in the room is helpful to some children. The thermostat should be set at about 70°F because higher temperatures decrease the humidity in the atmosphere. Appropriate clothing should be discussed. Antibiotics are ineffective against viruses.

Although a cold may last 1 to 2 weeks, it is important for parents to be aware of complications that might indicate a need for the child to return to the clinic or the physician's office. A persistent high-grade fever, an earache, or a continuing deep cough usually requires medical attention. Teaching parents about the symptoms of the cold, what to do for them, and when to seek professional care enables many parents to take care of the child with a cold at home.

The CHN might visit a toddler for a common cold, pharyngitis, or bronchitis. In all cases of URI, she would check for fever, nasal congestion, sore throat, coughing, sneezing, and breathing distress. The CHN would examine the tympanic membranes and lungs to check for normal breath sounds; to rule out congestion; and to look for signs of otitis media and pneumonia, respectively.

If the child has pharyngitis, a throat culture is usually ordered to rule out a beta-hemolytic streptococcus infection. Recommended supportive measures are cool mist added to the surrounding air, bed rest, and extra fluid intake. He might need juices, soups, and jello in his diet. It is important that the child's caregiver be instructed in basics of asepsis, such as placing used tissues in a paper bag pinned to the bed and other measures, to avoid spreading the infection to other family members. Medications used are aspirin or aspirin substitute for fever or general discomfort, a decongestant and cough syrup. An antibiotic may be prescribed, because young children are particularly prone to bacterial infections that can complicate a viral URI. In cases of bronchitis, a cool mist to humidify the environment is always recommended. The humidifier should be washed with soap and water and rinsed thoroughly every 48 hours to decrease infections from the mist. Commercial cleansing products, such as "disinfectant bathroom cleaner" or any detergent, are effective.

Toddlers are not usually hospitalized for URI unless the condition persists beyond about 10 days or becomes a lower respiratory condition, such as pneumonia. After a hospitalization for pneumonia, the CHN may receive a referral to assist the family in the continuing recovery and to prevent a relapse.

*Otitis media.* Acute otitis media is another infection occurring in childhood. Swelling of the nasopharyngeal lymphoid tissue in a child with a URI and mucous may cause the eustachian tube to become blocked. Once the eustachian tube is blocked, air is absorbed in the middle ear cavity. A vacuum is created in the middle ear, which results in negative pressure. Fluid is then secreted from the membrane lining of the middle ear in order to fill the vacuum, and a good medium for bacterial growth is established.

Two pathogens cause the most cases of acute otitis media. The most common pathogen in all age groups is *S. pneumoniae*, which causes 40% of all cases. Symptoms include an acute onset, high fever, and severe ear pain. The second most common pathogen, causing milder symptoms, is *Hemophilus influenza*, type B; this pathogen causes 20% of all cases. Group A beta-hemolytic streptococcus is a less common cause, figuring in about 5% of all cases (Lewin, 1978).

The major symptoms are ear pain and fever. According to Lewin (1978), 75% of the children have earache, and 40–70% may have fever. A toddler may pull or rub his ear instead of complaining of pain; his activity and appetite may also decrease. Hearing can be impaired. In a physical assessment, the CHN would establish that the following criteria are present for a probable diagnosis of otitis media: (1) redness, injection, and induration of the tympanic membrane(s); (2) bulging tympanic membrane; and (3) absence of the light reflex, with disappearance of the bony landmarks, in the tympanic membrane. Confirmation of the findings should be made by a physician.

Diagnosis is made on the basis of the otoscopic examination. Culturing the middle ear fluid is not routinely done. In acute otitis media, the tympanic membrane is inflamed and bulging and resembles a ripe tomato. There is a lack or decrease in mobility of the tympanic membrane. Occasionally the tympanic membrane may perforate. The parent may have noticed a bloody, purulent discharge on the pillow when the child wakes up in the morning. At that point, the child may no longer complain of pain, because the spontaneous rupture of the tympanic membrane is followed by an instant decrease of acute pain. Discharge may also be noted in the canal. It is usually not necessary to clean out the canal.

Treatment of acute otitis media includes a 10- to 14-day course of a broad-spectrum antibiotic. Ampicillin and amoxicillin are two of the most commonly used, since both are effective against the three pathogens mentioned above. If the child is too ill to take medication by mouth, the mother should take the child to the clinic for an antibiotic injection. Penicillin and other antibiotic injections are not given in homes by the CHN because of the possible allergic reactions that could occur after she leaves.

Auralgan ear drops may be used for pain, and children's aspirin or another analgesic may be used for reduction of fever and pain. In addition to ear drops, nose drops and cold packs to the ear are associated measures to relieve ear pain. Supportive therapy includes fluids and rest. The parents need to be told that the fluids aid in decreasing the fever, mucous blockage, and infection. The mother may need to hold the child in her lap to help him drop off to sleep because of irritability due to the ear pain (Chinn, 1974).

There are several areas to discuss with the parents concerning antibiotics. Often the child will improve greatly after 2–3 days of treatment, but it is important to stress to the parents that the child needs to finish the entire course of antibiotics to eradicate the infection. It is also important to remind the parents not to save the rest of the medication for another episode or to give it to another member of the family.

It is generally a good idea to telephone the family 2–3 days after the home visit to inquire about the child, reinforce the instructions, and answer questions. Additional home visits may be required, or the parent may need to be reminded of a clinic appointment. A child should be seen by a nurse practitioner (NP) or a physician after the completion of the antibiotic therapy to make sure the infection has been eliminated.

*Rashes.* Another common ailment is a rash, which can cover any body part and may indicate an allergic reaction, heat reaction, or communicable disease. The CHN is frequently requested by a mother to visit to observe a rash. The nurse should take the child's temperature or instruct the mother to do so to check for infection. She should note the time of onset, the location, the extent, the type of rash, and when the fever (if any) started. Rashes may be described as macular (discolors the skin, but is not raised), papular (a raised rash), vesicular (lesions that contain clear fluid), pustular (lesions that contain pus), or crusted (lesions in the healing stages). If possible, the suspected cause for the rash should be noted, because it may be a communicable disease— chicken pox, roseola, or scarlet fever. Immunizations for rubella and rubeola have decreased the incidence of these viral rashes. All known communicable diseases and their treatment are discussed in *Control of Communicable Diseases in Man,* published by the American Public Health Association (Beneson, 1981); this book is an invaluable aid to the CHN.

Additional nursing measures consist of keeping the skin clean and dry. Ointments are not recommended unless prescribed. If the child has a fever, itching, or pain, appropriate nursing measures should be instituted. Extra fluids are encouraged, and referral to a physician may be necessary if the rash continues or becomes infected. The CHN should alert the parents that automatic washers should not be overloaded (i.e., they should not be more than two-thirds full of dry clothes at the beginning of the cycle), and only the suggested amount of detergent should be used. If clothing is not rinsed properly, it can delay the healing process of an existing rash or can cause one.

*Gastrointestinal disorders.* Gastrointestinal disorders are usually caused by a virus and result in diarrhea and dehydration. The mother may need assistance to assess how serious the diarrhea and dehydration are. If the child has from six to eight or more stools in a 24-hour period, decreased urinary output, continued vomiting, or weight loss, a physician should be notified promptly. Diarrhea stools are loose (little or no formed substance), smell foul, and are usually greenish in color. Fluid replacement and medication to control the diarrhea are essential. Fluids are required to restore the electrolyte balance and control infection. The CHN must impress upon the parents that the fluid loss can be life-threatening. Usually food is not withheld unless vomiting is present. Reduction of roughage in the diet is necessary; for example, white toast should be given instead of cracked wheat, and cooked fruits and vegetables should be substituted for raw. Although mild or moderate diarrhea can be treated at home, a child occasionally requires hospitalization to reduce the fever and curtail the diarrhea (Chinn, 1974; Hughes, 1977).

*Fractures.* Fractures are not uncommon acute illnesses during the toddler years. Home care of a toddler in a leg cast for a fracture of the femur, tibia, or fibula, which includes keeping the cast clean and dry, is a challenge. If the cast involves the perineal area, a small piece of clear plastic may be used to protect it from urine and feces. Parents should be aware of warning signs of a cast that is causing skin irritation or is too tight. Skin at the edges of the cast should be checked for irritation and redness, and the tight cast can be trimmed a bit. If the cast rubs, it can be padded lightly with cotton. When the skin distal to the cast has a bluish color, the cast is too tight and impeding circulation. In an arm or leg cast, fingers or toes should be exercised every hour to increase circulation to the area. Bathing, skin care, diaper care, and bowel elimination are important. The toddler should be prevented from dropping small objects such as pennies into the cast. Some toddlers in leg casts can be taught to use crutches to ambulate, and some cannot. After the cast is removed, a toddler requires assistance with ambulation and exercises to develop range of motion (Chinn, 1974; Scripien, Barnard, Chard, Howe, & Phillips, 1979).

### Chronic illnesses

Chronic illnesses are those that have a duration of 3 months or more; they can affect any of the body systems. Examples of illnesses from the integumentary (burns), nervous (hydrocephaly and lead poisoning), and musculoskeletal (fracture from child abuse) systems are highlighted.

*Burns.* Burns result from accidents and child abuse. If a CHN assists a parent with a burned toddler during the posthospital or rehabilitation phase, the CHN stresses (1) prevention of infection, (2) preservation of new tissue, (3) development of mobility, and (4) psychological support for the family. Adequate fluids and optimal nutrition are required to prevent infection and maintain the new tissue. The physician or CHN may teach the mother how to irrigate a healing wound, to apply an antibiotic ointment and sterile dressing, and to air-dry the site.

The sterile technique should be maintained as long as there is any break in the skin. Protective clothing, such as loose-fitting garments, may be required. Physical therapy may be initiated if the burn is on an extremity, in order to insure proper mobility. Cosmetic surgery may be needed if there is disfigurement. Continued psychological reinforcement with play therapy, referral to an occupational therapist, and support of the mother through counseling are also required (Scripien et al., 1979).

*Hydrocephaly.* Hydrocephaly is a neurological disorder that occurs in 3 per 1000 births and becomes apparent at birth or during infancy. It is characterized by accumulation of cerebrospinal fluid in the cranial vault, head enlargement, brain atrophy, mental weakness, and possible convulsions. A child with hydrocephaly is usually referred to a nurse while still an infant, after a shunting (a surgical procedure). However, the nurse's home visits may continue into the toddler phase. The CHN should regularly measure the head circumference. Positioning of the head when lying down (to prevent decubitus ulcers) and progression toward ambulation are important nursing measures. Braces to aid ambulation should not rub on any body part and will need adjustment and changes as the child grows. Psychological counseling for the family is done by the CHN to assist them in accepting a developmentally disabled child who is physically and usually mentally retarded and needs continual care. Referral to the bureau for handicapped children in the state of residence is usually done to insure financial aid as needed and continued follow-up (Vaughan et al., 1979).

*Lead poisoning.* Lead poisoning is usually a disease of children between 1 and 3 years of age who live in slum housing, where the source of lead is paint peeling from plaster walls. A child who has a craving to eat unnatural items (pica) often eats peeled wall paint. There are about 1200 new cases of lead poisoning diagnosed annually, and there are about 200 deaths each year. Federal laws now prohibit lead paint, but there still are older homes with lead paint on the walls and a few imported toys with lead paint. Other less common sources are brightly colored (red and yellow) paper, such as comic sections of newspapers and candy wrappers that children may chew on, or evaporated milk (plugs are soldered into the cans in the closing process). Emissions from automobiles can pollute the air or soil with lead (Lundgren, 1980). the CHN should alert parents to the causes of lead poisoning.

The Surgeon General recommends that a concentration of 40 micrograms of lead per 100 ml of whole blood is evidence of a toxic level of lead absorption. A concentration of 80 micrograms/100 ml signals grave danger, and treatment is required. Symptoms vary from mild gastrointestinal symptoms to several central nervous system (CNS) signs such as convulsions and coma, which can result in death. Early in the disease the child suffers anemia, and if the blood lead content continues and increases, irreversible CNS damage results.

Treatment includes removal of the lead source, medication to increase urinary excretion of the lead, an iron supplement, and treatment for CNS symptoms such as convulsions if present. Calcium disodium edetate (EDTA) and dimercaprol (BAL) are two of the medications that aid in urinary excretion of the lead. EDTA is given intramuscularly over a 5-day period, with urine and blood lead levels checked daily. BAL can be used in conjunction with EDTA. A repeat of the drug regimen may be required (*Physician's Desk Reference,* 1982).

Matching federal funds are available for lead poisoning programs, so many health departments have childhood lead prevention and screening programs; these consist of blood screening tests done in homes and clinics to check for *suspected* lead poisoning. If lead poisoning is suspected in a child after screening, the CHN can refer the child to a lead clinic to have the level of lead confirmed and for treatment as indicated. In addition, sanitarians can check homes for lead levels with a special portable X-ray machine; in some cases, paint and plaster samples are taken for chemical analysis (Lundgren, 1980).

If the CHN is working with a diagnosed case of lead poisoning from pica, she should warn the mother to stop the child's pica to prevent lead ingestion. If the mother works, the child may need to be placed in a nursery school temporarily. The symptoms and treatment of lead poisoning should be explained to the family.

*Child abuse.* Child abuse can occur at any age and in any social class. When a CHN visits a toddler, she should be alert to signs of child abuse. The CHN should know the personality traits that characterize abusing parents: immaturity, self-centeredness, low self-esteem, and hostility. Some typical observations made in the homes of abusers include (1) poor hygiene, (2) cramped living space, (3) parents who are isolated, (4) children kept in cribs when they should be exploring their homes, and (5) excessive demands made on the children. These parents also often have little knowledge of growth and development and concomitant unrealistic expectations for their children. The abuse can be physical or psychological, such as fractures, bruises, burns, or verbal punishment. *War of the Eggs* (Paulist Productions, 1972) is an excellent film illustrating parental abuse of a toddler.

The CHN is a key person in preventing child abuse, because she diagnoses symptoms and provides continued support, education, and evaluation of families. The CHN's role includes reporting child abuse when suspected, providing objective documentation of her observations with recorded facts, looking for strengths in the parents, demonstrating alternate ways of working with child behavior to parents, helping parents and children to express feelings, and providing referrals for treatment for the children and psychiatric counseling for the parents. There are telephone hotlines for abusing parents, as well as self-help groups in some communities.

## Nursing Care in the Clinic, Physician's Office, and Well-Child Conference

### Health Maintenance Visits

The toddler, with his parent(s), usually visits the primary care health professional three or four times between the ages of 1 and 3 years for routine assessments and immunizations. These visits to a clinic, physician's office, or well-child conference include a history, physical examination, health screenings, developmental assessment, anticipatory guidance, and any required immunizations. Children can be cared for in well-child conferences, which are usually sponsored by health departments through the preschool years.

### History and physical examination

The history is an essential part of the visit. An initial history is taken if the child has not been to the office or clinic before. This history includes information concerning the pregnancy, the child's birth, health history, growth and development, habits such as diet and sleep patterns, and any current problems or concerns. If the child has been seen regularly at the clinic or office, the history focuses on what has occurred since his last visit in terms of habits and current problems. During this time the CHN or pediatric nurse practitioner (PNP) has the opportunity to discuss with the parent(s) areas of health education and anticipatory guidance, such as toilet training, discipline, and so forth, as discussed earlier in this chapter. This is also a good time to observe parent-child interactions.

The examination includes measurements of temperature, pulse, respiration, height, weight, and head and chest circumference (for children aged 2 years and less), as well as a physical examination. Growth measurements are plotted on a growth chart to indicate growth progress over time. The history and physical examination detailed in Appendixes A and C at the end of this volume, and the guidelines for examining preschoolers given in Chapter 5, can be adapted for a toddler. A toddler is not likely to be cooperative during parts of the examination. He may be frightened if he remembers that the nurse gave him an injection on a previous visit. There are a few ways to help lessen his fears and enlist his cooperation. First, the examiner may try playing with the child; the examinations can be made a game. For example, the examiner can let the child feel the stethoscope in his hands, or can demonstrate what it is for by listening first to the parent or to a stuffed animal. At times, this may relax the child and make him less frightened. At other times, he may become so interested in the equipment that other forms of distraction are not necessary. Talking first with the mother often helps. The child sees that his mother trusts the examiner, and he may begin to do so himself. Another device is to delay the more intrusive parts of the examination. For example, the examiner should look in the mouth, throat, and ears last to delay the screaming and crying that can result.

### Developmental assessment

Psychomotor development is checked before or during the physical examination. One of the most commonly used tests in clinics and offices is the Denver Developmental Screening Test (DDST) (Frankenburg & Dodds, 1967), designed to identify delays in development. The test does not identify the cause of any delay and is not an IQ test. It is designed to screen children up to age 6 in four areas of development: gross motor, language, fine motor–adaptive, and personal-social. The test is quick and easy to use. There are 105 tasks on the entire test, and a child is tested on approximately 20 tasks or items at one time. A manual that explains the procedure and interprets the results accompanies the kit.

Factors such as fatigue or illness affect the child's willingness to cooperate. These factors are noted on the test paper. If an unexplained delay is noted, it is best to have the child return in 2 weeks for reevaluation. If any delay in development is noted on the DDST, it is mandatory that the child return for rescreening.

### Immunizations

Immunizations are usually given at the end of the examination. At this age, the child is scheduled to receive two immunizations if he is up to date on the previous ones. At 15 months of age, he needs the measles-mumps-rubella (MMR) vaccine. This one is given subcutaneously in the deltoid area. At 18 months, he needs the first diphtheria-pertussis-tetanus (DPT) booster. This one is usually given intramuscularly in the vastus lateralis. Currently there is controversy regarding pertussis immunizations.

It is best to discuss reactions to the immunization with the parents before giving it. Having written instructions to give to the parent on possible side effects and what to do for them is helpful. The MMR vaccine may cause a slight rash and/or low-grade fever 7–10 days after the injection. The rash is not communicable. The site at which the DPT booster was given may become sore and reddened; the child may also develop a fever that night. Parents are advised to give baby aspirin or liquid acetaminophen for the fever and warm compresses for the site. If symptoms are severe or persistent, parents are advised to call the clinic or office.

*Anticipatory guidance*

The CHN or PNP plays another essential role in the well-child assessments during toddlerhood. In addition to taking the history and making physical and other assessments, she clarifies procedures for the mother, recommends dietary measures, and explains the effects of prescribed medicines. She interacts with the toddler and his parents in many ways during clinic visits to make the experience beneficial and satisfying.

The areas of anticipatory guidance for home visits that are discussed earlier in this chapter should be reinforced in the clinic, office, or well-child conference. There may need to be communication between the nurse in the clinic and the CHN who visits the home in order to accomplish necessary guidance. For example, if the toddler is found to have an iron deficiency in the clinic, the CHN who goes to the home is actually in a better position to evaluate the diet, especially if she visits at mealtime.

Keeping a toddler well by bringing him to a clinic for wellness supervision should be emphasized periodically. The CHN in the clinic provides many types of health education for parents in order to promote and maintain wellness in these early years after infancy.

## Acute Visits

Toddlers average three to five clinic visits a year for acute care. These children are brought to a clinic, a physician's office, or possibly to an emergency room if they are not regularly followed in a well-child conference. URIs are the most common cause of illnesses in infancy and toddlerhood.

If the CHN on a home visit suspects an otitis media, she should discuss her findings with the mother and encourage her to set up an emergency clinic appointment. The toddler needs to be seen by an NP or physician to establish the diagnosis, and the antibiotic must be prescribed by a physician. The clinic personnel will also answer any questions the mother has, clarify instructions, and be supportive of the toddler and the mother in eliminating the infection and relieving the associated pain.

## Chronic Visits

Examples of chronic problems—burns, hydrocephaly, lead poisoning, and child abuse—are discussed earlier in this chapter. Both home visits and clinic visits are necessary in these conditions to insure proper interventions and supportive measures for the parents. Toddlers with chronic problems will probably not receive the care intended unless the parents are supported in their efforts by the clinic personnel. Very often, referral to specialists such as orthopedists are made in the clinic. Finances are another necessary aspect with which parents may need direction and assistance if a child is chronically ill. Although the PNP collaborates with the physician in the care of toddlers with chronic conditions, her advent into the health care system has greatly enhanced the care. It has been particularly well extended in places where there was a lack of care for toddlers in the past.

# References

Barton, F. Personal communication, June 1979.

Beneson, A. S. (Ed.). *Control of communicable diseases in man* (13th ed.). Washington, D.C.: American Public Health Association, 1981.

Brazelton, T. B. *Doctor and child.* New York: Delacorte Press/Seymour Lawrence, 1976.

Center for Disease Control. *Morbidity and mortality weekly report* (Vol. 31, No. 22). Atlanta: Author, 1982.

Chinn, P. L. *Child health maintenance.* St. Louis: C. V. Mosby, 1974.

Cratty, B. J. *Perceptual and motor development in infants and children.* London: Collier-Macmillan, 1970.

Dale, P. S. *Language development: Structure and function.* Hinsdale, Ill.: Dryden Press, 1972.

Dales, J. Motor and language development of twins during the first three years. *Journal of Genetic Psychology,* 1969, *114,* 263.

Dallman, P. R. New approaches to screening for iron deficiency. *Journal of Pediatrics,* 1977, *90,* 678–681.

Erikson, E. H. *Childhood and society.* Harmondsworth, England: Penguin, 1963.

Frankenburg, W. K., & Dodds, J. B. The Denver Developmental Screening Test. *Journal of Pediatrics,* 1967, *71,* 181.

Gesell, A., Ilg, F., & Ames, L. B. (in collaboration with J. L. Rodell). *Infant and child in the culture of today.* New York: Harper & Row, 1974.

Githens, J. H., & Hathaway, W. Hematologic disorders. In C. H. Kempe, H. K. Silver, & D. O'Brien (Eds.), *Current pediatric diagnosis and treatment.* Los Altos, Calif.: Lange Medical Publishers, 1976.

Helms, D. B., & Turner, J. S. *Exploring child behavior.* Philadelphia: W. B. Saunders, 1976.

Hughes, J. G. *Synopsis of pediatrics.* St. Louis: C. V. Mosby, 1977.

Lewin, E. B. Middle ear disease. In R. A. Hockelman, S. Blatman, P. A. Burnell, S. B. Friedman, & H. M. Seidel (Eds.), *Principles of pediatrics: Health care of the young.* New York: McGraw-Hill, 1978.

Lundgren, R. Personal communication, October 29, 1980.

Paulist Productions (Producer). *War of the eggs.* Pacific Palisades, Calif.: Producer, 1972. (Film)

*Physician's desk reference.* Oradell, N.J.: Medical Economics, 1982.

Richmond, P. G. *An introduction to Piaget.* New York: Basic Books, 1970.

Scripien, G. M., Barnard, M. U., Chard, M. A., Howe, J., & Phillips, P. J. *Comprehensive pediatric nursing* (2nd ed.). New York: McGraw-Hill, 1979.

Shelton, P. G. Nursing-bottle caries. *Pediatrics,* 1977, *59,* 777.

Vaughan, V. C. III, McKay, R. J., Jr., & Behrman, R. E. (W. E. Nelson, Sr. Ed.). *Nelson textbook of pediatrics* (11th ed.). Philadelphia: W. B. Saunders, 1979.

Waechter, E. H., & Blake, F. G. *Nursing care of children.* Philadelphia: J. B. Lippincott, 1976.

White, B. I. *The first three years of life.* Englewood Cliffs, N.J.: Prentice-Hall, 1975.

# 5

# The Preschooler at Home, in the Clinic, and in Nursery School

*Dorothy D. Petrowski, Karen E. Miles, and Patricia Kachelmeyer*

## Introduction

The preschool period covers the span from toddlerhood to school age (i.e., the third through the fifth years). During this time, the child matures in various ways. He becomes less dependent on adults to meet his needs and seeks the companionship of peers. Play is probably his most important daily activity. The preschool child has a uniqueness that his parents, teachers, and nurses describe as very refreshing and rewarding. At times his self-awareness and insight amaze adults; at other times his subjective view of things leads him to believe dreams and fantasies are real.

One way to describe the behavior of this group would be "the age of curiosity." The preschooler has an intense interest in and curiosity about life and people. He may ask as many as 250 to 300 questions a day, many of which are frequently difficult to answer because they may be considered philosophical in nature (Pillitteri, 1977). Examples include "Why is the sky blue?" "How do babies get born?" "Why did Mr. Smith die?" Even though adults are sometimes overwhelmed by such questions, it is important to remember that a child at this age should receive answers that are at his level of understanding.

The child's world has grown beyond his home environment and immediate family, even though he still spends the majority of his time in the home setting. The community health nurse (CHN) or nurse practitioner (NP) may come in contact with him in the home, in the clinic, and in nursery school. This chapter discusses nursing of the preschool child in these three settings and in three care areas: (1) growth and development; (2) well-child care; and (3) common health problems.

## Growth and Development Overview

The preschool-age child gains only about 5 pounds a year. His growth in height is also minimal, approximately 2 to 2½ inches per year. Although his size changes very little, his body contour changes quite significantly. He becomes thinner, but still retains a sturdy-looking appearance. His trunk stays the same, while his legs become more elongated. A 3-year-old has attained one-half of his adult height (O'Dowd, 1982).

In terms of development, there is a wide variation in the tasks that 3-, 4-, and 5-year-olds accomplish. Therefore, development is briefly reviewed according to age, encompassing motor, cognitive, and language development.

### The 3-Year-Old

The 3-year-old walks up stairs alternating feet on the steps, but may still come down using both feet on a step. He is able to jump in place, climb a small ladder, and throw a ball; at times he may become unbalanced, but he is able to pedal a tricycle. His fine motor coordination and perception now allow him to hold a big crayon, draw a vertical line, and copy a circle. He can also build a tower of nine or ten cubes and can place raisins in a narrow-necked bottle (Whaley & Wong, 1979). He is able to undress himself and in most cases has bowel and bladder control during the day.

The 3-year-old is still at the beginning of Piaget's "preoperational phase," which is characterized by egocentrism, inability to conserve, and transductive reasoning. For example, he thinks he is always right, to the point of exasperating adults. He does not yet comprehend Piaget's concept of conservation (change in shape, but not volume); for example, he does not understand that two balls of Playdoh may be equal in amount, if one appears larger when flattened. The child at this age does not reason deductively and inductively, but transductively (a term coined by Piaget). For example, he associates dissimilar events, as when he states that it is morning because he has had his cereal. In addition, he is beginning to understand time and space by talking about past and future events (e.g., winter, Christmas) and about differences in location (e.g., inside and outside). He knows the meaning of taking turns and of words that affect him daily such as "tired," "hungry," and "cold" (Ginsburg & Opper, 1969; Yussen & Santrock, 1978).

A 3-year-old has a vocabulary between 600 and 1000 words. He talks and asks questions constantly and uses complete sentences of three or four words, often with plurals (Kaluger & Kaluger, 1974). He can usually state his full name and sex. If you show a child of this age a block in a primary (red, blue, or yellow) or secondary (e.g., green) color, he can recognize it. He may even identify several colors when asked to do so.

## The 4-Year-Old

The 4-year-old is able to walk up and down stairs, alternating feet on the steps, and can skip and hop on one foot. He can throw a ball overhand and catch it with both hands. His fine motor development and perception have matured; he is able to button some large buttons and cut out predrawn shapes. Of the five basic geometric shapes (square, triangle, circle, cone, and cylinder), he can copy the square, triangle, and circle. He is able to draw a person with three parts—head, body, and legs.

The 4-year-old has progressed into what Piaget calls the phase of "intuitive thought," but his reasoning is limited to his immediate perceptions and experience, and mostly to concrete situations (Lowrey, 1973). He believes he is the center of the world and thinks he has the ability to cause events. Therefore, he may experience guilt if "bad" things occur that he has wished. He is becoming less egocentric and has a better understanding of the concept of time, but he still does not have the ability to fully distinguish right from wrong.

The vocabulary of the 4-year-old grows to approximately 1000 to 1600 words, enabling him to ask many questions and tell stories in great detail (Kaluger & Kaluger, 1974). Though his stories are not always based on factual information, they are vividly described. He can identify several colors correctly. When asked, he will obey prepositional commands, such as "on," "under," and "in back of." He gives appropriate opposite words in analogies. For example, if you say "It is light in the daytime, but nighttime is _____," he will respond appropriately.

## The 5-Year-Old

The 5-year-old has good motor ability and is able to skip and hop on alternate feet; he can jump rope, throw and catch a ball, and walk a balance beam, and he begins to show an interest in group games. He can draw simple figures somewhat more sophisticated than those of the 4-year-old, can print his first name, and can probably tie his shoelaces.

He has a much better understanding of time than the 4-year-old does, and expresses it correctly (e.g., morning, afternoon). His memory of past events is surprisingly accurate (Lowrey, 1973). He is able to tell you when he eats breakfast and goes to bed, but probably cannot tell time. He is beginning to question events he hears his parents and other adults discussing, and he compares their versions to what his peers tell him. He is beginning to learn problem-solving techniques. Caregivers (parents, nurses, and teachers) must remember to show the 5-year-old that there is more than one way to solve problems. This is especially important since he follows the examples of his caregivers, who serve as role models for him in learning to do things the "right way."

The 5-year-old's vocabulary has grown to approximately 2000 words, and he uses all parts of speech in his sentence structure. Furthermore, he can identify a penny, a nickel, and a dime, as well as the days of the week and the months. He is able to define certain words when asked. For example, if asked what a dog is, he will state that it is an animal.

As can be seen, the development of the preschooler progresses rapidly during this 3-year period. The CHN who works with the preschooler must be aware of these factors in order to assess the needs of the preschool-age child and his family in order to stimulate his development. The Denver Developmental Screening Test (DDST), described in Chapter 4 in connection with toddlers, is an effective instrument for screening normal development and delays in this age group also. Other screening tools, as described by Stangler, Routh, and Huber (1980), are available for various other types of testing.

### Highlights of the Emotional Development of the Preschooler

In the preschool stage, the child is developing a sense of conscience. He must learn to solve his problems in such a way as not to feel guilty. To do this, he must be encouraged by his parents, teachers, and friends to use his knowledge and imagination to solve his problems. He will try very hard to learn about other people and the world—sometimes in unacceptable ways. He can be very noisy and may attack others on purpose or by accident during play (Marlow, 1977). When in a group situation, he will bid for the attention of others by teasing, questioning, and fabricating experiences. By the time he reaches 5 years of age, he will generally be more cooperative and less rebellious.

During this stage of development, the child forms a concept of his identity and family. He identifies with his parents (particularly the one of his own sex) by imitating parental behavior, which eventually becomes a part of his personality.

Other emotions besides guilt that the preschooler learns to adjust to include fear, jealousy, and aggression. Fears for the preschooler include fear of the dark, fear of imaginary creatures, fear of robbers, and fear of self-injury. A parent needs to be aware of and to respect these fears, and to assist the child to cope by listening and reinforcing reality. The most common form of jealousy for the preschooler exists when he realizes he must share his parents' love, particularly with siblings. To minimize sibling rivalry, parents should not show favoritism or compare one child to another (Helms & Turner, 1976). Consistent methods of discipline are of primary importance in helping the child cope with aggression, as well as in isolating the potential cause(s) of the behavior and establishing alternatives (e.g., substituting another activity for unattainable goals).

These sketches of a preschooler's growth and development can benefit CHNs when they observe and examine children and for counseling parents. Numerous textbooks exist if a CHN wishes to pursue the subject further.

## Nursing Care at Home

### Family Life

One of the major roles of parents is that of socializing their children. Because education in parenting is not a required part of the curriculum in our school systems, parents usually learn parenting skills from their own parents or by trial and error. Gordon's book *Parent Effectiveness Training* (1975) describes a basic course in parenthood and is one source that the CHN can recommend.

The preschool-age child spends the major part of his day at home or in day care. The family constellation is still the most critical factor in the physical, emotional, psychological, social, and spiritual development of the child. The well-developed preschooler is usually a very happy and independent child who listens to parents most of the time and enjoys the companionship of his peers, exhibiting few child-rearing problems.

However, there are some important needs of the preschooler that parents, caregivers, and nurses must recognize, such as supervision.

For example, parents may allow the preschooler to walk unattended to a neighbor's house, but only if it does not involve crossing a busy street. At this age, children have difficulty understanding that something is dangerous just because parents or an adult say it is, so continued reinforcement is needed.

Most parents enjoy their children at this stage of development because preschoolers are energetic, creative, and enthusiastic. Ideally, parents should provide a flexible environment. It may be difficult for some parents to allow their children the freedom they need at this period of development. For example, some parents have difficulty separating from their children and allowing the children to attend nursery school. The CHN can point out the benefits to both parents and children of this opportunity. Parents should encourage their children to become involved in outside activities, while still maintaining the quality of the home experiences. It is important for parents to continue to show an interest and to answer questions, in order to further language development, cognitive competence, and growth toward independence. Time between a parent and a child may be more meaningful for both of them if attention is given to specific activities (e.g., reading time).

Wellness Supervision

A routine visit by the CHN to the home may be made once or twice yearly for well-child supervision of the preschooler. This routine is established by a health department or visiting nurse association and does not preclude more frequent visits, which might be indicated in some situations. The CHN may also encounter a preschooler when she visits a home for another purpose, such as a prenatal visit to the mother. At this time, she may discuss areas that the mother mentions or concerns that the child presents. She may also discuss those problems that have been referred to her by a clinic, a private physician, or school personnel.

The CHN offers the mother or caregiver assistance with any concerns she might have at the present time, such as discipline. Also, she reviews the child's clinic care in the past 6 months and suggests appropriate literature, such as the government pamphlet, *Your Child from 1 to 6*. She may perform the DDST and then offer anticipatory guidance in the cognitive, motor, and affective domains.

Accidents, sexual development, play activities, discipline, and mental health counseling are common concerns; these are discussed in the following sections.

*Accident prevention*

Accidents are described in Chapter 4 in regard to poisons, burns, falls, and car safety; they are mentioned briefly here again, because they are one of the chief causes of morbidity and mortality in this age group. Motor vehicles, fire, poisoning, laceration from cutting or piercing objects, and drowning are the primary offenders. A 1977 study over a 12-month period in three counties of Pennsylvania reported that 77% of all childhood injuries occurred in the home, with the figure rising to 91% for children aged under 5 years (Davis, 1977).

The importance of teaching parents the relationship of growth and development to accident prevention is essential. The preschooler is particularly vulnerable to injuries from falls and cuts, since he is beginning to play outdoors. He can climb, ride a tricycle or bicycle, play ball, and use scissors—activities that have high accident potential. In addition, because he is curious, the preschooler has a tendency to investigate, taste, touch, and attempt to make things work. Because of this, the home needs to have "poison-proofing" and other kinds of child-proofing to keep the environment safe for the preschooler. The CHN can assist the parents in reviewing the safety of the home if requested. Safety principles include the following:

1. Posting the telephone number of the poison control center with other emergency numbers, so that neighbors or baby sitters have immediate access to it.
2. Storing cleaning supplies, paints, gasoline, lawn care products, and medicines (including vitamins and aspirin) in locked cabinets.
3. Keeping syrup of ipecac in the home in case of accidental ingestion of poisonous materials.
4. Providing safe toys and games for the child, as well as a fenced-in play area out of doors.
5. Being aware of physical dangers in the environment and ways to reduce them, such as getting rid of abandoned refrigerators.
6. Informing neighbors with outdoor swimming pools about the requirements for fencing these areas.
7. Impressing on the preschooler the dangers associated with busy streets, swimming pools, strange dogs and cats, and playing with matches.
8. Providing restraints when the child is riding in a motor vehicle, mandatory in many states.

*Sexual development*

One of the principal roles of the parents is to assist the preschooler in learning sexual identity and sexually appropriate behavior. The preschooler is very curious about his body and the bodies of others. He is aware of the differences between his parents, is beginning to ask questions about reproduction, and spends a great amount of time imitating sex-related roles. The parents should answer the child's questions in an open and honest manner, and should not punish the child for showing interest in the human body. The CHN can point out that this interest provides an opportunity for parents to foster the child's appreciation of the human body and to begin basic sex education. The CHN can offer the parents anticipatory guidance with appropriate literature and visual aids on human sexual anatomy. She should encourage open communication patterns in the family in order to enable the child and parents to discuss sexual questions freely and to assist the preschooler to accept and feel comfortable with his body. There are many excellent children's books that can help parents teach their children the basics of reproduction, such as the paperback *How Babies Are Made* (Andry and Sheppard, 1979).

*Play activity*

Another parental role is to encourage the child in imaginative or imitative play. The majority of the child's day is spent in many types of play activity, alone or with other children. It is not unusual for a child of this age to have imaginary playmates. He may tell his parents about something his imaginary friend has said or done to see what their reaction will be. He also works out some of his problems with imaginary friends.

Parents should encourage peer interaction by inviting playmates to come to the home, allowing the child to go to a friend's home, or enrolling the child in a nursery school. Selection of appropriate play materials is important. The CHN may want to review growth and development with the parents and offer guidance in the types of play materials that will be of benefit to the child's development, especially those that assist in developing his gross and fine motor skills (such as a tricycle, a wagon, and sports equipment for gross skills and clay, blocks, puzzles, and crayons and paint for fine skills). Because he spends a great deal of time in imitative play, a child of this age enjoys housekeeping toys, doctor kits, household tools, and dress-up clothes.

*Discipline*

Discipline, a primary responsibility of the parents, is frequently left out of well-child assessments. Nurses should initiate a discussion of discipline with parents, in order to prevent potential problems as far as possible. The CHN and the clinic NP, who are in a prime position to guide parents in discipline, are referred to the book *Between Parent and Child* (Ginott, 1965) for a good discussion of disciplinary styles and approaches. Parents who employ consistent discipline can avoid or overcome feelings of insecurity in the preschool-age child. In discipline, most authorities believe that the undesirable act and not the child should be disapproved. Love should be the motivating factor in discipline, and it should be expressed consistently. The CHN should stress that the objectives of discipline are to teach the child safe and socially acceptable ways of operating within his environment and to foster respect for parents and society, not to punish the child (Hymovich & Chamberlin, 1980). Children of all ages should be told why they are being disciplined, and a parent should be sure not to undermine a spouse's disciplinary style when interacting with a child.

*Mental health counseling*

Although preschoolers are generally healthy and well adjusted, certain situations may predispose the child to behavioral or emotional problems. Examples are the death of a parent or divorce. Two major developmental tasks of the preschooler are identification with his parents and the development of sex role; it is also known that preschoolers see death as separation, which they assess to be temporary. Intervention by a CHN who understands the dying and death process and the developmental needs of the preschooler may help prevent behavioral problems that could result from a parent's death (Sahler, 1978).

Grief and mourning are normal responses to loss, though the exact age at which a child is intellectually able to comprehend these concepts is not certain. Children do not talk about their feelings directly, but act them out in behavior and interactions with others.

The CHN working with the family who has experienced a loss should base her interactions on the following principles:

1. Be aware of her own feelings and attitudes about death and dying and divorce.

2. Encourage the child to talk about his feelings and be willing to listen to these feelings.
3. Educate the child's caregivers not to punish the child for the manner in which he acts out his grief.
4. Make sure the child and family are aware of available community resources, such as a child guidance clinic.
5. Have the family include the child in the ritual practiced by the family at the time of death, or explain the divorce process.

The role of the family in the mental health development of the child cannot be overemphasized. The CHN, who may be the one consistent person working with the family during a child's growing years, must recognize the importance of her counseling role in this relationship. She must be able to educate and provide anticipatory guidance for families, in order to help them recognize potential problems and deal with them before they become serious. She must also be able to refer them to the proper agencies for assistance.

Sickness Care

On occasion a CHN receives a referral from a clinic, a nursery school, the child's parents, the local developmental disabilities services or social welfare department, or a hospital to visit a child at home for an acute or chronic illness. Most of the acute illnesses are short-term infections, such as pneumonia or urinary tract infections (UTIs) (discussed later in this chapter). Chronic problems include lead poisoning, orthopedic problems such as "clubfoot," birth defects such as hydrocephalus or a meningomyelocele, and behavioral problems. Meningomyelocele is described in Chapter 3, and lead poisoning and hydrocephalus are described in Chapter 4.

In the event of an infection, the CHN should make sure that the mother knows the way to take a temperature, the need to force fluids, requirements for adequate rest, the importance of administering medication as prescribed, and the necessity to return to the clinic for further follow-up.

If the condition is chronic (i.e., of a duration of 3 months or more), the CHN should establish with the mother (by contract) the reason for her visit(s), what the nurse and the family can do for the child jointly, the expected outcomes, and the predicted frequency and duration of the CHN's visits.

## Nursing Care in the Clinic

### Routine Well-Child Examinations

The value of routine well-child examinations for the growing child is well documented. The preschool-age child should have at least yearly well-child visits. At each of these visits, there should be a history update to help confirm the child's health status, list complaints, and define areas for parental guidance and teaching. Guidelines for a preschool health history include the following:

A. Chief reason for visit

1. Well-child checkup, or
2. A specific complaint, such as an earache

B. Comments about the previous developmental periods

1. Prenatal (fetal, birth, newborn)
2. Infancy
3. Toddler

C. Family history

1. Well physically and mentally, or
2. Significant illnesses

D. Present history

1. Growth and development
2. Nutrition
3. Allergies
4. Accidents
5. Illnesses, operations, and hospitalizations
6. Attendance at day care or nursery school

The preschooler is usually very helpful and cooperative during a well-child physical assessment or examination. Suggested guidelines for a preschool physical examination include the following:

A. General appearance of child
B. Height, weight, and vital signs (temperature, pulse, respiration, and blood pressure taken with child's cuff)
C. Review of systems, using inspection, percussion, palpation, and auscultation (IPPA):
1. Head, eyes, ears, nose, and throat
2. Chest (lungs, heart, breasts)

3. Abdomen (bowel sounds, liver, spleen, kidneys)
4. Genitalia and rectal examination
5. Extremities—check pulses
6. Musculoskeletal system (gait and range of motion)
7. Neurological—check reflexes

The CHN should also refer to the general guidelines for a health history in Appendix C at the end of this volume.

A developmental assessment of the child should be done by the nurse while she is examining him. It is suggested that each CHN or NP develop guidelines of her own choosing. Although these may overlap the DDST, they are then readily available if combined with the examination. See Table 5-1 for suggested guidelines for the developmental assessment of the preschooler.

Preschoolers need certain laboratory screening and immunizations. A complete blood count and urinalysis should be done yearly. The 3-year-old needs a tine test for tuberculosis, and the 4-year-old needs immunizations for diphtheria, pertussis, and tetanus (DPT) and trivalent oral poliomyelitis vaccine (TOPV). (See Table 5-2 for immunization schedules.) Hearing and vision evaluations should be done at 4 and 5 years of age.

## Early and Periodic Screening, Diagnosis, and Treatment

One of the most vulnerable groups is that of the "children of poverty," the children of parents on welfare. Poverty and health status are interrelated. The CHN should be aware of the Early and Periodic Screening, Diagnosis, and Treatment (EPSDT) services that are available under Medicaid. This program is one of prevention, early detection, and treatment. It attempts to introduce eligible children into the health care system, and to make services available to these children before health problems become chronic and life-threatening. Although EPSDT is a program for the economically disadvantaged, it should be the prototype for all well-child care, regardless of economic status (Frankenburg & North, 1974). If the federal government curtails funds for this program, alternative ones will have to be found.

## The Clinic Nurse's Role

A major responsibility of the CHN is to educate the parents about the importance of regular well-child visits to a clinic. This is sometimes difficult, depending upon the cultural, socioeconomic, and ethnic practices

Table 5-1

Guidelines for the Developmental Assessment of a Preschooler

|  | 3-year-old | 4-year-old | 5-year-old |
|---|---|---|---|
| Gross Motor | Jumps in place<br>Pedals tricycle<br>Throws ball overhand | Hops on one foot<br>Walks a line<br>Catches a ball | Dresses self without help<br>Hops on one foot<br>Heel to toe walk |
| Fine Motor | Builds tower of 6 cubes<br>Places raisins in a narrow-necked bottle<br>Copies a circle | Cuts out predrawn shapes<br>Buttons large buttons<br>Draws a 3-part person | Prints his first name<br>Copies a square<br>Ties shoelaces |
| Expressive | Uses 3 to 4 word sentences<br>Asks "Why"<br>Uses plurals | Counts three objects<br>Knows his first and last names<br>Uses adjectives<br>Tells a story | Uses all parts of speech in a sentence<br>Asks questions about daily events<br>Uses language to exchange ideas |
| Receptive | Understands tired, cold, hungry<br>Understands what it means to take turns<br>Can name some fruits and vegetables | Repeats 8-word sentence<br>Responds to commands<br>Understands yesterday, today, and tomorrow | Understands opposites<br>Recognizes colors<br>Comprehends prepositions |

*Note.* Developed by Dorothy D. Petrowski and Marcia Etu.

123

Table 5-2
Immunization Schedules

IF YOUR CHILD IS TWO MONTHS OLD . . .

| Age | Diphtheria Pertussis Tetanus[a] | Polio[b] | Measles | Rubella | Mumps |
|---|---|---|---|---|---|
| 2 months | * | * | | | |
| 4 months | * | * | | | |
| 6 months | * | *(optional) | | | |
| 15 months | | | *[c] | *[c] | *[c] |
| 18 months | * | * | | | |
| 4-6 years | * | * | | | |

*Note.* From Center for Disease Control, *Parent's Guide to Childhood Immunization.* Atlanta: Author, 1977.

[a]Children should receive a sixth tetanus-diphtheria injection (booster) at age 14–16.

[b]Polio vaccine is oral.

[c]Measles, rubella, and mumps vaccines can be given in a combined form, at about 15 months of age, with a single injection.

of families. Its importance in primary prevention (health promotion, health education, and specific risk identification) cannot be overemphasized. The nurse in the clinic may have a variety of titles: clinic nurse, CHN, or NP. Each has the same basic job description: implementing the nursing process by performing health histories, providing direct nursing care (e.g., giving injections), counseling, giving anticipatory guidance, and teaching.

As discussed earlier in this chapter, sex education and safety prevention are good examples of areas in which health teaching and anticipatory guidance should be given by the CHN, irrespective of the setting. The CHN in the clinic should discuss these with the parents and reinforce what the CHN in the home has discussed. The clinic nurse should have audiovisual aids and pamphlets relating to health teaching and anticipatory guidance available for use with the parents on any of these subjects.

Nutritional guidance should be an important part of the nurse's role in every setting. A preschooler is usually not a big eater and may even be described as finicky. He is influenced by what others eat, imitating parents and friends. The nurse can assess in several ways whether the child is meeting his nutritional needs. The first is by looking at the child: Is he alert, active, and healthy-looking? The nurse can also ask the child's parents about his eating habits and general health status. His height and weight measurements are a good index. The recommended calorie intake for this age child is 1800 kcal per day. Using a 24-hour recall diary, the nurse can assist the mother in determining if the child's diet includes necessary nutrients. In addition, his blood work should indicate whether he is anemic.

The nurse should encourage parents to provide well-balanced meals and nutritional snacks for their preschoolers. A well-balanced diet includes foods from all four basic food groups. One question parents will ask is whether they should give their children supplemental vitamins; it is important to advise parents that a well-balanced diet usually provides the necessary vitamins and minerals. Parents should also be reminded to tell their preschoolers that vitamins and minerals are medicine, not candy. An overdose of a fat-soluble vitamin is one of the leading causes of poisoning among these children.

The nurse should know about growth and development, nutritional needs and common problems of the age group, and much more. Examples of common problems related to normal growth and development that nurses might discuss with parents include the normal fears of the 3-year-old (monsters, the dark) and the backtalk of the 4-year-old ("shut up," "you dummy"). Opportunities to explore areas of concern with the parent(s) aid the family in discovering what "normal" developmental behavior is and in obtaining information on handling problems that are not within "normal" limits.

## The Preschooler at Nursery School

### Impact of a Nursery-School Experience on a Preschooler

One of the most interesting and profitable experiences in the outside world for a preschooler is attending nursery school. The preschooler is usually ready for this experience and separates easily from his parents. Attending nursery school is a very important aspect of the socialization and social development of the preschooler. It provides stimulation for the child's motor, cognitive, language, social, and emotional development, and gives him an opportunity to interact with other adults as well as with fellow preschoolers. Interactions with peers create a tremendous influence on the child. Children become aware of many important things about themselves when they engage in play with peers that is not supervised by parents.

The preschooler often attends nursery school part of the day (morning or afternoon) either every weekday or several days a week. Association with peers in such a semistructured environment is an important experience in the total development of the child. The daily schedule at nursery school should include both individual and group activities, free play, outdoor play, quiet play, and snack and rest periods. A child's attendance at nursery school is an important activity that can aid in the development of those social skills necessary to get along well with peers (Biehler, 1976).

### Role and Functions of a Community Health Nurse in a Nursery School

The CHN's role in the nursery-school setting varies from limited involvement, such as infrequent visits to talk with the children about good health habits, to working with parents and the teaching staff as a resource person. She might teach good health practices, or she can acquaint the teachers with health literature and audiovisual aids. She can give the teachers classes on health-related topics (e.g., communicable diseases). Other activities may include assisting with administering health assessments and immunizations.

The nurse should be an astute observer of preschoolers in action to try to identify potential problems, such as visual and hearing deficits, orthopedic problems, or language problems. She should discuss these with the parents, teachers, and social worker, and should encourage the parents to seek medical advice.

Another role of the CHN may be that of "inspector" for the local health department. In some instances, CHNs and sanitary engineers from a county health department inspect nursery schools (including lunch and playground equipment) for safety and cleanliness, possibly taking samples for cultures if indicated. It has been suggested that federal safety standards be enacted for private and public playgrounds because many are unsafe ("Playground Safety Stressed in Report," 1980).

## Health Problems of the Preschool Child

During the preschool-age period the child has frequent, minor illnesses, about 80% of which are respiratory. There is an extremely low mortality rate for respiratory infections, except for pneumonia, which is a leading cause of death. The leading cause of death during this age is automobile accidents. Poisonings and falls are also significant as part of this age group's mortality rate (see Table 5-3) (Pillitteri, 1977).

The preschool-age child is susceptible to certain health problems as a result of his growth and developmental status. His gross motor capability has matured to the point where he is very active. He is ready to be more independent and freer of close supervision by his parents, and thus is particularly prone to accidental injuries. Also, the preschooler is exposed to communicable diseases and acute infections, because he is playing in groups and often attending nursery school.

The preschooler may react to illness or injury in a variety of ways. He may have a hard time understanding why and how he became ill. Illness is stressful and causes anxiety at any age. The preschooler worries about the threats that illness poses for him. He may or may not express his fears, either real or imagined. The nurse who is aware that the child of this age has certain fears and is able to educate the parent to assist the child in discussing them openly will help alleviate much of the anxiety of the preschooler.

The preschooler may fear coming to the clinic for a variety of reasons. He may have heard another child talk about how an injection hurt and made a "big red mark" on his arm. It must be remembered that a child of this age is particularly vulnerable to thoughts of anything that might harm his body. He may fear that he will have to be hospitalized, and thereby placed in an unfamiliar environment and separated from his parents.

In working with the ill preschooler and his family, the role of the nurse is to help them to understand that these anxieties and fears are a normal reaction. After she has accomplished this, she can begin to help the child work through these feelings and understand himself better through games and role playing. The preschooler's interest in "playing doctor and nurse" provides an opportunity to help him work through fears and anxieties by acting them out. The nurse should provide the child with the equipment necessary to "practice" on a doll or stuffed animal. Sometimes just being able to handle and play with the equipment (e.g., the reflex hammer) removes the threat of mystery and helps the child to be less anxious.

Table 5-3

Mortality for the 10 Leading Causes of Death for Children Aged 1–4 in the United States, 1979

| Rank Order | Cause of death | Number | Rates per 100,000 population |
|---|---|---|---|
| | All causes———————————————— | 8,108 | 65.6 |
| 1 | Accidents———————————————— | 3,349 | 27.1 |
| 2 | Congenital anomalies———————————— | 1,021 | 8.3 |
| 3 | Malignant neoplasms, including neoplasms of lymphatic and hematopoietic tissues——————— | 578 | 4.7 |
| 4 | Homicide and legal intervention———————— | 314 | 2.5 |
| 5 | Diseases of heart——————————————— | 265 | 2.1 |
| 6 | Pneumonia and influenza—————————— | 258 | 2.1 |
| 7 | Meningitis—————————————————— | 183 | 1.5 |
| 8 | Meningococcal infections————————— | 107 | 0.9 |
| 9 | Certain conditions originating in the perinatal period——— | 75 | 0.6 |
| 10 | Anemias——————————————————— | 73 | 0.6 |
| ... | All other causes————————————— | 1,885 | 15.2 |

*Note.* From National Center for Health Statistics, *Monthly Vital Statistics Report* (Vol. 31, No. 6, Suppl.). Washington, D.C.: U.S. Department of Health and Human Services, 1982.

## Infections

The acute or short-term conditions that frequently affect the preschooler include infectious diseases such as pharyngitis, otitis media (discussed in Chapter 4), and UTIs. The preschooler is also susceptible to long-term health problems and fatal diseases of childhood that are not addressed in this chapter.

### Pharyngitis

"Pharyngitis" refers to an infection involving any of the structures in the throat and surrounding area, including tonsillitis. Pharyngitis may be caused by either a viral or a bacterial agent; 15% of cases are caused by Group A beta-hemolytic streptococci, but the majority of cases are of viral origin. In order to make a definitive diagnosis, a throat culture should be done. This procedure can be done by the nurse in whatever setting she is practicing.

The clinical manifestations are very similar for viral and bacterial pharyngitis. The child with viral pharyngitis will usually complain of tiredness, lack of appetite, and headache for approximately 24 hours. Then he will begin to complain of a sore throat and to cough. The nurse, when performing a health assessment, will see a moderately ill child, usually with a low-grade fever. His pharynx will be slightly erythematous, with slightly enlarged tonsils and palpable cervical lymph nodes. Symptomatic treatments, such as rest and fluids, are all that are required in viral pharyngitis. Usually the child will prefer soft foods and fluids at this time, due to the soreness of his throat. Analgesic and antipyretic drugs, such as acetaminophen, are useful in reducing fever and discomfort. There is a new warning against using aspirin with children who have influenza and chicken pox, because it is associated with Reyes syndrome (Center for Disease Control, 1982). Also, sponging the child with tepid water may help reduce high fever (over 40°C or 104°F rectally). A cool mist vaporizer in his room, warm or cold compresses to the neck, and warm saline gargles will help relieve some of the throat soreness. Viral pharyngitis runs its course in 1 to 5 days.

The child with bacterial pharyngitis will usually complain of a severe sore throat. His fever may approach or exceed 40°C (104°F) rectally. The tonsils and pharynx will be edematous and will have white exudate on them, with firm and tender cervical lymph nodes. This child will need the symptomatic treatment described above, plus a 10-day treatment with an oral antibiotic such as penicillin. Many professionals ask that the child have a repeat throat culture after the antibiotic therapy has been completed, in order to be sure that the bacteria have been eliminated.

Tonsillitis sometimes becomes a chronic disease to the extent that tonsillectomy becomes the treatment of choice; tonsillectomy, however, has become a somewhat controversial subject, because many feel that this surgical procedure is performed too often and without proper justification.

Since the child with viral or bacterial pharyngitis will most likely be treated at home, nursing responsibilities include counseling the parents on giving the child symptomatic care, especially the importance of giving the medication continuously and on schedule for the entire 10-day period. Some parents may stop the antibiotic as soon as the child's condition improves. This may increase the child's chances of suffering from complications, such as rheumatic fever, that may arise from a streptococcal infection. The CHN should instruct the family to see that the child drinks at least 2000 cc of fluids in each 24-hour period.

### Urinary tract infections

UTIs are another health problem that the nurse working with preschool-age children will encounter. A UTI is most commonly defined as the presence of 100,000 bacteria per ml of urine in a properly collected urine specimen. The peak incidence of these infections occurs between 2 and 6 years of age. This does not include the infections caused from structural anomalies. Females have approximately 10 to 30 times greater risk than males of having a UTI. This seems to be attributable to the fact that the female urethra is much shorter than that of the male, and as well as to its proximity to the vaginal orifice; these factors make females particularly vulnerable to the organisms that cause UTIs.

A child may have a UTI without having any of the symptoms usually associated with UTIs. UTIs may be either acute or chronic, and the symptoms can be nonspecific and vary with age. The preschool-age child will usually exhibit the following symptoms: odorous urine, hematuria, abdominal pain, and vomiting (Stapleton & Linshaw, 1978). He may exhibit some of the more common symptoms such as burning on urination, frequent urination, and dysuria. However, these are not usually manifested until the school-age period.

The organism most likely to be the causative agent in UTI in females is *Escherichia coli*. In fact, the incidence of this organism as the causative agent is 75–85%. Other gram-negative organisms, such as *Pseudomonas aeruginosa* and *Serratia marcescins*, account for the remainder of infectious agents in females. In males, *Proteus mirabilis* has been identified as the most frequent organism, with *Staphylococcus epidermidis* as the next most frequent (Stapleton & Linshaw, 1978). These organisms enter the body by ascending through the urethra. The nurse should educate parents and children about identification of the presence of a UTI. Females between 2 and 6 years of age are a high-risk group. A routine urinalysis should be part of the yearly physical examination.

Certain predisposing factors have been identified in UTIs. The short urethra in the female has been mentioned. Another is vesicoureteral reflux, a retrograde flow of bladder urine into the ureters. When the child voids, urine is swept up into the ureters and then empties back into the bladder after voiding. Therefore, this residual urine is in the bladder, and the potential for infection is always present. Reflux can be either primary or secondary. Primary reflux is a result of a congenitally abnormal insertion of the ureters into the bladder, and secondary reflux comes about as a result of infection (Stapleton & Linshaw, 1978).

Chronic constipation has been identified as a predisposing factor in UTI. Probably this results from distention of the rectum, which in turn distorts the bladder (Whaley & Wong, 1979). Obstruction and urinary stasis then occurs. The use of stool softeners along with certain dietary measures should reduce the incidence of UTIs.

Treatment of the child with a suspected UTI includes obtaining a clean-catch specimen. The CHN may do this or teach the parent to do it. The nurse or parent should accompany the child to the bathroom, where the child should be told step by step what will be done. The perineum should be cleansed with an antiseptic solution on a sterile pad, wiping from front to back just once. After sterile water has been poured over the area, the child should void. After the child has begun to void, the midportion of the urine stream should be collected in a sterile container. The child should be praised at this time. Usually a repeat urine culture is done 4 to 7 days after the completion of the antibiotic therapy. Stapleton and Linshaw (1978) have developed a timetable for performing urine cultures following an initial UTI. This includes urine cultures 4 to 7 days following completion of antibiotic therapy at 6 weeks, at 3-month intervals for 1 year, and at 6-month intervals for 5 years thereafter. They also recommend that an intravenous pyelogram (IVP) be performed in all girls over 2 years old. One needs to evaluate whether an IVP is necessary following a single UTI, in view of present knowledge about hazards of radiation. If significant abnormalities are found, a voiding cystourethrogram should be done. Other measures in the management of the child with a UTI by his family include encouraging the child to drink generous amounts of fluids, especially cranberry juice, and to void regularly so that retention of urine does not occur.

The CHN can teach families certain basic hygiene principles to prevent UTIs. These include wiping from the anterior to posterior perineal area after voiding and defecation, and avoiding constipation. Parents should be alerted to avoid the use of bubble bath preparations that cause chemical irritation. In fact, the child who is susceptible to UTI should probably take showers, short tub baths, or sponge baths. If an IVP is done, it should be explained in order to prepare the child psychologically.

*Communicable diseases*

A "communicable disease" is defined as an illness caused by a specific infectious agent or its toxic products through a direct or indirect mode of transmission of that agent from a reservoir. In his expanded new environments and among his new acquaintances, the preschooler comes in contact with the organisms that cause communicable diseases. Chicken pox, "fifth disease" (erythema infectiosum), and scarlet fever are the most common ones that the nurse who works with preschoolers in an ambulatory care setting may encounter, and she may be the first person to recognize the signs and symptoms of a communicable disease. She should take immediate actions to isolate the child from other children. It is important to identify the causative agent, the incubation period, the mode of transmission, and the treatment for the particular disease. (See Table 5-4.)

Some of the first symptoms of a communicable disease may be a fever, a cough, or a rash. The CHN and NP should be able to identify the different types of rashes associated with communicable diseases, in addition to the prodromal symptoms associated with specific communicable diseases.

No matter what type of rash the child may have, he will complain about being uncomfortable and extremely itchy. To reduce discomfort, the CHN or NP can suggest a lukewarm bath with baking soda added. Aspirin (the usual dosage is 1 grain per year of age up to 10 grains) or aspirin substitute may be given for their analgesic effects. Calamine lotion can be obtained without prescription and will help relieve the itching. The child should be dressed in lightweight clothes, because heavy clothing and wool tend to make the rash more uncomfortable. His fingernails should be trimmed. Sometimes the physician may prescribe an antihistamine such as Benadryl to help reduce the itching.

Table 5-4

Communicable Diseases Common to the Preschool-Age Child

| DISEASE | CAUSATIVE AGENT | INCUBATION PERIOD | PERIOD OF COMMUNICABILITY | MODE OF TRANSMISSION | IMMUNITY | CLINICAL MANIFESTATIONS | COMPLICATIONS |
|---|---|---|---|---|---|---|---|
| Chicken pox (Varicella) | Varicella-zoster virus | 10-21 days | 1 day before rash to 6 days after appearance of vesicles | direct or indirect contact | no active & little passive placental immunity | low-grade fever; malaise; macular rash with progression to papules & vesicles which crust (concentration on trunk); rash extremely itchy | secondary infections of lesions, pneumonia, encephilitis |
| "Fifth Disease" (Erythema Infectiosum) | Virus | 6-14 days | unknown | direct contact | none | first symptoms: red, maculo-papular rash appearing on face; next day, rash appears on extensor surfaces of extremities; day later, rash on flexor surfaces & trunk | none known |
| Scarlet Fever | Beta-hemolytic streptococci-Group A | 2-5 days | throughout illness | direct & indirect contact | none | high fever, sore throat, headache & malaise at first; rash on skin & mucous membranes begins 12-14 hrs. after sore throat; tonsils covered with exudate; "strawberry tongue" | none if antibiotic (penicillin preferred) is administered, rheumatic fever, acute glomerulonephritis |

Another clinical manifestation of a communicable disease is fever. Teaching parents how to reduce high temperatures is an important role of the nurse. Administration of an antipyretic is recommended. Also, the child should be dressed in lightweight clothing. Heavy clothing will keep the heat close to the body and may even increase the temperature. A tepid sponge bath or tub bath will also aid in reducing the child's temperature. In rubeola the eyes may be affected (conjunctivitis), and the child may be irritated by bright light (photophobia). It is soothing to the child to keep the shades drawn and to use only soft, limited light until this symptom subsides.

The child with scarlet fever will require penicillin. Teaching parents the importance of administering this drug on a prescribed schedule for the entire 10-day course of therapy has been discussed earlier in this chapter. Occasionally another medication, such as cough syrup, is also prescribed. Symptomatic measures include adequate fluid and nutritional intake, rest, and perhaps diversional activities (Marlow, 1977; Waechter & Blake, 1976).

# References

Andry, A., & Sheppard, S. *How babies are made.* Alexandria, Va.: Time, Inc., 1979.

Biehler, R. F. *Child development: An introduction.* Boston: Houghton Mifflin, 1976.

Center for Disease Control. *Morbidity and mortality weekly report* (Vol. 31, No. 22). Atlanta: Author, 1982.

Davis, R. C. Prevention of childhood accidents through safety education. *Issues in Comprehensive Pediatric Nursing,* 1977, 1(6), 57–71.

Frankenburg, W. K., & North, A. F., Jr. *A guide to screening for the Early and Periodic Screening, Diagnosis, and Treatment Program (EPSDT) under Medicaid.* Washington, D.C.: U.S. Department of Health, Education and Welfare, 1974.

Ginott, H. G. *Between parent and child.* New York: Macmillan, 1965.

Ginsburg, H., & Opper, S. *Piaget's theory of intellectual development: An introduction.* Englewood Cliffs, N.J.: Prentice-Hall, 1969.

Gordon, T. V. *Parent effectiveness training.* New York: New American Library, 1975.

Helms, D. B., & Turner, J. B. *Exploring child behavior.* Philadelphia: W. B. Saunders, 1976.

Hymovich, D. P., & Chamberlin, R. W. *Child and family development: Implications for primary health care.* New York: McGraw-Hill, 1980.

Kaluger, G., & Kaluger, M. F. *Human development: The span of life.* St. Louis: C. V. Mosby, 1974.

Lowrey, G. H. *Growth and development of children.* Chicago: Yearbook Medical Publishers, 1973.

Marlow, D. R. *Textbook of pediatric nursing.* Philadelphia: W. B. Saunders, 1977.

O'Dowd, M. M. Personal communication, February 14, 1982.

Pillitteri, A. *Nursing care of the growing family.* Boston: Little, Brown, 1977.

Playground safety stressed in report. *Milwaukee Journal,* Feb. 10, 1980, p. 13.

Sahler, O. J. Z. (Ed.). *The child and death.* St. Louis: C. V. Mosby, 1978.

Stangler, S. R., Routh, D. K., & Huber, C. J. *Screening growth and development of preschool children: A guide for test selection.* New York: McGraw-Hill, 1980.

Stapleton, F. B., & Linshaw, M. A. Urinary tract infections in children: Diagnosis and management. *Issues in Comprehensive Pediatric Nursing,* 1978, 2(6), 1-10.

Waechter, E., & Blake, F. *Nursing care of children.* Philadelphia: J. P. Lippincott, 1976.

Whaley, L. F., & Wong, D. L. *Nursing care of infants and children.* St. Louis: C. V. Mosby, 1979.

Yussen, R., & Santrock, J. W. *Child development: An introduction.* Dubuque, Iowa: William C. Brown, 1978.

# 6

# Health during the School-Age Years

*Dorothy D. Petrowski and Charlene B. Tosi*

## Introduction

This chapter discusses the health of students from first grade through college age in the appropriate school setting for four age or grade groups: ages 6 to 11 (elementary school); ages 12 to 14 (junior high school); ages 15 to 18 (senior high school); and ages 19 to 24 (college or working). For each group, the chapter treats the promotion of wellness, minor problems, and major health concerns; first, however, the nurse's contributions are discussed.

## School Health Program

### The School Nurse's Responsibilities in Three Traditional Areas of School Health

The school health program has traditionally encompassed three main areas: health services, health education, and maintenance of a healthy school environment. Although health is an important goal, the school nurse must keep in mind that education is the main focus. School administrators, faculty, other staff personnel, students, parents, and others work with the school nurse to carry out the school health program.

The school nurse develops and implements a nursing program covering these three areas in collaboration with school personnel. In regard to health services, she provides clinical nursing care, including health assessments of students and supervision of the health activities of both students and school personnel. Within the broad program goal of health education, school nurses, administrators, and faculty assist in the development of a health education plan for the academic year. For example, many students learn about drug use and abuse, dental hygiene, and nutrition in the schools. Although her role in maintenance of the school environment is less than in the other two areas, she tries to ensure a safe, clean, and aesthetically pleasing setting in which to learn and teach, usually by coordinating her efforts with the sanitary engineers and sanitarians from a local (county or city) health department.

### The School Nurse's Roles, Functions, and Activities

The nurse in elementary school and high school usually functions in seven different roles, six of which are outlined by the American School Health Association and the American Nurses' Association in *Guidelines for the School Nurse in the School Health Program* (Knotts, 1974). The nurse's activities with students, teachers, administrators, parents, and the community can best be described by juxtaposing them with these seven nursing roles: (1) health manager, (2) provider of health services, (3) advocate, (4) health counselor, (5) health educator, (6) program evaluator, and (7) coordinator.

#### With students

The school nurse functions in the first four of the roles with students. As a health manager, she is responsible for organizing objectives and planning their accomplishment to benefit the students. In order to formulate relevant objectives, she often requests input from students via a questionnaire designed to determine their perception of health needs in the areas of physical health, mental health, sexuality, decision making, communication, and safety, as viewed from the perspective of children or adolescents. (See Appendix 6A for an example of a questionnaire of needs assessment for adolescents.) Because students' needs change, a needs assessment should be repeated every 3 to 5 years. The goal is to improve the students' health knowledge and habits.

Another aspect of the health manager role is maintaining health records on each student. At the beginning of each school year, the nurse reviews the records with the teachers who will be responsible for the students, discussing specific health problems. Together they can decide the best ways to further the health program. Usually the nurse meets with teachers after students have been dismissed. All student visits to the nurse are documented in the records. Other information includes screening results, physical examination results, immunizations, illnesses, excused absences from physical education, and communications from parents or school personnel. These records are confidential, legal documents, so they are kept in locked custody.

The nurse offers clinical nursing care to students in the role of provider of health services. New and transfer students are assessed by the nurse so that she may compile health records on them. During this assessment, the nurse inquires about any existing health problems and begins to establish rapport with each student. These sessions are scheduled on an appointment basis.

The nurse assesses any complaints as completely as possible. After assessment, she makes a nursing diagnosis based upon input from the student, and together they decide on intervention. The acquisition of physical assessment skills is strongly recommended for school nurses.

Medications, such as aspirin, may be dispensed if there are standing medical orders. Some schools provide a special form for the parents to sign to enable the nurse to give specific medication when needed, or to supervise a student's administration of medication such as insulin. Occasionally a school nurse visits a student's home to discuss a health problem with a parent or to assess a student's condition.

In the case of injury or accident, the nurse assesses the degree of injury and makes decisions based on her assessment. She may elect to call the parents and to detain the student for observation. In cases of severe or life-threatening injury, she may call for the community rescue squad. These activities obviously may require knowledge and skills that range from basic first aid to cardiopulmonary resuscitation.

Routine screenings, discussed later in this chapter, are also supervised by the school nurse. Usually the nurse teaches volunteers to do the initial screenings, and she rescreens and incorporates findings into student health records. If necessary, she notifies parents of the need for referral to a physician. It should be kept in mind that unnecessary referrals cost parents and students time, effort, and money; this is why the nurse rescreens pupils.

Health counseling is considered the school nurse's major role by many. It is accomplished on a one-to-one basis or in groups, depending on the needs of the students. Individually, a student or the nurse identifies a need, and together they explore the factors hindering the student from functioning at optimal level. To be an effective counselor, the nurse employs counseling techniques and knowledge about growth and development, health promotion and illness, and cultural differences. She must recognize when the student should be referred to another health professional, such as a mental health or psychiatric nurse clinician or someone specifically skilled in mental health counseling.

Group counseling is one way to allow students with similar concerns to express feelings and engage in problem solving. Topics for group discussions can be selected from the earlier needs assessment by the adolescents or from the nurse's observations of common student problems. Some suggested areas are student conflicts with parents, concern about alcoholic friends or parents, or chronic health problems of students. Despite possible conflicts with classes and after-school activities, group counseling may be organized with experimentation in timing, and often allows students to share their concerns in a safe, controlled environment.

Finally, the nurse contributes to the students' educational process as a health educator. There are multiple creative means of accomplishing this nursing activity. Poster presentations and the acquisition of other material on pertinent health issues may reach significant numbers of students. Team teaching with a teacher in a lecture-discussion format not only enables the nurse to contact a large number of students at one time, but also increases rapport with the teaching staff. The nurse usually takes the responsibility for making the initial contacts for these sessions, but not necessarily.

### With teachers and other school personnel

With teachers, the nurse performs in the roles of health manager, health counselor, provider of health services, and health educator. As a health manager, the nurse decides when to include the teachers or other professionals, such as guidance counselors and social workers, in the care of a specific student. This is often accomplished through team conferences initiated by the nurse or another health professional. The nurse is an active participant in these conferences, because health is vital to learning and influences many areas of student functioning. For example, students who are hyperactive may require specific health measures to promote their learning.

As a health manager, the nurse holds staff education sessions to discuss recent health legislation and to update policies and procedures about illness and injuries. For example, the nurse should interpret such laws as the Special Education Act of 1975 (PL 94-142), which requires that many students with handicapping conditions be mainstreamed into regular classrooms. These sessions offer an opportune time to discuss effects of certain handicaps and what can be done for students in the classroom. Teachers need a lot of support from the nurse in handling handicapped children. During these meetings, the school nurse might also discuss specific acute communicable diseases and the immunizations the state requires, as well as the policies and procedures of the specific school, such as when to exclude students from the classroom for health reasons.

The nurse has conferences with individual teachers to share information about students with chronic health conditions such as diabetes or epilepsy; this information may be vital to the teacher for understanding such crises as diabetic hypoglycemic attacks or epileptic seizures. When the teacher refers a student to the nurse, the nurse should report results to the teacher in order to facilitate the learning-teaching process in the system.

Communication is extremely important to ensure a good working relationship with the guidance department. Health counseling is a broad field; it is necessary for the nurse to clarify her counseling role with the guidance counselors and vice versa to avoid problems over "turf" issues. Possibly all school personnel who do counseling should establish guidelines together. It is not necessary to give detailed information about the counseling, but it is a professional courtesy to exchange basic information.

The nurse works with all people within the school walls on any given day. Therefore, the nurse provides health services to teachers and other personnel as well as to students. Building trust among the faculty population is as important as it is among students. Potential faculty health interests may include blood pressure screenings and stress reduction sessions during the lunch hour or after school.

Working with teachers in the role of health educator is a pleasant challenge, and requires that the nurse be both assertive and competent. The teachers usually involved are all elementary-school classroom teachers and those in high school who teach courses in physical education, health education, biology, family life, and child development. In order to select areas where input would be valuable, the nurse becomes familiar with each curriculum by attending area faculty meetings or by meeting with the teachers on an individual basis. In this way, she is able to identify areas of interest and to explain to the teachers what she can offer to benefit the school health program.

Fulfillment of the educator role is done in a number of ways. The nurse reviews current materials that relate to a particular health area and circulates pertinent information to interested faculty. Also, the nurse evaluates new health education textbooks and recommends some to the health education teacher in accordance with the needs of the student population. The nurse also fulfills her educator role by correlating the screening procedures with the health or biology curriculum (e.g., presenting a class on the anatomy and physiology of the human eye and eye care a week or so before vision screening is done). A nurse can teach an actual class or can provide consultation to the teacher on a specific health issue. She may also act as a consultant to teachers by acquainting them with resources such as films on dental care, speakers from community health agencies, or pamphlets on nutrition.

To function effectively as a health educator, the nurse can benefit from courses in educational methods, curriculum and instruction, motivation, group dynamics, and growth and development. Continuing-education courses in drug abuse, adolescent sexuality, or depression can also increase the nurse's effectiveness. Membership in the American School Health Association provides certain benefits, such as a subscription to *The Journal of School Health*.

### With administrators

The nurse functions mainly as a health manager, health advocate, and program evaluator in her relationship with school administrators. She interacts with superintendents and principals and possibly with school board members in her *manager* role. The nurse communicates to them her short- and long-range school health program goals and the accomplishments of the existing program. In order to make significant changes in the existing program, the nurse usually must confer with the principal, especially if she is new to the system. She meets regularly with the principal and submits to him or her a monthly or semiannual report of her activities.

It is no small task for the school nurse to enter the school system and carry out a health program. Most often, one of the keys to success is gaining the approval of administrators. This is especially true if the nurse is employed by the health department and not by the school system. The lines of authority for her role are often not well defined, and she must often employ an unusual amount of diplomacy to work with administrators and teachers on their turf.

The nurse serves as an advocate by interpreting health needs of students to administrators. For example, any health legislation affecting the students is discussed with administrators, so that it can be effectively and efficiently implemented as intended by law. The school nurse also communicates advances in health information relative to children and adolescents, such as updates on the care of obesity and new drug information, to administrators.

In concert with pupils, teachers and other school personnel, and administrators, the nurse acts as an evaluator of the school health program. The outcomes are measured against the previously formulated objectives. For example, the results of the hearing screening program and the drug education sessions are reviewed, and the programs are revised if necessary.

### With parents

Parental influence is the single most important factor in helping or hindering students as they grow, develop, and obtain an education. Yet some students do not feel a strong parent-child relationship. The school nurse realizes the impact parents have on their children and attempts to foster in the parents an awareness of their responsibility, if it is absent. She also encourages and assists them in their parental role by providing information to them, and she seeks their advice about their children. In working with parents, the roles of health counselor and health educator are the most significant ones.

### With the community

School health is an integral part of community health. The initiative to identify needs and plan programs to meet these needs is ultimately the responsibility of the community (Nader, 1978). The nurse is one of the agents in the community who is assigned the task of improving the health of students through planned programs. The nurse is also a partner with the community, sharing knowledge and responsibility, receiving guidance from the community, and giving the community information. It is important for the nurse to know the community—to know its ideas about health and its health priorities. The nurse can discuss the school health program through community groups such as church groups, the Rotary Club, the local medical society, and the city council. This may be done together with one of the school administrators.

The nurse must also be familiar with community resources that can serve students, such as drug and alcohol treatment centers, the Planned Parenthood Association, homes for runaway adolescents, free health clinics, clinics for venereal diseases, and dental clinics, to name a few. In many ways the school nurse acts as a coordinator between the school system and the community.

The School Nurse Practitioner in the School System

Various types of nurse practitioners (NPs) are mentioned in Chapter 1. The school nurse practitioner (SNP) ideally should have a background in pediatric and community health nursing. The University of Colorado conducts a School Nurse Practitioner Program, in which the SNP is taught to do physical assessments, diagnose and treat students who are ill or injured at school, and counsel handicapped children, among many other activities.

The Pennsylvania Department of Health conducted an extensive study of their school health program in the mid-1970s and made recommendations for role changes in the program. School nurses were educated to become SNPs. School nurses were required to take classes in basic pediatrics; physical examinations and use of medical instruments; psychosocial assessment, including growth and development; interviewing skills; process recording; and problem management planning. School health aide/technicians were trained to provide the screening tests, first aid, and clerical functions that the school nurses provided previously.

The Pennsylvania experience demonstrates that SNPs can successfully accomplish many functions that had been assigned previously to physicians with such activities as physical assessments, immunizations, and tine tests, although consultant pediatrician services were continued (Commonwealth of Pennsylvania, Department of Health, 1973–1974).

Medical Direction and Legal Aspects for the School Nurse

*Medical direction*

The school nurse is employed either by a board of education or by a local health department (city or county) and is responsible to her employer. If a school system employs a medical doctor, the nurse can work with the doctor's medical orders. If not, she can work with standing medical orders that have been approved by the local health officer (if he or she is a licensed physician) and the Board of Education. These standing orders, which should be updated annually, mainly cover emergency care, such as first aid for accidents and analgesics (aspirin, acetaminophen) for minor pain such as headaches or menstrual cramps.

Some health conditions and illnesses require attention during school hours. If a pupil has a chronic illness such as diabetes or epilepsy, the parents and family physician can make arrangements *in writ-*

*ing* for necessary health supervision in school hours. This might include administering medication, checking to insure that the student has taken medicine, or observing the student for signs and symptoms of impending trouble such as epileptic seizures. Some health conditions or acute and short-term illnesses (acne, pregnancy, fractures) require attention from the nurse also. The school nurse might make arrangements for teenagers to wash their faces with a special soap during school hours for acne, or to have a special diet for pregnancy; she might also teach crutch walking for a student who is in a leg cast following a fracture.

*Legal aspects*

A school nurse at her place of employment has an obligation to render professional services and is required to exercise the judgment of a reasonable person in employing her knowledge and skills. If a student is seriously ill, she may *not* neglect him until a physician, ambulance, or hospital takes over. If her professional judgment should ever be questioned, professional nurses with similar educational and work backgrounds could act as expert witnesses. Good Samaritan statutes should encourage school nurses to render reasonable emergency services.

Both the principal and the school nurse are responsible for the school health program and should be familiar with local, state, and federal school laws, regulations, and recommendations. The school nurse is expected to exert leadership to insure that the school health program is an integral part of the community's health program and priorities (Creighton & Squaires, 1974).

## Health Care by Age Group and Grade Level

Health promotion, minor and major illnesses, and nursing care are discussed for the various age groups or equivalent grade levels. Health promotion, which is first-level prevention of illness, comprises much of a school nurse's activity, as does caring for minor and major illnesses of students. Nursing intervention for specific minor and major health problems are described. Screening programs are also discussed.

### Health Care in Childhood or Grade School

A thorough knowledge of normal growth and development patterns is essential for all school nurses. For a review of the growth and development at each age level, the reader should refer to a current book on the subject.

### Health promotion and minor health concerns in childhood

*Promotion of wellness.* Health promotion in grade school is done in the classroom, as well as in group and individual discussions with the school nurse. The importance of diet, exercise, body cleanliness, recreation, and good interpersonal relationships; avoidance of smoking, alcohol, and drugs; and knowledge of human sexuality are some health topics that should be emphasized. Audiovisual aids are available from local and state health departments and libraries, as well as from the American Cancer Society and other agencies. These may be used to supplement other learning activities.

*Screening programs in school.* Health screening of children and teenagers accomplishes two purposes: It teaches students about the parts of their bodies and how to keep them functioning optimally, and it facilitates the early detection of defects. For example, the study of normal dentition can be paired with dental screening and oral hygiene. The screenings to be discussed here are those for height and weight, vision and hearing, scoliosis, dental problems, and blood pressure; the general physical examination, including the athletic physical examination, is also discussed. All screening programs are included here, although only one, the screening for scoliosis, is specific to the elementary grades. (Athletic physical examinations are done primarily in high schools.)

HEIGHT AND WEIGHT. Height and weight are measured annually by volunteers who are taught by the school nurse. These figures are recorded in each child's health record, and percentiles are plotted and compared with previous years. If the nurse notes any abnormal trend, such as lack of growth or obesity, she refers the problem to the parents and to the physician if indicated.

VISION AND HEARING. The school nurse organizes vision screenings annually in selected elementary-school and high-school grades. Volunteer mothers usually do the screening procedures in the classroom. The nurse rechecks questionable screening results before referral to parents. Measurement of 20/20 vision on a Snellen chart is an indication of a normal eye and optic pathway. Measurement of less than 20/20 vision in either eye indicates a refractive error or other optic disorder. Referrals of students with a visual defect of 20/30 or more in either eye is recommended. NPs can perform a more extensive examination, which includes an opthalmoscopic examination. The nurse also instructs students in proper care of eyes and care of glasses and contact lenses.

Hearing loss can result from various things such as infections, trauma, or noise pollution (especially high-frequency sounds, loud amplifiers, and live music in close quarters). Cursory hearing tests can be done by whispering into one ear at a distance of from 1 to 2 feet, with the other ear occluded with the examiner's hand; or by holding a wrist watch a few inches away. If hearing loss is present, a tuning fork is used to distinguish between sensorineural or bone conduction deafness (Rinne test). The fork used should provide 512 to 1024 cycles per second. If the student has a loss of 30 decibels or more in the range from 500 to 2000 cycles per second, he should be retested on a different day and then referred to an ear, nose, and throat specialist. Screening of hearing helps locate those struggling to cope with a hearing loss, yet unaware of what is truly causing such problems as lack of concentration and poor interpersonal relationships (Malasanos, Barkauskas, Moss, & Stoltenberg-Allen, 1977).

SCOLIOSIS. Scoliosis is a curvature of the spine often related to rapid growth, muscle weakness, and poor posture in children. It may also occur as the result of a genetic defect. Screening for scoliosis is done mainly in elementary-school and middle-school grades, but ninth-grade girls are often screened routinely. The screening is done by looking at each student through a grid in two positions: (1) standing, and (2) bending forward at the waist. Unequal shoulders or hips when standing and a "rib bump" when bending are reasons for rescreening or referral. Some schools contract with an orthopedic specialist for rescreenings, thus relieving the parents of a financial burden if scoliosis should not be present to a degree requiring treatment.

DENTAL PROBLEMS. Screening for dental problems is done on an annual basis in some schools by a dental hygienist or a dentist. Decayed, missing, or filled (DMF) teeth, malocclusion, gum problems, other mouth problems, and the need for dental work are noted. Referral slips are sent to parents. At the time of the dental screening, the hygienist or the school nurse teaches the students the correct way to brush and floss their teeth. Brushing and flossing are equally important.

BLOOD PRESSURE. It is recommended that a blood pressure program be set up in the school system, because children 3 years old and older should have blood pressure readings done yearly. The Federal Task Force on Blood Pressure Control in Children suggests that a school is an appropriate setting for such a program.

Prior to establishing a blood pressure program in a school, it is suggested that the nurse do the following:

—Meet with the superintendent, principals, teachers, parent groups, medical community, and students to explain the blood pressure program, gain cooperation and answer questions.

—Develop educational materials for display and distribution. (These are available from the National High Blood Pressure Educational Program, Landow Building, 13th Floor, 7910 Woodmont Avenue, Bethesda, Maryland, 20012.)

—Develop a referral system and referral forms.

—Avoid labeling any children as hypertensive as a result of a screening program. A physician must make a definitive diagnosis.

Blood pressure levels (obtained on at least three separate occasions) above the 95th percentile for a specific age group should be considered abnormal and referred to a physician. (See Figure 6-1.) It is necessary to have appropriate-size cuffs for children in order to obtain correct readings. The inflatable bladder should completely encircle the arm without overlapping. The examining area should be quiet, and each child should be reassured. Ideally, this program should be an integral part of the school health program; for example, it could be done at the same time as vision screening.

If a physician diagnoses hypertension in a student referred to him, he may request that the school nurse follow up assessments and interventions at school. This might consist of placing the student on a program of weight reduction and a moderate, salt-restricted diet (5 gm/day of salt for teenagers, less for younger children); encouraging discontinuance of cigarette smoking (or not starting); monitoring the blood pressure; and administering medicine. The parents would also be involved. The school nurse should have written orders updated at least every 3 months for the care of a hypertensive student (National Heart, Lung, and Blood Institute's Task Force on Blood Pressure Control in Children, 1977).

PHYSICAL EXAMINATION, INCLUDING ATHLETIC PHYSICAL EXAMINATION. Some schools require annual physical assessments done by a physician or NP. (See Table 6-1 for guidelines.) The history and physical assessment for athletes is performed by a doctor or SNP. A urinalysis and a check for hernia or other abnormalities that may be aggravated by participation in sports should be noted.

*Minor health problem in childhood: upper respiratory infections.* Usually grade-school children have at least one upper respiratory infection (URI) each school year. If a child comes to the nurse's office, she should note any general malaise; take his temperature, pulse, and respiration (TPR); check nasal discharges; examine the pharynx; and auscultate the lungs. If there is an elevated temperature, the student should be excluded from the classroom, and the parents should be notified. The

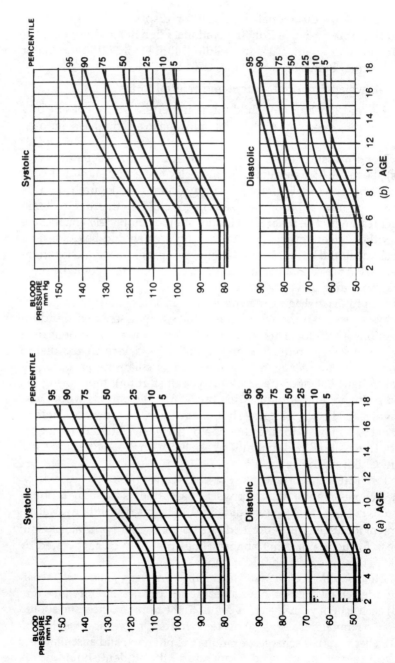

Figure 6-1. Percentiles of blood pressure measurement in (a) boys and (b) girls (right arm, seated). (From National Heart, Lung, and Blood Institute's Task Force on Blood Pressure Control in Children, "Report of the Task Force on Blood Pressure Control in Children." *Pediatrics,* 1977, 59(5), Part 2, 803.)

Table 6-1

Guidelines for Physical Examination by the School Nurse, Adapted for the School-Age Child and the Adolescent

| Use the basic adult physical examination with these modifications: | |
|---|---|
| Grade-school child | 1. Take TPR in consideration of a possible communicable disease or infection. |
| | 2. Assess growth and development. |
| |   a. Take height and weight. |
| |   b. Note particular problems such as scoliosis, obesity and emotional problems. |
| | 3. Take blood pressure with a smaller cuff. |
| | 4. Eye examination is always done using a Snellen chart; view the external eye and do an ophthalmoscopic examination. |
| | 5. Hearing tested with whisper test and/or tuning fork. |
| | 6. Examine mouth, noting DMF teeth to ascertain need for referral to dentist. |
| | 7. Check for scoliosis. |
| | 8. Pelvic is almost never done. |
| Junior- and senior-high-school student | 1. Do the above, and in addition: |
| | 2. Check for acne vulgaris. |
| | 3. Check posture for scoliosis. |
| | 4. Check pubertal development in both sexes. |
| | 5. Pelvic is not done routinely, but is done if student is sexually active or has menstrual problems, vaginal discharge or suspected pregnancy. |
| | 6. Check for signs of drug or alcohol abuse. |

nurse should recommend extra fluids, bed rest, decongestants, and an analgesic. (See the section on streptococcal pharyngitis later in this chapter.)

*Major health problems in childhood*

Although middle childhood is generally considered one of the healthiest periods of a person's life, there are certain major health problems in this period that may concern the school nurse. Among them are obesity, hypertension, dental caries, scoliosis, acute communicable diseases, and vision and hearing deficiencies; discipline problems, obesity, dental caries, and acute communicable diseases are discussed in detail here.

*Discipline problems.* There are various ideas about methods of child discipline, and child discipline is viewed differently in different social classes. Usually lower-class parents are more concerned with training their children to conform to external standards, while middle-class parents want the child to control his own behavior (Hanson & Reynolds, 1980). In the "Spock era," after World War II, discipline was pursued essentially according to the latter concept: The child was to be consulted about his actions, take part in the decision regarding how he would be punished, and practice self-control. This concept has influenced American disciplining of children even into the 1980s.

Disciplining is basically physical (spanking the child, having him sit on a chair) or psychological (removing privileges, reasoning), or a combination of both. Physical discipline is effective on very young children because their reasoning processes are not fully developed. Many experts, however, feel that physical discipline creates hostility in the child and/or constitutes child abuse by the parent.

In the school system, psychological discipline is used; physical discipline (hitting of any kind) is not permitted. On occasion, the classroom teacher may consult the school nurse about a specific student's discipline problem. The nurse should be alert to the fact that inattention and unruly behavior can be related to a physiological health problem, such as a hearing loss or hyperactivity.

*Obesity.* It has been estimated that from 3 to 20% of school-age children are obese, depending on the definition of "obesity." Generally, "obesity" has been considered weight 20% over the 95th-percentile weight for a particular child. However, the use of skin-fold calipers has recently promoted the method of calculating the percentage of total body fat by measuring skin-fold thickness in millimeters to define obesity (Neumann, 1977).

The immediate physical effects of obesity in the school-age child are usually not serious, but the psychosocial effects can be devastating. The obese school-age child suffers from a poor self-image and from feelings of inferiority and rejection. With the ridicule and teasing of peers, the obese child develops even greater feelings of rejection and inferiority.

School-age obesity may continue into adulthood because of the increased numbers of fat cells deposited in response to the excessive intake of calories. The prime age of this hyperplasia is between 7 and 11 years of age, or possibly even before age 7. At particular risk are those children whose diet is high in starch and "junk" food, and who have limited physical activity or abuse of TV viewing. Occasionally, childhood obesity may be a reflection of a child's response to stress. The school nurse should consider this possibility in her assessment of the problem.

The initial assessment of an obese child, or a child with an over-eating problem, should determine the following:

1. Family history of obesity or associated diseases.
2. Onset of the weight problem, with emphasis on the precipitating factors or events.
3. A feeding history, including the child's birth weight and a record of the child's height and weight for the first year of life.
4. The family's concept of a "healthy child," including the family's philosophy about food and feeding and their perceptions of what quantity of food a child should eat.
5. The family relationships and the degree of dependency, maturity, motivation, and self-image of the child.
6. A 24-hour food recall to identify quantities and patterns of food consumed by the child.
7. Family meal or food intake patterns.
8. Food allergies and/or intolerances.

The nurse should gain the cooperation of the family and school personnel. She should then plan a program that focuses attention on the child's whole person, not just the weight problem. The program should modify the child's environment and make the child aware of his food intake and ways to manage it. The *Recommended Dietary Allowances* (National Research Council, 1980) should be used as a guideline for childhood and teenage nutrition. If the child is to be on a specific calorie reduction diet, the family physician usually writes a diet prescription that specifies the number of calories and the grams of carbohydrates, fat, and protein.

It is especially important to deal with obesity in children because of the health implications of obesity for adulthood. Routine height and weight screening is done in approximately 80% of all schools, giving the nurse the opportunity to identify those students needing intervention (National Education Association, 1973; Neumann, 1977).

*Dental caries.* Although it is estimated that dental caries affect 98% of the U.S. population, school-age children are particularly susceptible to them. By age 12, 90% of all American children have one or more caries. Carious teeth can be troublesome, incapacitating, and expensive, and they can also lead to infection, facial disfigurement, speech or chewing impairment, or malnutrition; these are important health concerns. Caries can affect the child's emotional well-being.

The school nurse can present a three-part dental hygiene program. Parental involvement in the program should be strongly encouraged, as it is in the home where most dental health practices are undertaken. The first part should focus on the prevention of dental caries and gum disease and should cover the following:

1. Adequate nutrition—especially adequate amounts of protein, Vitamins A, D, and C, calcium, phosphorus, and fluoride.
2. Snacking habits—mainly limiting sugar intake at and between meals. A discussion of the content of junk foods will help to illustrate the necessity of controlled snacking. (Also, fibrous food snacks that promote salivary flow and the buffering capacity of saliva should be promoted.)
3. Self-care procedures, including proper brushing and flossing techniques.
4. Emphasis on prophylactic care by the dentist—for example, routine examinations and topical application of fluoride.

Generally, "dental health" is a combination of tooth vulnerability, heredity, the nutrient nature of the diet (especially sugars, starches, and fiber), the buffering capacity of the saliva, local factors such as fluoridation or brushing practices, and the virulence of bacteria in the oral cavity. The school nurse, by promoting prevention and early treatment of dental caries, can instill the basis for optimal dental health (Nizel, 1977).

The second, or treatment, phase of the dental program includes referral to a dentist if dental care is needed. The third, or maintenance, stage is continued dental follow-up to ensure maintenance of the teeth and gums that the dental hygienist and dentist have cared for.

*Communicable diseases and immunizations.*   The prevention of communicable disease is done mainly through immunizations. School-age children in most states are required by law to have immunizations for diptheria, pertussis, and tetanus (DPT); rubeola (red measles), mumps, and rubella (German measles) (MMR); and poliomyelitis prior to entry into first grade, with boosters for some at specified intervals. Initially, DPT is given in infancy, MMR at 15 months of age, and poliomyelitis before age 2; children who have not had these early childhood immunizations require them later. The school nurse must become familiar with regulations in the state in which she is working. It is suggested that the nurse or teacher discuss communicable diseases in health and science classes, so that the students will learn the significance of prevention. The school nurse should consult the paperback *Control of Com-*

*municable Diseases in Man* (Beneson, 1981) for discussions of causes, prevention, and treatment for these diseases. She should assist teachers in excluding sick students, and she should assist parents in their return to school.

Rubeola (measles), varicella (chicken pox), and streptococcal pharyngitis are discussed in this section because these are fairly common diseases in schools. At present, measles is seen in schools because some parents do not have their children vaccinated, and the herd immunity is at a low level in the susceptible population. There is no vaccine for chicken pox or streptococcal pharyngitis. Both measles and streptococcal pharyngitis can result in serious complications, such as otitis media, pneumonia, and acute encephalitis.

RUBEOLA (RED MEASLES). Measles is an ancient viral disease, acute and contagious, with an incubation period of 10 to 11 days. Fever and malaise appear first, followed by coryza, conjunctivitis, and cough in the first 24 hours. A body rash, erythematous maculo-papular eruption, appears on the fourth day, and Koplik's spots invade the buccal and labial mucosa on the sixth day. The child feels the worst between the second and third day of the rash. The rash subsides in about 6 days. Petrowski has seen many cases of blindness from corneal ulceration in children after measles in Zimbabwe, Africa. This is a complication not seen in the United States (Krugman, Ward, & Katz, 1977).

VARICELLA (CHICKEN POX). Varicella or chicken pox is an acute generalized viral infection with a sudden onset of slight fever, mild constitutional symptoms, and a skin eruption that becomes vesicular in about 4 days, leaving scabs. Lesions tend to be more numerous on the covered portions of the body. Complications in childhood are rare. Varicella is caused by a primary infection with varicella-zoster (V-Z) virus. Herpes zoster (shingles), usually an adult disease, is probably caused by the activation of latent V-Z virus (Krugman et al., 1977).

STREPTOCOCCAL PHARYNGITIS (STREP THROAT). Although the peak incidence of streptococcal pharyngitis is seen in the preschool years, the school nurse may be asked to take a throat culture if this disease is suspected. (See Chapter 5 for a discussion of streptococcal pharyngitis.) The treatment is the same for preschool and school-age children. Parents should be instructed to keep the child out of school until the throat culture is negative. They should also be instructed that the child must take the complete 10 days of the penicillin. This treatment ameliorates the acute illness and sore throat and prevents the development of acute rheumatic fever and acute glomerulonephritis, which can be complications of this disease.

Health Care in High School

*Introduction to adolescent students*

The term "adolescence" is derived from the Latin verb *adolescere*, which means "to grow into maturity." The period of life from 12 to 14 years of age is often considered the first half of the transitional stage from childhood to adulthood, or "early adolescence." The term "older adolescent" generally refers to those in the ages of 15 to 18.

In ancient Rome, the changeover from puberty to adulthood was signaled by the wearing of a toga. Puberty rites still exist in some primitive cultures, such as the Masai in East Africa, the Hopi Indians in Arizona, and the aborigines of Australia. Today, confirmation in Christian churches and the Bar or Bas Mitzvah in the Jewish faith give American children some identity with the adult world. But children today no longer fit into the job market at age 14–16, because more training and education are required to function in an industrialized society. This has resulted in a greatly extended and very visible adolescence (Kaluger & Kaluger, 1974).

Late adolescence is a time when young people grow and develop physically, psychologically and in other ways. It is a time of great experimentation with ideas and activities, such as religion and morality, or driving a car and dating. Most adolescents complete high school at about age 18.

As previously suggested, the school nurse needs a sound background in the understanding of normal growth and development. Many adolescent health concerns arise out of the rapid physical and psychological changes that commonly occur during this time of life. The school nurse assists adolescents in their development through providing screening programs, monitoring of communicable diseases, counseling about puberty and menstruation, and participating in a myriad of other health concerns.

*Minor health problems in adolescence*

Teenagers are typically concerned about their bodies because they are changing so rapidly. They ask questions about their bodies and show concern about health practices, but may not follow the advice they are given. A school nurse should be aware of health areas that are of concern to teenagers and should counsel accordingly.

*Personal health concerns.*

PERSONAL HYGIENE.   Because of body awareness, adolescents are often overly conscientious about personal care. Girls may wash their hair daily and insist on a clean set of clothing each day when getting ready for school. One eighth-grade girl whom Petrowski observed wore the same stylish overalls to school each day, but washed them each evening. She was concerned about cleanliness and being in style. Both sexes try many types of shampoo, toothpaste, deodorants, bath soaps, and mouth washes. A few teenagers, going to the other extreme, become personally very "sloppy" and seem to want to provoke comment from parents and teachers by this action; this may be due to a feeling of need for peer acceptance.

CLOTHING. Most teenagers tend to follow the crowd, their peers, when it comes to dress. When a child cannot trust his body, it is reassuring to be dressed like everyone else. Those adolescents who work often spend all of their income on clothes. Parents need to understand why teenagers focus on clothing and clothing fads, and must be flexible in their advice. They can understandingly admonish their child to save some earnings for items other than clothing; such advice may be heeded at some later time, if not immediately.

FATIGUE. So many adolescents complain periodically about fatigue that it may actually be a normal characteristic of this age group. Their diets, sleeping, and activity patterns contribute to increased fatigue. Occasionally a young person complains about fatigue to avoid unpleasant school work or a trying social situation. Nevertheless, the school nurse should take a careful history if fatigue persists. She should be aware of the possibility of such problems as depression or anxiety as causative factors in cases of persistent fatigue. Referral to a physician may be in order to check the hematocrit for anemia, to do a complete blood count to test for mononucleosis, or to do a tuberculin skin test.

POOR POSTURE. Poor posture (round shoulders and shambling, slouchy gait) is exhibited by so many adolescents that it is considered a problem of this age group. Females may slouch to hide developing mammary glands, or to be shorter than boys they find attractive. Both sexes may bend over and shuffle when they walk because they are not accustomed to their new height. The skeleton grows faster than the muscles, and this growth imbalance accounts, in part, for the poor posture of adolescents. A poor, or rapidly changing, self-concept may also account for poor posture in some teenagers. It is difficult to stand or sit up straight when one does not feel "good" or is uncertain about oneself.

ACNE VULGARIS. Acne vulgaris, most commonly known as acne, is the most common disorder of the early adolescent years. In fact, though it does not affect all teenagers, it may be the most common teenage problem. In preadolescence, the sebaceous glands are small and relatively inactive. In puberty, as the androgen level rises in both sexes, the sebaceous glands become active. Because not all of the sebum, the sebaceous gland secretion, can be eliminated through the skin surface, some gets trapped in the glands. It darkens from dirt that has accumulated in the pores and hardens, forming comedones (blackheads). If bacteria collects as well, pustules form. The scalp, face, external ear, back, and upper arms are the usual sites for acne. Emotional stress or menstrual periods can produce flareups of acne.

Treatment for acne includes washing the affected areas at least three times daily with a sulphur and salicylic acid soap, such as Acneveen, Basis, Aveeno Bar, or Fostex. Arrangements should be made by the school nurse for badly affected adolescents to wash at school as well as at home. A teenager is more likely to do this if the physiology of the sebaceous glands during early adolescence is explained in a health class or with a movie. There are various external and systemic medications that the physician orders in severe cases. Severe cases of acne should be referred to a dermatologist. If acne is untreated, roughened, unsightly skin can result; this condition may necessitate a surgical planing (surgical removal of the scarred skin surfaces) later on.

MENSTRUAL IRREGULARITIES.   Many teenagers experience irregular menstrual periods during the first year after the menarche. If this irregularity continues into the second year when ovulation begins, a gynecologist should be consulted. Girls who are obese, malnourished, or emotionally upset tend to have more irregularity. The emotional climate of the home may also affect the menstrual cycle. Occasionally a girl does not start menstruating at the expected age, 12 to 14. If this absence of the menarche persists after her 15th or 16th birthday, a gynecologist should be contacted.

Mild analgesics (aspirin 650 mg or acetaminophen 325 mg) should be included in the school nurse's standing orders, so she can dispense these to students who complain of menstrual cramps. This allows these girls to continue their classes. A very few may require referral to a gynecologist. The reasons for the menstrual cramps should be explained to these students: They are caused by the congestion of blood in the pelvic vessels and mild uterine contractions. Discomfort occurring between menstrual periods is often related to ovulation and is termed "mittelschmerz," from the German word for intermenstrual pain. The nurse should reinforce the understanding that menstruation is a very normal body process. This can be done using diagrams of the female pelvic and reproductive organs, which are available from several commercial sources, such as Tampax, Inc. (Pillitteri, 1977).

*Minor illnesses.*

HEADACHES. If a student complains of a headache, the nurse should try to establish the cause. Although there may be numerous causes, one of the most frequent is stress. Nonprescription analgesics may be given if there are standing physician's orders. If eye strain is suspected as the underlying problem, the school nurse should do an eye examination using the Snellen chart. If the same student returns frequently with headaches, the parents should be contacted. It is well to remember that most minor illnesses, such as influenza, have other symptoms in addition to a headache. It is also a good idea to check a student's TPR, as well as any visual symptoms described by the student.

CUTS, BRUISES, AND SPRAINED ANKLES. A teenager most often becomes injured at school during physical education classes or sports activities. The nurse should have a well-equipped first aid kit to care for cuts and bruises. The setting up of a first aid kit is an excellent project for a health class or service club. The nurse should review with junior-high students and their teachers, especially in physical education classes, the procedure for treating cuts and bruises, so that they can care for an injured student in her absence. Other injuries, such as a seriously sprained ankle or a suspected fracture, should be referred immediately to a physician; the school nurse then provides follow-up care such as bandaging, cast care, or lessons in crutch walking.

*Wellness promotion in adolescence*

The school nurse can be instrumental in the promotion of wellness for the adolescent. This is best accomplished by individual counseling and by teaching health education classes for adolescents.

*Individual wellness.*

NUTRITION. Except for infants, adolescents require more nutrients per pound of body weight than any other age group. The recommended daily caloric allowance for the 15–18 age group is 3000 for males and 2100 for females (Mercer, 1979). If the calorie intake is not met, the body burns protein for energy instead of using it to build and maintain body tissues. This can hamper the normal process of growth. Nutrition information can be provided to students along with the lunches in the school cafeterias; it can also be provided in informal group discussions or classes.

SELF-ESTEEM. Promoting wellness by fostering self-esteem is an important need of changing, developing adolescents. It is important for the school nurse to accept each adolescent as a unique individual with many needs, to listen to what he is saying, and to be flexible in her interactions. If the nurse feels the adolescent is not being honest, she should tell him so. An effort to hide her feelings of mistrust shows in her body language and other behavior. The nurse should not accuse the adolescent by saying, "You are lying to me." Instead, she should say, "I'm confused. What you say doesn't add up." This latter statement allows the nurse to "own the problem" without destroying the adolescent's trust in himself.

To foster self-esteem, the nurse builds trust by allowing the adolescent to become an active participant and decision maker in his own health care. The adolescent's cognitive ability is developed to the extent that he can appreciate the nurse's assessment and decide what alternative is best for him. The nurse should not accept a decision that would be harmful or unhealthy, however.

*Wellness in relationships with others.*

RELATIONSHIPS WITH SCHOOL PERSONNEL.    Adolescents spend most of their time in school relating with six to ten adult professionals in the course of the day. How do these relationships affect their level of wellness? The most important factor affecting a student's progress in and adjustment to school is how he relates to his individual teachers. If a student expresses difficulty with a teacher, the nurse should help him devise a plan of action for resolving the conflict with the teacher. This is one way a student learns to communicate negative feelings and resolve conflicts without acting out in unacceptable ways. Life is full of stressful relationships, and helping the adolescent develop skills to handle negative feelings and conflicts is valuable for an adolescent's wellness, life style, and growth.

RELATIONSHIPS WITH PARENTS.    Separation from parents is a normal part of achieving independence from home. Conflicts with parents are usually in two areas: Adolescents want more independence than the parents think they should have, or they act more dependent and childish than the parents can tolerate. Often they vacillate between these two stances.

To facilitate wellness in this area, the nurse's role is to stress the need for open communication between parent and teenager. An excellent resource for the school nurse in working with adolescents is T. Gordon's book, *Parent Effectiveness Training* (1970). The principles in this book can be taught to adolescents as well as to a group of parents.

RELATIONSHIPS AT WORK.    Another expression of an adolescent's independence is getting a job outside the home. Along with working come adult responsibilities and possibly stress. The nurse should be aware of the working adolescent's schedule. An after-school job com-

bined with classes, homework, and extracurricular activities may put
too much stress on the student, causing physical complaints such as
headaches, stomachaches, and so on.

The nurse's role in dealing with work relationships is to help the
teenager decide which activities are the most important. The nurse may
also teach the teenager how to relax through breathing and other stress
reduction exercises. These exercises can be put on a cassette recorder
and listened to while resting in the health room. If the nurse believes
that the adolescent needs to talk with other school personnel, a referral to the guidance department may be in order, especially if the school
courseload is heavy.

RELATIONSHIPS WITH THE OPPOSITE SEX.    A high-school adolescent is
seeking to feel comfortable not only as a person, but as a sexual person with desires, feelings, and physical changes that are often hard to
understand or accept. Much agony and frustration can come from a relationship with a member of the opposite sex.

By late adolescence, teenagers are double- or single-dating, as opposed to the group dates of early adolescence. "Going steady" is a very
common practice and offers security. Occasionally a student wants to
"break up" a quite long-lasting relationship and needs to talk about
how to accomplish this. Problems also arise when a teenager dates too
many persons, wants to date but is not invited out, or is rejected when
asking for a date.

Another common problem is wondering how sexually involved
to become. A model for sexual decision making is provided by Juhasz
(1975). He first poses the alternatives of virginity or intercourse. If intercourse is chosen, the alternatives are children or no children. If no
children are desired, alternative methods of birth control are discussed,
and one is chosen. In case of pregnancy, the alternatives are delivery
or abortion. If delivery is chosen, the alternatives are to keep the child
or give up the child for adoption. If abortion is chosen, the alternatives
are legal or illegal. If the child is kept, the decision is whether to marry
or stay single. Presenting this model to adolescents makes them aware
of the consequences of their sexual behavior. Other alternatives to intercourse for the adolescent are masturbation and abstinence.

*Major health problems in early adolescence*

*Adolescent pregnancy.*    Adolescent pregnancy is a serious and
growing health, social, economic and moral problem in this society
and the world. *The main concern is that it is a health problem!* Adolescent
pregnancy jeopardizes the health and life of the young woman and her

newborn. Other problems, which are numerous though not necessarily life-threatening, are out-of-wedlock births; increased incidence of sexually transmitted diseases; increased incidence of abortion; interrupted schooling; and no means of financial support.

STATISTICS ON ADOLESCENT SEXUAL ACTIVITY, PREGNANCY, BIRTHS, AND CONTRACEPTION. There are 29 million young people in the United States between the ages of 13 and 19. About 12 million of these are estimated to engage in sexual intercourse—7 million males and 5 million females. Although 18% of males and 6% of females aged 13 to 14 years have had sexual intercourse, the proportion does rise sharply with increasing age. Evidence suggests that this phenomenon of early sexual activity is present in all socioeconomic classes.

There are about 1.1 million adolescent pregnancies yearly. The 18- to 19-year-olds account for 685,000 pregnancies yearly; 15- to 17-year-olds account for 425,000, and girls younger than 15 account for 30,000. About 10% of these young women do marry before they deliver. Another 51% terminate their pregnancies before birth (through abortions and miscarriages), leaving 39% of these adolescents to deliver after conception. Of these, 17% marry after delivery (or near delivery), and 22% have out-of-wedlock births. The end result is that approximately one-fifth (554,000) of all U.S. births each year are to adolescents.

Nearly two-thirds of the sexually active adolescents do not practice contraception or use a contraceptive method consistently, although only 9% desire to conceive. The use of contraception does increase with age. Teenage females appear to be informed about the various male and female contraceptive devices, but lack knowledge about the biology of reproduction. For example, many do not know that ovulation occurs in the middle of the menstrual cycle, but think it occurs immediately before, after, or during the menstrual period. Many think they are too young to conceive, and there is considerable taking of chances even by adolescents who understand reproduction (Guttmacher Institute, 1981).

CAUSES OF ADOLESCENT PREGNANCIES. The reasons for the increased numbers of teenage pregnancies are varied, starting with the sexual freedom of present-day society. Many attribute this increase in sexual activity to changing societal mores, greater availability of "the Pill," and increased female independence. In spite of this climate of permissiveness, parents and schools do not provide adequate education in the areas of sex and birth control. As a result, many teenagers do not understand human reproduction and the use of contraceptives. Some teenagers were themselves born out of wedlock; their self-esteem in some instances is low, and they conceive in order to have someone to love. Yet another factor is that girls do not prepare themselves for sexual behavior: The best oral contraceptive is "no," but teenage girls are not taught to answer the boys' "lines" (S. Gordon, 1979). (See S. Gordon's 1978 book, *You Would If You Loved Me,* for a collection of "lines" used by boys to seduce girls.) Some girls seduce boys. Experts list many other reasons for teenage pregnancies.

CONFIRMATION OF PREGNANCY. When a teenage girl comes to the school nurse to announce that she is pregnant, or that a friend thinks she is pregnant, the nurse should listen and use crisis intervention skills. The first step is to determine whether the girl in question is, in fact, pregnant. Equipment for pregnancy testing can be obtained at Planned Parenthood for a nominal charge. Counseling about the alternatives to the pregnancy is offered at agencies such as this, giving the adolescent responsibility for a choice between abortion, adoption, or keeping the baby. Listening without making judgments or decisions is very important in order to keep communication open. Parental involvement is a real concern, and referral of the girl to the guidance counselors may be helpful in dealing with the parents.

If the girl decides to stay in school during pregnancy, the school nurse can be a very valuable source of prenatal counseling and teaching. Prenatal care needs to be encouraged. Specific prenatal teaching can be found in Chapter 2.

CONSEQUENCES OF EARLY CHILDBEARING TO THE MOTHER AND INFANT. The physiological demands of pregnancy are accompanied by emotional adjustments. Pregnancy, birth, and the care of an infant necessitate major changes in life style. Most school-age females are not developmentally ready to accept such changes. When the increased nutritional demands of pregnancy are added to the heavy food requirements for an adolescent, the mother and the fetus both may suffer. Many teenagers, because of their eating habits, are in a poor nutritional condition when they become pregnant. A young woman still requires a great deal of parental nurturing, and when she becomes pregnant, her psychological needs are thwarted. Her formal education is likely to be either truncated or terminated. Society's negative attitude toward teenage pregnancy adds additional stress. A financial burden may exacerbate these psychological adjustments. In short, the pregnant adolescent has undertaken the development of another human being before her own body and mind are mature. Her well-being and potential contributions to society may be affected all her life.

162 Handbook of Community Health Nursing

Complications associated with pregnancy are far more frequent with teenagers than with older women, except for the 40-and-older age groups. Such complications include toxemia, anemia, prolonged labor, increased maternal and infant mortality, increased prematurity, and lower birth weights.

Infant mortality for mothers aged 15 to 19 is twice as high as for older women. The risk of having a preterm baby or one with low birth weight is about 39% higher among adolescents. Low birth weight decreases the overall survival rate and adversely affects development. These babies may have lower IQs, more perceptual and motor disturbances, increased speech problems, and greater psychological problems, in addition to being shorter and weighing less. It should be pointed out that mothers aged 17 and under and those aged 18 to 20 represent two distinct groups; the latter are mostly high-school graduates, who usually have normal infants and are able to care for them adequately (Guttmacher Institute, 1981; Jensen, Benson, & Bobak, 1981).

*Alcohol and drug abuse.* The abuse of alcohol and drugs is continuing at an alarming rate, yet most people are not fully aware of the magnitude of the problem and of its destructiveness to individuals and families. Because of this, alcohol and drug abuse should be dealt with in the school population on three levels of prevention.

The primary level focuses on drug prevention programs, which should be started in the first three grades and should be extended to parents as well as all students through the twelfth grade. Information giving should peak at the junior-high-school level, where most drug experimentation begins. A program of peer counseling can be carried out by trained high-school students as a primary preventive measure in grade and junior high schools.

The role of the school nurse in the area of primary prevention should be in the areas of health education and counseling. The nurse can offer her teaching services and knowledge to science, health, or physical education teachers by participating in classes that focus specifically on the drug and alcohol problem. A preventive measure undertaken with parents could be classes on improving their communication skills with their adolescent children, aimed to bridge the generation gap in discussing alcohol and drug use.

In dealing with adolescents who are using drugs, the school nurse needs to understand the difference between experimentation and chemical abuse or dependence. Adolescents experiment for a variety of reasons: to yield to peer pressure, to gratify curiosity, to model adult behavior or to separate themselves from adult standards, to experience pleasure, or even to add excitement to a boring day. When an adolescent begins abusing drugs, the problem is more serious, and intervention is needed. Abuse is seen when behavior changes in a way that interferes with the adolescent's normal development and/or functioning. His behavior could also be affecting his family and others around him in a harmful way.

It is the nurse's role to become familiar with the clinical manifestations of alcohol and various drugs, and to observe and record behaviors that are indicative of drug and alcohol use—whether it is experimentation, abuse, or dependency. To go one step further, it is important that the nurse confront the student with observable behaviors, and ask the student in the process of interviewing whether he has been drinking alcohol or using any other drug. Denial is usually very strong, and the student will probably not admit abuse in one confrontation, but the nurse's continued concern should make it clear that his conduct is not appropriate.

The nurse's next step is to discuss her observations with teachers, counselors, and principals to inquire whether they have also noticed unusual behavior changes. In some schools this is done by referring the case to a core group, which gathers data from all people in contact with the student. The data is compiled and, if the evidence indicates abuse, an intervention is made with the student; this intervention constitutes a secondary level of prevention.

When an adolescent is referred to a treatment center for alcohol- or drug-related behavior and is recovering, the tertiary level of prevention begins. At this stage, the school nurse needs to cooperate with the counselors in order to provide ongoing support to the adolescent returning to school and to his parents. This support can be generated by a group composed of returning students. The group explores the feelings and changes that they face upon returning to the same environment with a different life style. This support is crucial to the recovering adolescent and needs to be provided in addition to any aftercare program. The adolescent may also attend a community-sponsored support group such as Alcoholics Anonymous.

Another tertiary preventive measure needed in our schools is the formation of student groups concerned about alcoholic family members other than the students themselves. These Alateen groups are sponsored by Alcoholics Anonymous; they allow adolescents to develop ways of dealing with their feelings about the alcoholic family members as well as themselves. The nurse's role should be to facilitate such groups. There are numerous other resources available to anyone requesting material and information. A partial list is included in Appendix 6B at the end of this chapter.

*Major health problems of later adolescence*

*Sexually transmitted diseases.*   The term "sexually transmitted disease" (STD) replaces the older one, "venereal disease," because it is more encompassing. Even this term is misleading, because many of the 20 to 30 diseases in this group can also be transmitted by other means. Among STDs, only gonorrhea and syphilis are reportable diseases (i.e., there is a legal requirement to report each case to the local health department). It is estimated that 5 million Americans contract some type of STD each year, making it one of the nation's greatest public health problems. These diseases are as prevalent as the common cold, but with much more serious consequences.

Gonorrhea, syphilis, *Herpesvirus hominis*, and trichomoniasis are discussed in this section. All are at near-epidemic proportions, and all are found mostly in young people. The nurse's involvement with STDs in the school system is discussed relative to all STDs (Medical Datamation, 1976).

GONORRHEA.   Gonorrhea ranks first among reported communicable diseases in the United States. In 1977 a total of 1,000,177 cases was reported, of which teenagers (15–19 years of age) accounted for 25%, and young adults (20–24) accounted for 39%. *Neisseria gonorrhea*, the causative bacteria, survive only in a moist, warm environment. It is usually contracted only through sexual intercourse, though a newborn can contract it in the vagina during birth. Gonorrhea is diagnosed by microscopic examination or culture of discharges. Symptoms appear in the male in 2 to 9 days with painful urination and a yellowish discharge. In females, 80 to 85% have no early symptoms. Pelvic inflammatory disease, acute or chronic, is a frequent complication of gonorrhea in females and can lead to chronic abdominal pain, permanent sterility, ectopic pregnancy, and even death. Other complications include conjunctivitis, disseminated gonorrheal infection, and the male complications of epididymitis, prostatitis, and urethral stricture. Recommended treatment is penicillin with probenecid (Center for Disease Control, 1979; Jerrick, 1978; McCoy & Willbelsman, 1978; Rein, 1975).

SYPHILIS.   Syphilis ranks third (exceeded only by gonorrhea and chicken pox) among reported communicable diseases in this country, with young adults having the highest incidence. In 1977, there were 64,473 reported cases in all stages in the United States. The infecting agent is the spirochete *Treponema pallidium*, usually diagnosed by a blood test, the Venereal Disease Research Laboratory (VDRL) test. The VDRL test is required in most states and the District of Columbia before a marriage license is issued, because of the serious nature of congenital syphilis.

Within a few weeks of the appearance of the primary skin lesion, the chancre, the infection spreads rapidly. The chancre disappears in about 2 weeks, but a secondary stage occurs if the client goes untreated. This stage resembles influenza, with fever, but with the addition of an extensive red body rash. Then the disease enters a latent stage, usually with occasional flareups. In the tertiary stage any body organ can be infected, which is why syphilis is called the "great imitator." If the disease is still untreated, the nervous or cardiovascular system are usually irrevocably damaged in this last stage. A few individuals are cured without treatment. Penicillin is used to treat syphilis at any stage of the disease (Center for Disease Control, 1979; Medical Datamation, 1976).

HERPESVIRUS HOMINIS GENITAL INFECTION.   Two types of *Herpesvirus hominis* commonly infect humans. The common cold sore is caused by Type I, and Type II infects the genital area. In 1978, the Center for Disease Control estimated the prevalence of genital herpes to be about 1 million cases, roughly comparable to that of gonorrhea (Himell, 1981). The incubation period is from 3 to 7 days, after which the client notes burning and pain in the genital area, as well as small, grouped blisters that develop on the external genitalia, vaginal wall, or cervix and ulcerate. Associated with these lesions are extreme pain, adenopathy, and fever. The primary infection persists for several weeks, heals spontaneously, and then may recur. There is little doubt of a connection to cervical cancer. Neonatal infections can cause permanent brain damage or death. There is no vaccine or cure, and only one medication that is palliative. In 1982, Zovirax (acyclovir) Ointment 5% was produced for topical application; it alleviates symptoms only. It is more effective for males than for females. Other symptomatic therapy exists: applying topical viscous Xylocaine or petroleum jelly, spraying the external genitalia with cool water, or taking warm sitz baths two or three times daily (Burroughs Wellcome Company, 1982; Center for Disease Control, 1976, 1979; Weisser, 1976).

TRICHOMONIASIS.   Trichomoniasis is a frequently acquired STD, with 2.5 million cases occurring annually. The prevalence among women attending gynecology clinics is 13–23%. It is caused by the protozoan *Trichomonas vaginalis* and can be transmitted by means other than sexual contact, such as sharing douche equipment or communal bathing. The incubation period is from 4 to 28 days, with pruritus and discharge the common symptoms. The discharge is often yellow, copious, frothy, and foul-smelling. It is treated with oral metronidazole

(Flagyl). Alcohol should not be consumed during treatment, because metronidazole has an effect similar to that of Antabuse in the presence of alcohol. Sexual partners should be treated simultaneously. Trichomoniasis is an important STD, because it is thought that it predisposes its victims to malignancy of the cervix (Rein & Chapel, 1975).

OTHER SEXUALLY TRANSMITTED DISEASES. Other STDs that young people acquire include *Pediculosis pubis* (crabs), *Condyloma acuminata* (genital warts), nongonococcal urethritis, and scabies (Center for Disease Control, 1979).

The nurse's role in a high school is mainly to educate students about the symptoms and complications of the varius STDs prevalent today. The nurse must recognize the reality of sexual relations among adolescents and should talk openly about prevention and intervention; facts should be presented in classes. Trust should characterize the nurse-student relationship, so that a student can openly discuss fears and realities of STD with the nurse. Often, small-group discussions are the most effective means of allowing students to question the nurse openly regarding their concerns. (Audiovisual aids are available from the Center for Disease Control, Attention: Technical Information Services, Bureau of State Services, Atlanta, Georgia 30333.)

In addition to her role in the school, the school nurse should also become a part of the national community action program to eradicate STDs. A community group should provide the following services: (1) a telephone counseling and referral service, (2) a speakers' bureau, and (3) special campus projects. If a hotline is not available in the community and an STD is suspected, information can be obtained from the national "Operation Venus" hotline; the toll-free number is 1-800-523-1885. This service, which operates out of Philadelphia, supplies STD diagnostic and treatment information. The school nurse may need to supply this national hotline information to school authorities. She can offer to present facts about STDs to faculty, parents, and community leaders. The nurse, teachers, and school counselors may also organize a high-school project to display STD information, or may conduct a school survey to determine the level of knowledge about STDs. STDs are so prevalent and so serious that the Center for Disease Control conducts local, interstate and international surveillance (Center for Disease Control, 1978).

*Infectious mononucleosis.* Infectious mononucleosis, caused by the Epstein-Barr virus, occurs predominantly in children and young adults. It is believed that students who are fatigued are more susceptible. The disease is characterized by persistent fatigue, anorexia, low-grade fever, headaches, pharyngitis, generalized lymphadenopathy, and splenomegaly. Sometimes a fine, red rash is present. If infectious mononucleosis is suspected by the nurse, the student should be referred immediately to a physician for diagnosis. The disease is confirmed by a laboratory test that reveals an increase in atypical lymphocytes and a high titer of the heterophil antibody in the serum.

In general, the prognosis is excellent. The treatment for this disease is predominately rest and aspirin. The length of bed rest varies from 1 week to 1 month, and the time for full recovery can take as much as 6 months. Reassurance by the nurse is important in aiding the adolescent and his family in full recovery and reestablishment of normal functioning (Krugman et al., 1977).

*Bone and muscle injuries.* Many older adolescents are very active in sports, and athletics-related injuries involving the muscles and joints are very commonly seen in the school nurse's office. It is important for the nurse to distinguish between what can be treated with ice or heat, and what should be referred for further evaluation. Consulting with the coach or physical education teacher is very helpful in determining how the injury occurred.

A "strain" is a muscle injury, and a "sprain" is an injury of the ligaments. In both, swelling often results, and the I-C-E (ice, compression, elevation) formula is necessary to prevent adhesions from forming around the joint. Ice and compression will constrict the blood vessels, and elevation will reduce swelling. After the first 48 hours, moist heat treatment is recommended to speed the healing process (McCoy & Willbelsman, 1978).

Knee injuries are very common in the adolescent age group. The Osgood-Schlatter disease, caused by the rapid growth of legs and knees, is often seen in the 9–15 age group. The tibial tubercle is inflamed, so the client has pain when squatting, running, or kneeling. This discomfort is often referred to as "shin splints." Supportive treatment is immobilization and heat. Symptoms subside when the epiphyseal growth is complete. The nurse's role is to explain the nature of his disease to the student and his parents, refer the student to a physician, and monitor his progress when he returns to school (Hughes, 1975).

*Depression and suicide.*

STATISTICS AND CAUSES. The nurse working with adolescents is exposed to a wide range and depth of their emotions. The adolescent ego is under pressure to adapt to the physical changes of puberty and to the family's and society's expectations of responsibility. The sensitivity of the nurse can allow her to distinguish the fleeting problems from those that can be destructive and ongoing. The feeling of being "down" or "blue" is common in adolescence. Depression, however, is of great concern because of the propensity of teenage depressives to maintain a depressive outlook through adulthood, the severe emotional discomfort that accompanies depression, and the rising suicide rate among our youth. Suicide ranks as the eighth leading cause of death in the 5–14 age group for both sexes. It is the third leading cause of death in the 15–24 age group, and it is on the increase (National Center for Health Statistics, 1978).

Depression is often associated with a perceived significant loss. Some common losses among adolescents are the loss of a boyfriend or girlfriend, parental divorce, death of a close relative, death of a pet, an abortion, moving to a new neighborhood, or even a loss of health due to an illness such as infectious mononucleosis or diabetes. Breaking away from parents, a normal separation, can generate feelings of loss that produce loneliness, guilt, or lowered self-esteem. The depressed person perceives himself as lacking something essential for his happiness.

NURSING ASSESSMENT AND INTERVENTION WITH DEPRESSION. The nurse needs to recognize that depression in the adolescent may trigger latent feelings linked to depression in herself. Being aware of what is happening is usually enough to help the nurse gain control of her feelings and focus her attention on the distressed subject.

The nurse's major activities in working with depression are to distinguish between normal mood swings and severe depression, to assist in the treatment of minor cases, and to refer the severely depressed. A health history helps determine whether the adolescent has recently experienced a loss. She is in a strategic position to be helpful to adolescents if she remains sensitive to their feelings. She needs to establish an open and nonjudgmental environment in order to help students recognize their feelings in her presence.

Behaviors in a student that could indicate depression are drinking alcohol or taking drugs, promiscuous behavior, running away, psychosomatic complaints, school phobia, aggressiveness, hyperactivity, and crying. Reading the nonverbal expressions of depression—flat tone of voice, decreased talking, slumped posture, and slow gait—can give clues. Depressed persons express feelings (either verbally or nonverbally) of sadness, loss of control, boredom, restlessness, isolation, inadequacy, rejection, and loss of interest.

The school nurse can schedule counseling sessions with a student who exhibits symptoms of depression; these sessions can help him to recognize his problem and feelings. She can intervene by discussing ways to fill the loss he has suffered. For example, if he is failing in a subject, a different schedule could be arranged with the teacher. If inter-personal relationships with peers are troublesome, the student can be guided into a peer group that accepts him more readily. Some students need referral for psychiatric help outside the school system.

NURSING ASSESSMENT AND INTERVENTION WITH SUICIDAL THREATS.   With any depression, including a suicidal one, the nurse should determine the source of the depression by allowing the student to talk without interfering. Through active listening, the nurse may sense that the student is suicidal. Most persons who commit suicide announce their lone-liness and intention, so prevention is possible in most cases. The most frequently noted symptoms in an adolescent are these:

1. Fatigue and insomnia
2. Sudden and continued loss of appetite
3. Severe mood swings
4. Increased drug and alcohol use
5. Heavy smoking
6. Significant decline in school work
7. Writing many letters to friends
8. Giving away prized possessions

The nurse should instruct the teacher to refer suicidal students to her, the school psychologist, or the student's family physician if the above symptoms are evident in a classroom ("Suicide Rate for U.S. Teens in Steep Rise," 1979).

If suicide is a possibility, the nurse should ask the student if he has a plan for taking his life. She should stay with the student and tel-ephone a parent, a counselor, or another friend of the student to alert them of the student's need. The nurse should always call in front of the student, never behind his back. *A suicidal person should never be al-lowed to wander out of the office,* whether the nurse feels he is faking or is seriously disturbed. If the adolescent is suicidally depressed, a referral should be made to an agency where the student can receive intensive counseling and guidance by a professionally trained mental health worker. The nurse needs a list of such agencies in order to be ready for a crisis situation. If the student is not suicidal, and only needs ac-ceptance from a nonjudgmental person, the relationship should still be continued if possible. The nurse has a responsibility to inform the teachers and other school personnel about the general problem of de-pression and suicide in adolescents, and also about specific cases, if ap-propriate.

*Conclusion*

Myriad school health issues face a school nurse each week. The ones discussed above are typical of the problems encountered, with proposed guidelines for their solutions. Fortunately, most teenagers in the United States and in most of the world are healthy.

## The Young Adult in College or Working

*Introduction*

There are 30 million people in the United States between the ages of 18 and 24, or about 13% of the 226 million persons in the United States today (U.S. Bureau of the Census, 1981). This segment of the overall population is often ignored when planning for health care needs, partly because young adults are essentially healthy, have few chronic diseases, and seek health care mainly for crisis intervention after problems develop.

The community health nurse (CHN) encounters the young adult in the same places as she does older adults, with the exception of the college health service. Young adults are most often seen at places of employment, in clinics, or in their homes (at times when they are pre-natal clients or have a chronic disease such as multiple sclerosis). This section focuses on their developmental stage, the causes of mortality and morbidity in this age group, wellness in this group, and the university health services. Prenatal care and occupational health are dis-cussed in Chapters 2 and 7, respectively. The primary role of CHNs and other health professionals with young adults is the promotion of wellness.

*Developmental stage*

In order to plan for health needs and to work effectively with young adults, a CHN should be aware of the more prominent elements associated with this developmental period. Approximately 28% of the population aged 18–24 are studying at institutions of higher education. For this segment of the population, total independence is often post-poned ("How They Stack Up," 1977). They frequently maintain close ties with their families through both psychosocial and financial sup-port systems. This leaves approximately 72% of this population in a variety of other roles, such as employment, marriage, childrearing, mil-itary service, and even crime.

A factor in successful self-identity is liberation from family control. This does not mean that family ties are severed, but that the individual must establish himself independently. This task is difficult since these young people often need financial assistance. Many cannot find employment; some begin families and find that the cost of establishing a household exceeds their means; and some choose to continue schooling.

Probably one of the biggest hurdles of this period is the sexual transition. Biological maturation is complete for both the male and the female. Sexual intimacies are a part of this transition, but the ability to form intimate relationships entails more than just sexual intercourse. Erikson (1960) believes that intimacy involves the ability to blend one's identity with that of another without fear of losing one's self. Without this, the ability to form meaningful and/or lasting relationships is unlikely.

D. L. Farnsworth (1966), a noted authority on health concerns of college students, has compiled a list of six tasks associated with this developmental period. Counselors at West Virginia University Student Counseling and Psychological Services Center (1977) have added two more. These tasks, although developed from observations of college students, are similar for all young adults. They are as follows:

—Changing from relations of dependence upon one's parents and other people to those of independence.

—Dealing with authority.

—Learning to deal with uncertainty and ambiguity, particularly in matters involving the balance between love and hatred.

—Developing a mature sexuality.

—Finding security, developing feelings of adequacy or competence, and attaining prestige or esteem.

—Developing standards and value systems.

—Learning how and whom to trust.

—Learning to accept responsibility for one's own behavior.

*Health concerns*

*Psychosocial problems.* Many young adults do encounter difficulty with the transition from childhood to the adult role. A list of the most common causes of death in this age group reflects the nature of some of the difficulties (see Table 6-2). More than half of the deaths in this

Table 6-2

The Most Common Causes of Death in the 15–24 Age Group
(Rates per 100,000)

| | | |
|---|---|---|
| 1. Accidents | | 58.4 |
| Motor Vehicles | 39.3 | |
| All Other Accidents | 19.1 | |
| 2. Homicide | | 12.5 |
| 3. Suicide | | 10.5 |
| 4. Malignant Neoplasms | | 7.5 |
| 5. Major Cardiovascular Disease | | 3.7 |
| 6. Diseases of the Heart | | 2.0 |
| 7. Influenza and Pneumonia | | 1.3 |
| 8. Cerebrovascular Disease | | 1.3 |

*Note.* From National Center for Health Statistics, *Provisional Statistics: Annual Summary, 1977.* Rockville, Md.: U.S. Department of Health, Education and Welfare, 1977.

age group result from various accidents. Almost a quarter of the deaths among this population are from homicide or suicide; violent deaths suggest stress and depression as mental health problems in their lives.

Depression, anxiety, and feelings of inadequacy are potential problems for all young adults, but they may be increased for college students who are away from home and under pressure to get good grades. A Boston study (Dunn, Lanning, Patch, & Sturrock, 1980) reported that depression and anxiety are the two most common reasons why college students seek mental health counseling. Of the sample, 49% were depressed, and 27% exhibited symptoms of anxiety. They frequently complained about "friendlessness," academic problems, and concerns about identity, self-image, and self-satisfaction. In the frenetic 1970s, underlying personality pathology was often masked by drug effects. Although today illicit drug use has subsided, alcohol use and abuse has not declined in this population (Dunn et al., 1980).

The young person's exploration in order to establish a sexual identity is essential. But at times it can create problems, such as (1) a rapid increase in the number and types of STDs; (2) more cases of cystitis, vaginitis, and urethritis; (3) an increased number of abortions; (4) an increased number of teenage pregnancies, and (5) an increased divorce rate. The main communicable diseases in this age group are the STDs, with the 20- to 24-year-olds having the highest incidence of gonorrhea and syphilis (Center for Disease Control, 1979). Birth rates among unmarried females aged 18–19 are now higher than among those aged 20–24, reversing a trend of the early 1970s (Planned Parenthood Federation of America, 1976). The liberation of sexual relationships has also increased the number of alternatives to marriage. This may be good, but it has also created some psychological turmoil for a number of young people.

*Physical problems and illnesses.* Physical health problems of this age group are varied, and there is not always a sharp demarcation between physical and psychological health problems. All forms of cancer, especially leukemia, account for a substantial number of deaths in older adolescents. Examples of other physical problems are URIs, dermatological problems, dysmenorrhea, and musculoskeletal injuries such as fractures from skiing accidents.

### Nursing functions

*Assisting with physical and psychological problems.* The CHN's basic understanding of the developmental tasks these people are experiencing is helpful as she plans for their health care needs. Probably the major task for young adults is to define and incorporate an identity of their own. CHNs can assist these clients through this period by opening up lines of communication. The nurse should capitalize on their strengths; this helps to build self-confidence and establish self-esteem, so that they can accept the responsibilities associated with adulthood.

It is important that CHNs make themselves available for assistance with physical problems as well as psychological support. This might be best accomplished through screening and educative processes in places of employment, schools, and community groups, and at times on a one-to-one basis. Types of health education in which CHNs could be involved are family planning information, information on control of communicable diseases, self-help seminars, child-rearing classes, information on how to use the health care system, and crisis intervention centers. Other ways the nurse can help with physical concerns include teaching good nutrition, emphasizing regular physical exercise, and stressing avoidance of harmful habits—all parts of a healthy life style.

*Self-help and self-care practices.*   Young adults show an interest in the health care they receive. It is a wonderful opportunity to introduce or encourage self-help and self-care skills. Actually, most health care is provided by lay people themselves and not by professionals, and studies show that self-care practices before medical contact are 90% relevant (Levin, 1979).

It is also very important that these individuals be included in the care planned for them, as in explanations of offered treatments and expected outcomes, inclusion of both parents in childbirth classes, provision of rationales for drugs prescribed, and explanations of signs and symptoms of various diseases. This is also a time to impart the need for preventive health measures. Discussions about the need for pelvic examinations and breast self-examinations; cancer warning signs; sexual concerns of both male and female clients; nutritional needs of adults and children; and hypertensive screening are of extreme relevance.

### Focus on wellness promotion in the emerging adult

The main health care for the 18–24 age group should be a focus on wellness. If they learn how to care for themselves and stay well, they may enjoy life more fully and avoid many of the problems associated with chronic illness later in life. Wellness promotion includes knowledge and practice of an adequate diet; physical fitness, and stress control; avoidance of alcohol, drugs, and cigarettes; and personal growth and fulfillment. The nurse can provide information about these topics on a one-to-one basis when she encounters these clients in clinics, in university health services, and at work. She can reach groups of them if she is willing to give talks in the community.

There are numerous sources of free or inexpensive literature on wellness concerns. The United States and Canadian governments both publish booklets on physical fitness, available at a nominal fee. The booklet, *Adult Physical Fitness—A Program for Men and Women*, is available from the U.S. Government Printing Office (President's Council on Physical Fitness, 1980), and *The Royal Canadian Air Force Exercise Plans for Physical Fitness* is published by Pocket Books (1972). The National Clearinghouse for Alcohol Information of the National Institute on Alcohol Abuse and Alcoholism publishes literature on all types of alcohol problems. The American Cancer Society, in addition to publishing pamphlets about smoking, conducts free classes (or requests a $5.00 donation) on how to stop smoking. Information on personal growth and fulfillment comes from many sources, including public libraries, churches, the U.S. Government Printing Office, and state health departments.

*Health problems in university health services*

*The health care program.* The health care in a university health service is based on student needs, spanning a variety of physical and psychological concerns. The health care programs of university health services include (1) treatment and rehabilitation, (2) prevention, and (3) health promotion. Treatment and rehabilitation can be either acute or chronic, physical or mental, inpatient or outpatient, and general or specialized. Prevention encompasses immunizations, risk appraisal, early detection and screening (specific and general), family counseling, antismoking therapy, and genetic counseling. A client can receive a vaccination for rubella, blood pressure screening, or contraceptives. Health promotion includes health education, life style awareness, mental and physical health management (exercise, diet, and stress management), rap lines, information clinics, self-help, and self-care. Mental health sessions on stress control, relaxation, breathing, thought control, and behavior modification are popular with students. Rap sessions about human sexuality are conducted in many universities. Frequently, students are involved in conducting these sessions (Stuehler & O'Dell, 1979).

*The college nurse practitioner.* A few educational programs have been developed to prepare NPs for college health work. These programs expand the skills of registered nurses to assume responsibility for primary health care. These NPs must have advanced skill in the assessment of the biopsychosocial and health or illness status of these clients. As the consumer's advocate, or primary health care trustee, the nurse provides preventive care, maintenance, coordination of care, and restorative aspects involved in the physical and emotional health of individuals (American Nurses' Association, 1975). An NP's duties in a college health service are similar to those of the school nurse, discussed earlier in this chapter.

# Appendix 6A: Needs Assessment for Adolescents

Listed below are areas where you may need more information, understanding, or help in learning how to accept or deal with health-related situations. Please indicate your needs by circling YES, NO, or UNSURE.

A. *Physical Health*
   I need:
       1. to understand better how my body
          functions                   YES   NO   UNSURE

2.  help in understanding physical
    changes that happen to my body          YES    NO    UNSURE
3.  to know what my blood pressure is        YES    NO    UNSURE
4.  to lose weight                           YES    NO    UNSURE
5.  to gain weight                           YES    NO    UNSURE
6.  to know what to do about acne (pim-
    ples)                                    YES    NO    UNSURE
7.  to understand why I feel tired all the
    time                                     YES    NO    UNSURE
8.  to know more about athletic injuries,
    how to prevent them, and what to do
    for them                                 YES    NO    UNSURE
9.  help in understanding why I have a
    chronic disease such as diabetes, asth-
    ma, or epilepsy                          YES    NO    UNSURE
10. support to quit smoking                  YES    NO    UNSURE
11. to understand more about how alco-
    hol and drugs can affect me              YES    NO    UNSURE
12. to determine whether or not I am us-
    ing drugs or alcohol too much            YES    NO    UNSURE

B.  *Physical Health: Sexuality Aspects*
    I need:
    13. to learn how to examine (girls) my
        breasts or (guys) my testicles for
        lumps (cancer)                       YES    NO    UNSURE
    14. to understand more about masturba-
        tion                                 YES    NO    UNSURE
    15. (girls) to talk with someone about my
        problems with menstruation (e.g.,
        cramps, irregularity)                YES    NO    UNSURE
    16. (guys) to talk with someone about
        erections, wet dreams, and sexual
        fantasies                            YES    NO    UNSURE
    17. (girls) to understand what happens
        during a pelvic examination          YES    NO    UNSURE
    18. to understand more about my sexual-
        ity (anatomy and feelings)           YES    NO    UNSURE
    19. to learn the difference between sex
        and sexuality                        YES    NO    UNSURE
    20. to learn how to make decisions re-
        garding my sexual activity           YES    NO    UNSURE
    21. more information about birth control  YES    NO    UNSURE
    22. more information about venereal dis-
        eases                                YES    NO    UNSURE

23. to know where to go to get a preg-
nancy test                                 YES    NO    UNSURE
24. more information about abortions      YES    NO    UNSURE

C. *Decision Making and Communications*
I need:
25–29. to learn how to communicate better
        with peers/friends               YES    NO    UNSURE
        with the opposite sex          YES    NO    UNSURE
        with my parents                YES    NO    UNSURE
        with teachers and other adults    YES    NO    UNSURE
        to learn how to ask nurses or doc-
        tors questions about my health    YES    NO    UNSURE
30. to learn how to deal with peer pres-
sure                                      YES    NO    UNSURE
31. to learn how to say ''no'' to my
peers, so I don't hurt their feelings   YES    NO    UNSURE

D. *Mental Health and Stress*
I need:
32. to discuss problems in my family that
are bothering me                 YES    NO    UNSURE
33. to learn how to handle all the pressures of school, home, work      YES    NO    UNSURE
34. to become less fearful of failing in
school                               YES    NO    UNSURE
35. reassurance that I am normal     YES    NO    UNSURE
36. to feel less tense and upset in my
stomach                             YES    NO    UNSURE
37. to know what causes my frequent
headaches and what to do about them   YES    NO    UNSURE
38. to learn to stand up for what I believe   YES    NO    UNSURE
39. to understand my mood swings    YES    NO    UNSURE
40. help in understanding my feelings of
depression                        YES    NO    UNSURE
41. to discuss my feelings of suicide with
someone                           YES    NO    UNSURE

E. *Safety*
I need:
42. to be more careful when I am driving   YES    NO    UNSURE
43. to learn how to save a drowning per-
son                                     YES    NO    UNSURE
44. to learn how to save someone who is
choking                            YES    NO    UNSURE

45. to learn cardiopulmonary resuscitation
(CPR)                                                  YES   NO   UNSURE

F. *General*
I need:
46. to understand what a school nurse
can do to help me be a healthier per-
son                                                    YES   NO   UNSURE

G. Please comment on something you feel may have been left off the list:

_____

_____

Thank you.

Student's Name (optional): _____

# Appendix 6B: Addresses for Information on Alcoholism and Drug Use

1. National Institute of Alcohol Abuse and Alcoholism
5600 Fishers Lane
Rockville, MD 20857
(301) 468-2600

2. National Council on Alcoholism
733 Third Ave.
New York, NY 10017

3. Alcoholics Anonymous World Services, Inc.
Box 459
Grand Central Station
New York, NY 10163

4. Al-Anon Family Group
Headquarters, Inc.
P.O. Box 182
Madison Square Station
New York, NY 10010

5. National Clearinghouse for Drug Abuse Information
P.O. Box 1635
Rockville, MD 20850
or
5600 Fishers Lane, Room 10A-56
Rockville, MD 20857

6. Prevention Branch
   Division of Resource Development
   National Institute on Drug Abuse
   5600 Fishers Lane, Room 10A-30
   Rockville, MD 20857

# References

American Nurses' Association. *Guidelines for short-term continuing education program for college and university health nurse practitioners.* Kansas City, Mo.: Author, 1975.

Beneson, A. S. *Control of communicable diseases in man* (13th ed.). Washington, D.C.: American Public Health Association, 1981.

Burroughs Wellcome Company (Medical Division). *New antiherpes agent* (circulars). Research Triangle Park, N.C.: Author, 1982.

Center for Disease Control. *Treatment of genital herpes infection* (mimeographed guidelines no. 00-2906). Atlanta: Author, 1976.

Center for Disease Control. *What you and your community can do* (DHEW, Publ. No. (CDC) 78-8268). Atlanta: Author, 1978.

Center for Disease Control. *STD fact sheet* (DHEW Publ. No. (CDC) 79-8195). Atlanta: Author, 1979.

Commonwealth of Pennsylvania, Department of Health. *Report on the school health program of the Department of Health.* Harrisburg: Author, 1973–1974.

Creighton, H., & Squaires, G. N. School nurses: Legal aspects of their work. *Nursing Clinics of North America,* 1974, *9,* 467–474.

Dunn, R. F., Lanning, J. R., Patch, V. D., & Sturrock, M. D. The college mental health center: A report after ten years. *Journal of the American College Health Association,* 1980, *28,* 321–325.

Erikson, E. H. Youth and the life cycle. *Children,* 1960, *7,* 43–49.

Farnsworth, D. L. *Psychiatry, education, and the young adult.* Springfield, Ill.: Charles C Thomas, 1966.

Gordon, S. *You would if you loved me.* New York: Bantam Books, 1978.

Gordon, S. Coming to terms with your own sexuality first. *Journal of School Health,* 1979, *49,* 247–250.

Gordon, T. V. *Parent effectiveness training.* New York: Peter H. Wyden, 1970.

Guttmacher Institute. *Teenage pregnancy: The problem that hasn't gone away.* New York: Author, 1981.

Hanson, R. A., & Reynolds, R. *Child development: Concepts, issues, and readings.* St. Paul, Minn: West, 1980.

Himell, K. Genital herpes: The need for counseling. *Journal of Gynecological Nursing,* 1981, *10,* 446–450.

How they stack up. *Newsweek,* October 10, 1977, p. 67.

Hughes, J. G. *Synopsis of pediatrics* (4th ed.). St. Louis: C. V. Mosby, 1975.

Jensen, M. D., Benson, R. C., & Bobak, I. M. *Maternity care: The nurse and the family* (2nd ed.). St. Louis: C. V. Mosby, 1981.

Jerrick, S. J. Federal efforts to control sexually transmitted diseases. *Journal of School Health,* 1978, *48,* 428–432.

Juhasz, A. M. A chain of sexual decision-making. *Family Coordinator,* 1975, *24,* 45.

Kaluger, G., & Kaluger, M. F. *Human development: The span of life.* St. Louis: C. V. Mosby, 1974.

Knotts, G. R. (Ed.). *Guidelines for the school nurse in the school health program* (pamphlet). Akron, Ohio: Hiney Printing, 1974.

Krugman, S., Ward, R., & Katz, S. L. *Infectious diseases of children* (6th ed.). St. Louis: C. V. Mosby, 1977.

Levin, L. Self-care: New challenge to individual health. *Journal of the American College Health Association,* 1979, *28,* 117–119.

McCoy, K., & Willbelsman. *The teenage body book.* New York: Wallaby Pocket Books, 1978.

Malasanos, L., Barkauskas, V., Moss, M., & Stoltenberg-Allen, K. *Health assessment.* St. Louis: C. V. Mosby, 1977.

Medical Datamation. *Venereal disease* (pamphlet). Bellevue, Ohio: Author, 1976.

Mercer, R. *Perspectives on adolescent health care.* Philadelphia: J. B. Lippincott, 1979.

Nader, P. R. (Ed.). *Options for school health.* Germantown, Md.: Aspen Systems Corporation, 1978.

National Center for Health Statistics. *Facts of life and death* (DHEW Publ. No. (PHS) 79-1222). Washington, D.C.: U.S. Department of Health, Education and Welfare, 1978.

National Education Association. *Department-wide study of school nurse practices.* Washington, D.C.: Author, 1973.

National Heart, Lung, and Blood Institute's Task Force on Blood Pressure Control in Children. Report of the Task Force on Blood Pressure Control in Children. *Pediatrics,* 1977, *59*(5), Part 2, 799–810.

National Research Council (Food and Nutrition Board, Committee on Dietary Allowances). *Recommended dietary allowances* (9th ed.). Washington, D.C.: Author, 1980.

Neumann, C. G. Obesity in pediatric practice: Obesity in the preschooler and school-age child. *Pediatric Clinics of North America,* 1977, *24,* 117–121.

Nizel, A. E. Preventing dental caries: The nutritional factors. *Pediatric Clinics of North America,* 1977, *24,* 141–143˙and 153.

Pillitteri, A. *Nursing care of the growing family: A child health text.* Boston: Little, Brown, 1977.

Planned Parenthood Federation of America. *11 million teenagers: What can be done about the epidemic of adolescent pregnancies in the United States?* New York: Alan Guttmacher Institute, 1976.

President's Council on Physical Fitness. *Adult physical fitness: A program for men and women* (Publ. No. 040-000-0026-7). Washington, D.C.: U.S. Government Printing Office, 1980.

Rein, M. F. *Gonorrhea* (Tx. Doc. No. H758.8 G589, 1975) (pamphlet). Distributed by Texas Dept. of Health Resources, Venereal Disease Div., 1975.

Rein, M. F., & Chapel, T. A. Trichomoniasis, candidiasis, and the minor venereal diseases. *Clinical Obstetrics and Gynecology,* 1975, *18,* 73–76.

*The Royal Canadian Air Force Exercise Plans for Physical Fitness.* New York: Pocket Books, 1972.

Stuehler, G., & O'Dell, S. T. The manageable approach to college health service planning, Part II. *Journal of the American College Health Association,* 1979, *28,* 98–108.

Suicide rate for U.S. teens in steep rise. *Milwaukee Journal,* June 26, 1979, pp. 1 and 4.

U.S. Bureau of the Census. *Statistical abstract of the United States 1981* (102nd ed.). Washington, D.C.: U.S. Department of Commerce, 1981.

Weisser, R. N. *Sexually transmitted diseases.* Paper presented at the Second Annual Hal Wanger Family Practice Conference, West Virginia Medical Center, Morgantown, West Virginia, September 16, 1976.

West Virginia University Student Counseling and Psychological Services Center. Handout relaying the developmental tasks of college students (no title). Unpublished material, 1977.

# 7

# Young Adults in the Clinic, in Occupational Settings, and at Home

*Dorothy D. Petrowski and Charlene C. Ossler*

## Introduction

The young adult aged 25 to 39 has completed the process of maturation and moved to an exciting period of peak mental and motor functioning. Community health nursing services for these clients are concentrated in clinics and occupational settings, with a few cared for at home. Health care needs of the young adult population are related to developmental, psychosocial, moral, and physical changes. This chapter emphasizes the prevention and treatment of coronary heart disease (CHD), the leading cause of mortality in the United States and the second in this age group for males.

## Health Care Needs of the Young Adult Population

### Developmental Needs

The healthy young adult becomes other-centered while maintaining and enhancing his own personal identity, as described by Erikson (1968). He strives for meaningful relationships with others that may culminate in marriage or another form of a long-lasting relationship. The individual usually creates a new family and assumes responsibility for maintaining that unit. At the same time, the young adult continues to mature in his ability to adapt to an increasingly complex world. He learns to recognize and satisfy his needs and to interact socially with little effort and discomfort. Able to tolerate frustrations, he makes choices that enable him to maintain a high level of adaptation and harmony within his personal, social, and business groups. Career goals are set and modified as the individual acknowledges his potential and limitations.

## Psychosocial Needs

Psychosocially, the young adult develops in three areas: cognitive, emotional, and moral. He usually completes any advanced education and training and makes choices about the direction of his career. Decisions may become stressful and complex when there are competing values. For example, the two-career family may be confronted with the dilemma of being forced to foster one partner's career at the expense of the other's. As the individual progresses through this period, he develops skills to solve problems creatively and demonstrates an accelerated ability to do this abstractly.

The young adult experiences an increased number of in-depth interpersonal relationships. If he has not already done so, he may select a partner with whom he shares his life. Childbearing and child-rearing become central concerns for the majority. The young adult achieves a new standing of adulthood within his family of origin and often moves from his community of birth for reasons of education and employment.

## Moral Needs

Many young adults begin to question their moral values and belief systems. Religion may become more important as people probe the meaning of life; making commitments to a spouse or partner, a career, and an employer implies an ethical willingness to abide by those commitments. Individuals often face some of life's most difficult moral dilemmas during this period and may need the assistance and support of health, social, and religious professionals.

## Physical Needs

Physically, the young adult is most often "well." Physical maturation is complete, and all body systems usually function at optimal levels. Illnesses are usually of an acute, nonserious nature, and health is taken for granted. In the 1976 Health Interview Survey (National Center for

Health Statistics, 1978b), the leading diagnostic category for this age
group was acute upper respiratory infection (URI). Yet is is also during this time that individuals develop habits or life style patterns that
can lead to diseases later. A typical disease that can begin now is CHD,
which is included later in this chapter. Accidents are the chief cause
of death among Americans aged 25 to 44, especially males (National
Center for Health Statistics, 1978a). Venereal disease and hepatitis are
common communicable diseases on the rise in this age group. Also,
toward the end of this age period, cirrhosis due to alcoholism is beginning to appear as another frequent cause of morbidity and mortality
(1975 National Conference on Preventive Medicine, 1976).

   The major emphasis in health care for the young adult is on education for prevention (i.e., teaching people to maintain and enhance
a high level of wellness). Nursing approaches to this type of care are
outlined in books such as Diekelmann's *Primary Health Care of the Well
Adult* (1977). Clinics, occupational health, and home care for the young
adult are discussed in this chapter.

## The Clinic

### Types of Clinics

Although they are an important source of health care for many Americans, clinics are discussed here primarily because they provide many
young adults with a substantial portion of their follow-up care, and
clinics are the setting in which young adults usually encounter the community health nurses (CHNs) or nurse practitioners (NPs). Official clinics are those established and maintained by a government (federal,
state, or local). Private clinics are usually operated for profit by groups
of physicians, hospitals, or other investors. Voluntary clinics are non-
profit and are often formed in response to particular needs of a special
group in the community. The nurse is an essential care provider in clinics, with the CHN especially essential in governmental clinics.

#### Official clinics

*Local health department clinics.*   These official clinics function under
a legal mandate of the state to safeguard the health and welfare of its
citizens. The characteristic organizational structure for official clinics
is within a city or county health department. Traditionally, these clinics reflect the major health concerns of the local health department: venereal disease detection and control; maternal and child health; serv-

ices for handicapped children; family planning; treatment for substance abuse; and, less frequently, general medical and surgical services. These services, provided from a central location, are usually supported by a department of community health nursing, which staffs the clinics and follows clients for home health care.

Clients who wish to use the official clinics must usually meet eligibility requirements of local residency and low income level. The income requirement may be waived by some clinics for venereal disease and family planning. Since the clinics are supported by taxes from the local population, services are restricted to those who reside in the area. The majority of official clinic consumers are low-income families and elderly people on fixed incomes. This pattern may differ in rural areas, where the official clinic may be the only source of health care.

*Public health service and Veterans Administration facilities.* Exceptions to the local health clinics are two types of direct health services offered by the federal government. One group is under the control of the U.S. Public Health Service and includes the Public Health Service facilities, the National Institutes of Health Clinical Center, and Indian Health Services. The other group is the vast array of clinics supported by the Veterans Administration (VA).

## Private clinics and health maintenance organizations

Private clinics are often referred to as "group practices" and include the newer concept of "health maintenance organizations" (HMOs). Physician group practices began in the first quarter of this century, when doctors banded together for the economic benefits of sharing the costs of a medical practice and to promote better coverage of clientele by sharing "on-call" responsibilities.

These private endeavors, notably Kaiser-Permanente and the Health Insurance Plan of Greater New York, were successful. They grew in number and began to demonstrate savings in the cost of health care without a decrease in the quality of care or comprehensiveness of coverage. Because of an emphasis on prevention and ambulatory versus acute hospital care, they have become known as HMOs, a term coined in the United States. The Health Maintenance Organization Act of 1973 provided monies to initiate and expand such services (Health Maintenance Organization Act of 1973, 1974).

An HMO is defined as an organized system of health care providing comprehensive services to a voluntarily enrolled population for a per capita prepaid fee (Bates, 1972). It can be public or private. Comprehensive services include the entire continuum from primary health care to emergency, acute in-hospital, and rehabilitative care. The HMO must be able to provide directly or arrange for all those health services considered to be necessary to maintain the health of a defined population group. Some HMOs offer a complete health care package for a set fee; others use copayments or deductibles for certain services such as dental care and pharmaceutical products.

The employer-run clinics are also examples of private clinics where the CHN works. In large industries, they are part of the total occupational health program.

### Voluntary clinics

Voluntary clinics proliferated especially during the 1960s, as "free clinics" became established in neighborhoods where people were unlikely to use the traditional health care delivery systems. Frequently they developed in response to young people who rebelled against "the establishment" or who perceived the available services as unresponsive and too authoritarian. For example, the Haight-Ashbury Free Medical Clinic in the "hippie" area of San Francisco still operates. It currently focuses on drug or drug-related problems and women's needs (Smith, 1981). Many of these clinics, however, have closed for lack of providers and funds.

### The Nurse's Role and Function in the Clinic Setting

Young adults receive routine history and physical examinations, treatments for minor conditions such as URIs, or for more serious illnesses like hepatitis or injuries from automobile accidents in clinics. Because many young adults are becoming more health-conscious, teaching about diet, exercise, cigarette smoking, or drinking alcoholic beverages is frequently included by the CHN when clients present in the clinic with acute conditions. Refer to Appendixes A–C at the end of this volume for guidelines on the history and physical examination.

Traditionally, clinics have depended upon the expertise of the professional nurse to organize and coordinate health services as well as to supply them. Nurses also provide primary health care, health education, counseling, assistance to the physician, and continuity of care. The use of the professional nurse for primary care in the clinic setting has accelerated as more nurses are prepared to take on this role. NPs perform routine history and physical examinations for healthy people such as young adults, women with uncomplicated pregnancies, well children, and those with stabilized chronic illnesses. Working with a health team, the NP consults with the physician, nutritionist, social worker, or other team members and refers clients when appropriate.

Nurses have always had the primary responsibility for client advocacy in clinic settings. After the physician-client interaction, the nurse offers clarification of the physician's findings and prescribed regimen and provides health education oriented to prevention of a decline in health status. Regardless of the clinic nurse's functions, her role of ensuring holistic care that meets the needs of the client and family is paramount.

## Occupational Settings as a Place of Health Care

### Need for Occupational Health Services

Young adults, the largest portion of the work force, spend a quarter of their time at work. Many jobs may expose the worker to diseases or hazards, which result in illness, injury, or a shortened life span. Employers acknowledge the importance of a health care program as a determinant of an effective, productive work force. Bernhardt (1976) cites six positive results of such programs: control of absenteeism; increase in worker efficiency and quality of the product; safer work practices; decrease in workers' compensation costs; decreased group health insurance premiums; and intangible benefits such as the employee's positive response to management's apparent concern with his health and safety.

Recognition of this interaction between work and health has led to the development and expansion of health care at the site of employment. This movement has been stimulated by the Occupational Safety and Health Act of 1970, federal legislation that mandates the protection of the health and safety of workers (Occupational Safety and Health Act of 1970, 1971). The extent of health care services to employees varies, according to the nature and size of the business and the type of occupational health professionals hired by the employer. The need for occupational health services, the occupational health team, and the components and services of an occupational health program are discussed in the following section.

#### Incidence of occupational health problems

The incidence of reported occupation-related illnesses and injuries has been increased as work becomes more mechanized; as exposure to harmful agents becomes more frequent; and as more problems are reported. The reporting is also influenced by employees' increased job security and level of sophistication. The statistics are still thought to be incomplete, but according to the Departments of Labor and Health, Education and Welfare (Gordon, Akman, & Brooks, 1971; U.S. Department of Health, Education and Welfare, 1976), more than 9 million injuries occurred at the workplace. Of these, 2.2 million meant temporary or permanent disability for the employees involved. It is estimated that 14,000 were killed in work-related incidents and that 300,000 new cases of occupationally induced illnesses developed that year.

Allowing for the suspected large number of cases that remain unreported, it is estimated conservatively that one of every 11 workers in the United States experiences a work-related illness or injury annually (Stellman & Daum, 1973). These data do not include the largely unknown effects of long-term exposures to noise, temperature extremes, vibrations, and emotional stress that are part of many workers' jobs; continued loud noise, for example, can cause deafness. A group of workers who warrant special attention are women of childbearing age. Over half of American women are now in the labor force, and the effect of work exposures on fertility and pregnancy outcome is still largely unknown (Hricko & Brunt, 1976).

As can be seen in Table 7-1, a great proportion of reported occupational illnesses are skin disorders, followed by pulmonary diseases. The listing "All other occupational illnessess" in the table includes such diagnoses as eye disease and trauma, chemical burns, hearing loss, and digestive and cardiac symptoms due to exposure to toxic materials.

### The Occupational Safety and Health Act of 1970

The need for health and safety programs at the workplace prompted the Williams-Steiger Occupational Safety and Health Act of 1970 (1971). The law reads that the programs are "to assure so far as possible every working man and woman in the nation safe and healthful working conditions." Covering all businesses that conduct interstate commerce and have one or more employees, the Act has been implemented by two federal agencies. The National Institute for Occupational Safety and Health (NIOSH) under the Department of Health, Education and Welfare (since 1980 the Department of Health and Human Services, or DHHS) recommends standards, researches potential hazards, provides educational programs for occupational health personnel, and teaches employers and employees prevention of occupational injury and illness. NIOSH is decentralized into 10 regional offices ac-

Table 7-1

Distribution of Occupational Illnesses by Category of Illness, Private Sector,
United States, 1978 (Numbers in Thousands)

| Category of Illness | Illnesses | |
|---|---|---|
| | Number | Percent |
| Total ............................ | 143.5 | 100.0 |
| Skin diseases or disorders | 65.9 | 46.0 |
| Dust diseases of the lungs | 1.6 | 1.1 |
| Respiratory conditions due to toxic agents | 13.6 | 9.5 |
| Poisoning | 5.6 | 3.9 |
| Disorders due to physical agents | 16.7 | 11.6 |
| Disorders associated with repeated trauma | 20.2 | 14.1 |
| All other occupational illnesses | 19.9 | 13.8 |

*Note.* From U.S. Bureau of Labor Statistics, *Occupational Injuries and Illnesses in the United States by Industry, 1978* (Summary Report No. 586). Washington, D.C.: U.S. Department of Labor, 1980.

cording to the DHHS regions. One of their most recent endeavors has been the establishment of Educational Resource Centers (ERCs) in each of their regions for the education of occupational nurses, physicians, industrial hygienists, and safety engineers.

The other enforcer of the Act is the Occupational Safety and Health Administration (OSHA) under the Department of Labor. OSHA may conduct inspections of the workplace and has the right to issue citations for violations of standards and to assess penalties if the violations are not corrected. OSHA's functions are carried out by state- or federal-level OSHAs that have been approved by the federal administration. OSHA is available to the employer for consultation and advice about compliance with the law. The effectiveness of the 1970 OSHA legislation is currently under study.

The Act requires employers to keep records and to report periodically on all work-related injuries, deaths, illnesses, and exposures to toxic agents, except for minor injuries. A schema for determining which incidents are reportable has been formulated by OSHA. An illness, injury, or death to an employee that results from an accident or exposure in the work environment must be recorded in the OSHA Log. Recordable injuries must involve medical treatment beyond first aid, loss of consciousness, restriction of bodily motion or work activities, or transfer to another job. OSHA requires that accidents resulting in hospitalization of five or more employees or in death be reported to them by telephone or telegraph within 48 hours. The assessment, treatment, and reporting of these incidents are performed by the occupational health team. In addition, the law mandates certain health examinations and screenings for specific exposures. These are described in NIOSH publications for each of the agents for which there is an approved standard.

## Objectives and Types of Occupational Health Programs

The objectives used as a basis for occupational health programs are listed in the American Medical Association's *Scope, Objectives and Functions of Occupational Health Programs* (1971). They are as follows:

1. To protect employees against health and safety hazards in their work situation.
2. Insofar as practical and feasible, to protect the general environment of the community.
3. To facilitate placement of workers according to their physical, mental, and emotional capacities in work which they can perform with an acceptable degree of efficiency and without endangering their own health and safety or that of others.
4. To assure adequate medical care and rehabilitation of the occupationally ill and injured.
5. To encourage and assist in measures for personal health maintenance, including the acquisition of a personal physician whenever possible. (p. 6)

The extent to which these objectives are achieved in creating an occupational health unit in a given company depends upon the size and nature of the company, its profit margin, its employees' specific needs, and the company's interest in an occupational health program.

In the United States, occupational health programs range from those that minimally meet the first objective to comprehensive programs exceeding the listed objectives. The minimal programs, usually found in smaller businesses, may consist of an individual or group of workers trained in first aid or a one-nurse unit whose primary responsibility is to maintain records for the OSHA and insurance forms. Examples of comprehensive programs such as the Kimberly-Clark Health Management Program ("Kimberly-Clark Health Management Program

Aimed at Prevention,'' 1977), with its preventive focus and extensive physical exercise facilities, are newer and smaller in number. Other types of programs include part-time contracted services of professionals from a local health department,· hospital, industrial clinic, or HMO (Plant, 1978; Ralston, 1973).

## The Occupational Health Team

The objectives of an occupational health program are carried out by the occupational health team and, of course, by the employees. Many occupational injuries and illnesses can be prevented, as is true of other causes of illness and death among this age group. Such prevention is the goal of a full occupational health team comprised of nurses, physicians, industrial hygienists, safety engineers, psychologists, and others concerned with human factors and work, such as ergonomists. While the nurse is the predominant provider (and the only provider in a third of all companies) of occupational health care, each of the other team members can provide valuable expertise. The team also performs treatment as indicated.

*Occupational health physician, industrial hygienist, and safety engineer*

Depending on the size and needs of the business, an occupational health program may have a full-time physician director with a medical staff, a full- or part-time company physician, or a physician who is available for on-call advice and consultation. A well-prepared occupational physician has completed a residency in that field, or has otherwise been trained in public environmental health, occupational diseases, and toxicology.

The role of the industrial hygienist is that of recognition, evaluation, and control of hazardous environmental factors. The industrial hygienist is familiar with all equipment and processes of the plant and is capable of surveying the work environment; monitoring equipment; analyzing all physical, chemical, and biological stresses in the workplace; and advising appropriate control techniques. His educational qualifications may range from a baccalaureate up to a doctoral degree in industrial hygiene or engineering. The American Industrial Hygiene Association provides a certification process to accredit industrial hygienists.

The safety engineer or specialist assists the rest of the team by identifying and controlling industrial hazards. Most concerned with accident prevention and safety education, the safety engineer may also perform the functions of an industrial hygienist in some industries.

### Occupational health nurse

There are approximately 24,000 nurses employed as occupational health personnel, and the majority of these are employed in manufacturing industries (American Nurses' Association and U.S. Department of Health, Education, and Welfare, 1979). Dolinsky (1974) estimates that a shortage of 19,000 nurses would exist if all companies were to provide an occupational health program. The majority of occupational health nurses are prepared at the diploma level and have received no formal education in occupational health care. With the advent of the Educational Resource Centers, however, industry is beginning to seek the employment of baccalaureate- and master's-level nurses, as well as occupational health NPs.

*Definition.* The American Association of Occupational Health Nurses (1976) defines occupational health nursing as "the application of nursing principles in conserving the health of workers in all occupations." This organization is independent of the American Nurses' Association. Occupational health nursing is concerned with prevention, recognition, and treatment of illness and injury and requires special skills and knowledge in the fields of health education and counseling, environmental health, rehabilitation, and human relations. Because of the comprehensiveness of this role, it is recommended that nurses interested in occupational health first gain experience in emergency room care, community health nursing, ambulatory care, and NP skills. Occupational health nurses can be certified after successfully passing an examination by the American Board of Occupational Health Nursing. Currently, only 1500 occupational health nurses are certified and may use the title Certified Occupational Health Nurse (American Association of Occupational Health Nurses, 1976). In the late 1970s, a few universities added master's programs in occupational health nursing.

*Functions.* An important reference for the occupational health nurse is Lee's publication, *The New Nurse in Industry* (1978). Subtitled *A Guide for the Newly Employed Occupational Health Nurse,* this book provides an introduction to the concepts and principles of an occupational health program and occupational health nursing. Lee describes 15 specific functions of the occupational health nurse:

1. Collaborate with management to plan and administer a nursing service which gives the best possible nursing care to employees.
2. Provide primary nursing care for occupational and nonoccupational injuries and illnesses, based upon nursing assessment, nursing diagnosis, and medical directives.
3. Supervise the transportation of ill or injured employees to a hospital, clinic, or physician's office for appropriate care.
4. Make health referrals and coordinate plans for continued care and follow-up measures with community health services.
5. Develop and maintain a system of health and safety records and reports that conform to reporting procedures within the company.
6. Develop and update a nursing policy and procedure manual for the nursing service.
7. Assist with [or perform] physical examination[s] . . . , obtain health and work information, perform screening measures, collect biological samples, interpret the findings, and make appropriate referrals and recommendations about positive results.
8. Counsel distressed employees and intervene to assist in resolving personal and emotional problems.
9. Teach employees about good health and safety practices and motivate individuals to improve health practices.
10. Identify health needs of workers, develop objectives, and implement programs in health promotion, maintenance, and restoration.
11. Collaborate with the occupational health team to explore ways of promoting an environmental surveillance and to provide continuous medical monitoring for workers exposed to potentially harmful substances.
12. Be aware of current standards for health and safety legislation and legal statutes pertinent to the practice of nursing and medicine in occupational health.
13. Periodically evaluate the nursing service planned programs and activities for appropriateness, adequacy, effectiveness, and efficiency.
14. Participate in professional nursing organization and community health activities.
15. Assume self-responsibility for professional growth and development. (pp. 9–10).

Along with these guidelines, the occupational health nurse should implement the nursing process for any employee seeking care.

The actual functions performed by an occupational health nurse will vary, depending on employees' needs, the size of the occupational health unit, presence of other team members, the preparation of the nurse, and the objectives of a given occupational health program. For example, she may do individual mental health counseling or teach breast self-examination in a group.

194 *Handbook of Community Health Nursing*

Components and Services of an Occupational Health Program

There are six components of an occupational health program: preplacement examinations (PPEs); care for acute and chronic work-related illnesses and injuries; evaluation and care for illnesses and injuries that are nonoccupational in nature; surveillance; mental health services; and environmental surveys. Each of these components has several services that combine to create a comprehensive occupational health program.

*The preplacement examination*

Previously thought of as a method of excluding the incapable worker, the PPE is now considered the source of adequate information to enable the employer to fit an employee into an appropriate job. The PPE becomes a preventive health assessment when it is used to achieve a fit between an employee's limitations and the requirements of a specific job. The PPE also provides a baseline against which to measure changes in health status of an individual possibly due to work. The PPE is often the only health assessment received by healthy, asymptomatic young adults and frequently is the point at which treatable medical conditions are first detected. Strasser (1979) reports that a recent survey of 150 PPEs at one company disclosed 50 abnormalities.

The type of PPE performed is determined by company policy, the characteristics of the applicant pool, the anticipated hazards and exposures associated with the work in question, and the occupational health personnel who provide the examination. Some OSHA standards—for example, those for working with asbestos—require a PPE to include particular assessments, such as pulmonary function tests. The PPE may also differ according to the physical status and abilities required for a particular job. Guidelines for a PPE include the following (Bernhardt, 1982; Lee, 1978):

1. Personal and family medical history (including life style).
2. Occupational health history, which includes all past job exposures, part-time employment, and hobbies.
3. Reproductive history for female employees.
4. Screening tests—height and weight measurements, vision test, blood pressure examination, hearing test, spirometry, selected blood tests, electrocardiogram (EKG), urinalysis, chest X-ray.
5. Physical assessment with attention to body systems potentially under stress on the job (e.g., integumentary, respiratory, and musculoskeletal).
6. Psychological assessment as indicated.

The occupational health nurse is often the professional who conducts this examination, so she has the opportunity to use the PPE as an introduction to provide health counseling and education to the worker. The nurse may detect health deficits or special risks from previous employment; these require a referral to the community health care system or further follow-up by the occupational health unit if the applicant is hired. Refer to Appendixes A–C at the end of this volume for guidelines on the history and physical examination.

### Care for work-related problems

The occupational health professionals who are employed on site or in nearby contracted facilities are responsible for the diagnosis and treatment of illness and injury that is work-related. First-line assessment of such incidents is usually conducted by the nurse. The degree of this responsibility may range from administration of first aid for a superficial skin laceration to emergency referral to a physician or hospital for a serious injury. The health professional determines the ability of the worker to return to his job and must be aware of the necessity for restrictions if these are indicated by the nature of the job or the illness/injury. Recording of these visits in the occupational health unit is crucial for follow-up of the client, legal protection of the employer and nurse, and identification of potential problem areas in the plant.

### Care for nonoccupational illnesses and injuries

The basic function of the occupational health nurse in relation to this component is the evaluation of workers who become ill during working hours or who return to employment after an illness or injury that has occurred off the job. When an employee becomes ill at work, the nurse and client decide what the problem is and plan the intervention. He may only need an analgesic for a headache, or may be so ill that he must go home. When a worker returns after an absence, the nurse must determine whether he is capable of resuming his former work without any restrictions. She may have to recommend a temporary assignment to a different position. The nurse may also determine that a returning employee will need some health supervision, education, or counseling from the occupational health unit. A newly diagnosed diabetic, for example, may come to the health unit when he experiences symptoms of glucose imbalance. (See Chapter 8 for a discussion of diabetic care.)

Currently, employers are investing more in preventive occupational health programs that address some of the major nonoccupational illnesses. At present, there is a major drive to teach cardiopulmonary resuscitation to all line supervisors and a critical number of employees. The American Red Cross will provide classes in this life-saving technique at no cost. Larger companies are developing extensive in-house programs that provide annual physical examinations, health education, and facilities and equipment for employees to maintain physical fitness. Fielding (1979) describes the comprehensive health program for employees provided by the Gillette Company. He estimates that, considering the cost of nonoccupational illnesses covered by the company health insurance policy and the cost in work time when an employee receives treatment outside the work site, the company saved over $1 million in 1976 by providing a comprehensive on-site health maintenance service.

### Surveillance

The frequency of periodic assessments may be based upon the age and health status of each employee. Some companies provide periodic assessments to those over 40 and/or to employees with long seniority. The longer an employee stays with a company, the greater the investment that company has in him. An example of this type of assessment is the "executive physical," which is a complete examination provided for top management personnel at work or at an outside facility at company expense.

### Mental health services

Companies may provide special components such as mental health, alcoholism, and drug abuse services in their occupational health programs. The latter services may be called "employee assistance programs" to minimize stigma. The National Institute on Alcohol Abuse and Alcoholism estimates that 10% of the employed work force are alcoholics. This poses a serious problem in efficiency and absenteeism for management. Alcoholism and drug abuse have been of such concern in some companies that the companies require new applicants to consent to an alcohol and drug screening as part of the PPE.

Psychosocial problems may interfere with a worker's productivity to a greater extent than physical illness may. Acknowledging this, some employers hire a part-time or full-time mental health staff. This may consist of a psychiatrist, a psychologist, and/or a psychiatric mental health nurse clinician. IBM has found that group therapy and family therapy provided on site are two services in high demand by their employees.

*The environmental survey*

The environmental conditions that affect worker health and safety are monitored by the industrial hygienist. The industrial hygienist does this by conducting evaluative surveys of the work site and subsequent samplings of the work environment. The survey includes a review of all raw materials, products and by-products, sources of air contaminants, types of physical agents used, and control measures in use (Brief, 1975). Sampling is done with a variety of instruments at the breathing zone of the worker, in the generalized breathing space of the room, and at the site of particular operations. For the major contaminants, there are standards for permissable levels, which are known as "threshold limit values."

The nurse will be collaboratively involved with the industrial hygienist and will use his data and recommendations to provide care to employees. The nurse can play a vital role by incorporating safety teaching and encouraging the use of personal protective equipment (ear plugs, safety glasses, and hard hats) when she counsels well, injured, or ill employees. The nurse may need to interpret company policy here as well.

Although all occupational health nurses should be aware of factors in the workplace that endanger the health and safety of employees, this information becomes especially important to the professional who operates a one-nurse unit in small plants. A technique employed to gather such information is termed the "walk-through survey," a periodic on-site visit to the workplace. Tinkham (1972) and Serafini (1976) have developed tools to assist the nurse in this task.

All of the above services must be carefully documented in the occupational health unit's records. Establishment of a record system that is easy to use, accurate, and useful for surveillance and epidemiological studies is a primary objective of an occupational health program. An OSHA regulation guarantees that employees have the right of access to their individual and exposure records. Retention of health records for 30 or more years is required, and larger firms are employing electronic data systems to store health information.

## Conclusion

Thus far, we have considered the health needs of the young adult population, usually a well group of individuals. Two sites for health care of this population have been included. The clinic setting has been described as either official, private, or voluntary. Health care at the workplace has been presented as a unique service that draws upon general community health theory and practice.

The nurse has essentially the same role with most young adults, regardless of the specific type of setting. Occasionally a young adult receives the services of a CHN at his home. The care for a client with CHD is described next, because specific disease prevention related to life style during the young adult years is crucial. Home care and clinic care for CHD are also discussed.

## Coronary Heart Disease: Prevention in the Young Adult Years Can Help

### Introduction to Coronary Heart Disease

CHD is the principal cause of death in the United States, and the third cause for this age group. The underlying causative factor, atherosclerosis, accounts for approximately half the deaths in the Western world. Although the client with CHD is usually over 40, he may be in his early 30s or even 20s. More important, the life style habits that contribute most heavily to CHD in later years are formed during young adulthood. Therefore, prevention of the risk factors during the young adult years is essential in order to decrease the incidence of this disease. Treatment and rehabilitation of CHD are included in this chapter to increase continuity for the readers. CHNs frequently give home care to those who survive an acute attack of CHD (Health Services Administration, 1977; Kannel & Dawber, 1972).

### Etiology

CHD is caused by a narrowing of coronary arteries, resulting in a reduced blood supply to the myocardium. Figure 7-1 is a schematic drawing of a normal heart, detailing the myocardium and coronary arteries; the inset shows the most common sites of myocardial infarction (MI). In most cases, the narrowing of the arterial lumen or obstruction of it is caused by atherosclerosis. Atherosclerosis is a form of arteriosclerosis with localized accumulation of lipid-containing material in the blood vessels. As this condition develops, fatty deposits of mostly cholesterol collect in plaques in the arterial walls, causing them to become calcified and thickened, and to lose elasticity. This can cause angina pectoris, a temporary anorexia of the myocardium, or a complete loss of blood supply to the myocardium, as in MI (Beeson & McDermott, 1975).

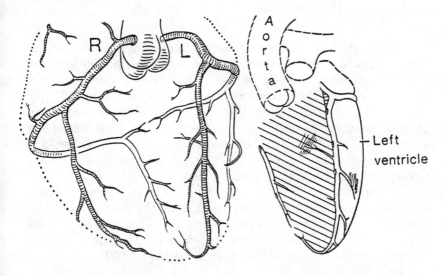

Figure 7.1.   Schematic drawing of the heart with the right and left coronary arteries and their branches. Inset shows left ventricle and intraventricular septum, which are common sites for acute MIs. (Artist: Barbara Gould, Manager of the Biomedical Illustration Department, Medical Center, West Virginia University, Morgantown, West Virginia.)

The onset of an MI is characterized by precordial pain, more intense than angina pectoris, with changes in an EKG and a rise in certain serum enzymes. An infarct (necrosis) develops in the myocardium, usually the result of ischemia (lack of blood supply) following occlusion of a coronary artery.

## Morbidity and Mortality Statistics

### *Morbidity*

The incidence of CHD is extremely high. Each year there are about three-quarters of a million (750,000–800,000) new cases, and at least another 500,000 repeat attacks. Therefore, the total yearly incidence is approximately 1.25 to 1.3 million.

Adding those who survive from the above total to the existing cases, one arrives at the estimated prevalence, the total living with CHD, which is about 4 million Americans (Thom, 1980).

*Mortality*

Although there has been a decline in the death rate from CHD in the past decade, it is still the main cause of death in the United States. The 1978 estimated mortality rate for CHD, based on a 10% sample of all death certificates in the nation (641,140 deaths), was 294 per 100,000 (Thom, 1980). Table 7-2 shows that CHD, also called "ischemic heart disease," is by far the largest single cause of cardiac death. About 90% of the mortality from all forms of heart disease is still attributed to ischemic heart disease (Health Services Administration, 1977; National Center for Health Statistics, 1982).

One-half of the deaths from CHD in initial or recurrent attacks are sudden, with another one-sixth termed early deaths (i.e., death occurs in the first 1 to 6 hours). Only about one-third of those who die from CHD ever reach the hospital; therefore, the first few minutes or hours are critical for survival (Kannel & Dawber, 1972).

*Females and coronary heart disease*

There is a substantial sex difference in the incidence of MIs, as demonstrated clearly by an analysis of data from 110,000 men and women aged 25 to 64 in New York City (Weinblatt, Shapiro, & Frank,

Table 7-2
Selected Death Rates From Heart Disease in the United States,
1972 and 1981 (Rates per 100,000 Population)

|  | 1972 | 1981 |
|---|---|---|
| Diseases of the Heart | 363.0 | 331.7 |
| Ischemic Heart Disease | 328.7 | 244.9 |
| Acute Myocardial Infarction (MI) | 171.9 | 128.3 |
| Other Acute and Subacute Forms of Ischemic Heart Disease | 2.2 | 1.8 |
| Old MIs and Other Forms of Chronic Ischemic Heart Disease | 154.6 | 114.5 |
| Angina Pectoris | 0.1 | 0.2 |

*Note.* The statistics in this table are drawn from Health Services Administration, *Vital Statistics of the United States, 1968–1973* (Vol. 2, *Mortality*) (Washington, D.C.: U.S. Department of Health, Education and Welfare, 1977); and National Center for Health Statistics, *Monthly Vital Statistics Report* (Vol. 80, No. 12) (Washington, D.C.: U.S. Department of Health and Human Services, 1982).

1973). For these adults under 65 with a first MI, the frequency was five times greater for men. These clients had been enrolled for at least 2 years in a prepaid comprehensive group practice, the Health Insurance Plan of Greater New York. On the other hand, the rates for both sexes have been found to increase markedly with age (Kannel & Gordon, 1974). The rate doubled for both sexes between the ages of 55 and 64; after 64, while the rate continued to double for males, there was a sevenfold increase for women.

There is a new problem for younger women, however. Evidence linking MI with oral contraceptives is convincing. A sizable study (Mann, Vessey, Thorogood, & Doll, 1975) based on a rough estimate of women hospitalized with MIs in two of the 15 hospital regions in England and Wales showed a 5.6 rate per 100,000 married women aged 30–39 who were on oral contraceptives, as opposed to a rate of only 2.1 for those not on "the Pill." In the next age group (40–44), the incidence increased to 9.9 for those using the pill. It appears that if one or more of the major risk factors (elevated blood cholesterol, hypertension, and smoking) is present in conjunction with the use of oral contraceptives, there is an increase in MIs (Oliver, 1974).

The overall decrease in CHD deaths in the United States parallels a general decline in every major cause of death except cancer and accidents from poisonings and violence. The age-adjusted death rate for all causes in 1976 was the lowest ever recorded. Speculative reasons for this overall decline in deaths include the following: no major influenza epidemic since 1968; life style changes, such as eating less fat, weight watching, exercising, and curbing smoking; and increased treatment of asymptomatic hypertension (Kannel & Gordon, 1978).

## Risk Factors

Strong evidence that specific variables (hypertension, hypercholesterolemia, obesity, cigarette smoking, and lack of exercise) introduce risk factors for CHD was established by the 20-year longitudinal epidemiological study of heart disease begun in Framingham, Massachusetts, in 1948, which studied 5209 men and women aged 30–62. Therefore, general hygienic measures indicated for the prevention of CHD are (1) stopping the cigarette habit, (2) reducing weight, (3) changing diet, and (4) exercising more. MIs develop twice as often in smokers as in nonsmokers. A diet low in calories is the key to weight control, and restriction of fats is an efficient way to accomplish this. Physical activity not only makes an MI less likely, but reduces the chances of a lethal outcome should there be one (Kannel & Gordon, 1974). Attention to these four specific risk factors, which are characteristics of life style, is particularly important in order for young adults to avoid CHD in young and older adulthood.

### Prevention at Places of Employment or in Neighborhood Groups

Measures for the prevention of heart attacks are necessary both for persons who have had one or more attacks and those who have had none. Preventive measures in industry are usually conducted by occupational health nurses or health educators. Industrial programs like the Kimberly-Clark health management program are directed at prevention of such diseases as atherosclerosis and hypertension. The programs include physical fitness, nutrition instruction, weight control, and smoking cessation; facilities for the programs are equipped with Olympic-size swimming pools, indoor and outdoor jogging tracks, and exercise equipment. Many companies have similar programs.

Group classes in a community setting or teaching via public television and radio are other avenues to promote prevention of heart diseases. The classes should discuss the above risk factors for MIs and ways to reduce them. Good nutrition can be taught by using the four-group food plan with visual aids from the National Dairy Council, which can be supplemented by describing foods low and high in cholesterol. The young adult can be a victim of American dietary habits—"fast" foods, convenience foods, fatty meats, refined sugars, pastries, and salty foods. These contribute to CHD because they can increase the blood cholesterol level, contribute to hypertension, and cause obesity.

The nature and amount of exercise could be patterned after Cooper's (1970) aerobics exercise research. Aerobic exercises are the foundation on which most exercise programs should be built, because they strengthen the muscles of respiration, increase the pumping efficiency of the heart, and tone up arteries and muscles. In short, they increase the body's capability for oxygen utilization, and consequently the person's physical endurance. A feeling of well-being also results. Examples of good aerobic exercises are jogging or running, swimming, cycling, and playing handball. Physical education in the school years emphasizes team activities that are often not possible after graduation. A young adult needs physical activities he can engage in alone as well as with others.

Prevention and self-care are preferable to medical care in saving lives. Research by Belloc and Breslow (1972) has shown that life expectancy and better health are significantly related to a number of simple basic health habits. These include the following:

1. Eat breakfast almost every day.
2. Eat between meals only occasionally.
3. Moderate weight.
4. Moderate exercise (long walks, bike riding, swimming, gardening) two to three times weekly.
5. Adequate sleep (7 to 8 hours a night).
6. No smoking.
7. No alcohol, or only in moderation.

Specifically, these researchers found that the physical health status of those who reported following all seven good health practices was consistently about the same as that of people 30 years younger who followed only one or two of these practices. Living a long and healthy life appears to be greatly influenced by one's life style and motivation for self-care.

## Management of a Client with a Myocardial Infarction at Home and in the Clinic

After a stay in the coronary care unit of 2 to 5 days and in a medical ward of a general hospital of 2 to 4 weeks, the MI patient is discharged to his home. The damaged heart muscle heals in 21 to 28 days (Phibbs, 1979). If the heart attack has been uncomplicated—that is, with no arrhythmias—the patient is discharged in about 2 weeks. If it has been complicated, the discharge is usually made 3 to 6 weeks after the onset. The referral to the CHN from the hospital should supply medical details for his care during the first few weeks at home.

### Physical and psychological factors

Discharge instructions should be written prior to discharge and should include recommendations for medication, diet, weight control, smoking, rest, exercise, recreation, sex, visits to the clinic or the private medical doctor, and the return to work and/or normal daily living. Psychological counseling may also be warranted. The treatment recommended when the client leaves the hospital varies with the severity of the attack, the physical condition and life style of the client, and the physician's preferences. Inasmuch as the healing process for the myocardial necrosis is usually complete in 6 weeks, care at home is directed toward rehabilitation of the heart muscle to a level of optimal functioning. After hospital discharge, the patient may experience problems of a physical nature, including angina and early congestive failure symptoms, and signs such as arrhythmias, elevated blood pressures, dyspnea, or syncope. Measures to decrease dyspnea, fatigue, and pain include the use of rest periods and medication (MacIntyre & Haywood, 1975).

Psychological manifestations such as exhaustion, insomnia, irritability, loss of powers of concentration and memory, and weepiness can further compound the existing physical problems. Post-MI depression is a reality for many patients, especially for those who are over 50 years of age and suffering a second MI. The attack itself is terrifying, and the patients may fear death. Later a patient may remark, "You know I was clinically dead," when describing the doctor's rushing in to save him.

Other emotional problems may arise when the client experiences angina pain following an MI. The CHN should explain that an angina attack is not damaging, that it is not another MI, and that it can be relieved by medication. The absence of a definite exercise or activity program after the initial phase of treatment can contribute to anxiety, as can uncertainty about returning to work. Family difficulties can arise from factors such as reductions in energy, libido, and income.

Research studies differ in their conclusions about the effect of a patient's reluctance to admit the physical problems and discuss them. One study (MacIntyre & Haywood, 1975) indicated that those who deny their problems have a greater mortality rate after hospital discharge; but another (Gentry & Haney, 1975) suggested that such denial may be a helpful coping mechanism, increasing the years of life remaining. All things considered, it would appear to be useful for the CHN to assist the client in verbalizing feelings and thoughts concerning the illness and anticipated outcomes. She should also provide specific information about the condition, in order to enhance the formation of realistic expectations concerning the physical condition and rehabilitation process.

### Medical regimen and self-care

*Medication.*   Medications vary greatly among physicians, and depend upon the extent of the infarct, complications such as cardiac failure, and the patient's age. Medications and their actions are discussed in a later section.

*Diet and weight control.*   Weight reduction is usually needed after the first MI, so a 1200- to 1500-calorie diet is often prescribed until optimal weight has been achieved. Dietary cholesterol should be reduced to less than 200–300 mg daily. It is desirable to have patients 15–20% below their pre-MI weight. The client must be involved in the decisions about his diet and weight control, so that he can understand and follow the guidelines (Jain, 1978).

*Smoking.* Smoking is prohibited, because cigarettes introduce nicotine and carbon monoxide (from inhaling), and cigars and pipes also contain nicotine. Nicotine-caused atherosclerosis of the coronary arteries will not progress if smoking is stopped. Though smoking is prohibited, many clients will not stop unless self-motivated to do so. The CHN and their families should assist and encourage them.

*Rest, exercise, and activities of daily living.* Daily rest periods are recommended after hospital discharge and even sometimes after the return to work. The client may have particular exercises that are preferred over others, and these should be considered in the discussion. The following is a list of recommended exercises and activities of daily living after hospital discharge (Flink, 1977; Jain, 1978):

*First week* (these instructions are similar to those for the client's last week in the hospital):

1. Stay at home.
2. Walk on the level—no stairs.
3. Take showers instead of tub baths.
4. Avoid strenuous exertion such as heavy lifting, sexual intercourse, or swimming.

*After 2 weeks:*

1. Can use stairs.
2. Can go outside, even drive a car, if accompanied by someone. Recommended: automatic shift, power steering, and short drives of no more than 10–15 miles.

*After 1 month:*

1. Can begin to increase daily walks gradually to the 4 miles noted below.
2. Can engage in sexual intercourse as the passive partner, but it must be geared to dyspnea, pain, and fatigue, and limited if angina pectoris is present.

*After 2 to 3 months:*

1. Can walk 4 miles.
2. Can usually practice sexual intercourse actively.

*After 6 months:*

1. Can walk, swim, or shovel snow, but should avoid undue fatigue or exposure to hot or cold weather.

*Home nursing care for a client
with a myocardial infarction*

Community health nursing care of the MI patient should begin before hospital discharge. The medical orders as outlined above should be explained to the patient, and he should be allowed to ask questions. The exercise program should begin with physical therapy at the hospital. A referral to the local visiting nurse association or health department should be made prior to hospital discharge; the initial referral should be done by telephone and confirmed in writing. Occasionally a CHN works in the hospital and serves as a coordinator for referrals, or the home care department of a hospital can do it. The Intake Record of the District of Columbia Visiting Nurse Association may be used by the CHN to record information telephoned in by a hospital, doctor, or another source. It includes identifying demographic data, diagnoses, medical orders, and other data. It is distributed by computer to the appropriate office in the city.

As soon as the patient arrives home, a nursing visit should be planned in order to assess the care to be given. The assessment of client care should include an examination of these factors: (1) the home environment; (2) medical orders; (3) medication; (4) diet; (5) rest, exercise, and activities of daily living; (6) plans for visits to the clinic or physician's office; and (7) plans for the return to work. Implementation and evaluation of the nursing care follow assessment.

*Assessment of client care.*

THE HOME ENVIRONMENT.   Assessment of the physical and psychological home environment is essential, because the environment has a great influence on the patient's recovery. If the client is a male and his wife works, a homemaker may be needed temporarily by the family; financial worry may be reduced if the wife is employed, however. If the client lives alone, Meals on Wheels may be needed. In a multistory, walk-up apartment, it may be necessary to ask a neighbor to bring mail from a first-floor box. A visit to the home by a professional health worker can assess the impact of the home situation and family dynamics on the recovery process. Psychologically supportive family members, neighbors, and friends are invaluable to the patient's progress.

MEDICAL ORDERS.   The medical orders are supervised by the CHN. On her first visit to the home she ascertains the client's understanding of them, reviewing them in detail. The family should be involved in this review, because they can often assist the client in his recovery. When a client and his family fully comprehend the orders and the reasons for them, client acceptance is much higher. Clients frequently question such items as medication, diet, and the amount of exercise and activity permitted. Occasionally instructions are omitted, such as what to do for the insomnia that often accompanies the anxiety of returning home after several weeks in the protected hospital environment.

Although the medical orders may be very detailed upon discharge, they may still be very unrealistic for the home, omit important elements, or cover an insufficient period of time. The CHN can be very instrumental in insuring that the plan is comprehensive enough for a particular client and fits the home setting. For example, she may need to telephone the physician to work out alternate plans of care based on the nursing assessment. The nurse's continued encouragement to the client and family is essential for recovery.

MEDICATION. The nurse should check that the client has prescriptions in the correct dosage, that he and/or his family can read and understand the instructions, and that the importance of taking them and the actions of the drugs (both positive and untoward) are understood. The CHN should also find out what other medications are taken, in order to encourage that they be taken or to check for negative synergistic effects. She must keep abreast of new medications for the client with an MI. The posthospital medications prescribed depend upon the extent of the MI, and the ones described here are those usually ordered.

If arrhythmias are experienced, procainamide hydrochloride (Pronestyl), quinidine sulfate (trade name identical), or propranolol (Inderal) are ordered. Because propranolol can cause difficulties in breathing, such as wheezing, it is not ordered for asthmatics. Calcium channel blockers, verapamil (Isoptin or Calan) and nifedipine (Procardia), are new drugs for ischemic heart disease. They have widespread use as antiarrhythmic agents, antianginal agents, or for coronary artery spasm. These drugs are nor equivalent in their clinical effects and must be selected accordingly (Zeldes & Verme, 1982). A pharmacological reference should be consulted for further information.

If angina pectoris is present, a rapidly acting nitrate such as nitroglycerin is administered sublingually immediately to terminate an acute attack. Nitroglycerin Systems (available in bandage form) can also be applied to any skin site (other than the distal parts of extremities) that is free of hair (a site may need to be shaved) and that is not subject to excessive movement; anginal symptoms can thus be relieved in 30 minutes. Unlike topical nitroglycerin, Nitroglycerin Systems deliver a premeasured drug dose at a steady rate for 24 hours and avoid the messiness of ointment ("New Drugs—Drug News: Transdermal Nitroglycerin Systems," 1982). Nitroglycerin improves blood flow to the ischemic areas in the myocardium by dilating coronary vessels. A momentary frontal headache and/or hypotensive episode is a manifestation that the drug is working—that is, that blood vessels have dilated. The headache also can indicate that the medicine is fresh. The patient and family and the CHN should be aware of this action, so that the drug is not discontinued.

The superiority of long-acting nitrates such as isosorbide dinitrate (Isordil) or pentaerythritol tetranitrate (Peritrate) over the rapidly acting nitrates has not been definitely established.

If congestive heart failure is present with an MI, digitalis and diuretics are ordered. Digitalis increases the efficiency of the heart muscle by increasing the speed and force of contraction. Digitalis intoxication from overdosage or depletion can cause nausea, vomiting, and life-threatening arrhythmias; this intoxication can occur because the difference between the therapeutic and toxic level is small. Moderate toxicity is manifested by nausea and vomiting, headache, and malaise; severe toxicity is signified by diarrhea, blurring of vision, and disorientation. Diuretics such as hydrothiazide hydrochloride (Hydrodiuril) are ordered to reduce salt and water retention. Because these agents not only increase renal excretion of salt and body fluid, but other electrolytes as well, replacement potassium is necessary to maintain the acid-base balance (and, additionally, to prevent digitalis toxicity).

The antianxiety effect of tranquilizers such as diazepam (Valium) is well established. The MI client sometimes uses these for sedation at bedtime. However, the patient should alter his life style and slow his pace, because of the danger of developing a dependency on this class of drugs. Because there is an association between MIs and hypertension (about one-fifth of MIs have hypertension), hypotensive drugs may also be given (Goth, 1976; Jacknowitz, 1982).

DIET COUNSELING AND WEIGHT CONTROL. The diet is one element of treatment that should be tailored to the home setting. In the hospital, the patient is instructed in a calorie reduction diet, with foods low in cholesterol and sometimes also low in sodium. When he arrives home, these instructions should be reinforced. He may have forgotten them, or perhaps he cannot read the written diet sent home with him. The client should be helped to understand why the objectives are a diet low in saturated fat and possibly restricted in sodium.

Diet counseling should begin with an inquiry into what the client is accustomed to eat and who cooks his meals, and an explanation of written guides sent home with him, using pictures if necessary to show kinds and amounts. All MI clients should be given a list of foods to avoid, such as those high in saturated fats and cholesterol. A discussion of food preparation is also in order, because an egg fried in butter, for example, has much more saturated fat than a soft-boiled one. If the client's wife buys the groceries and cooks his meals, she should be included in the discussion. If she works, the CHN may have to visit the home when she is there.

If the diet is for a specific amount of calorie reduction, the prescription should be taught to the client and his family. It would include a breakdown of the calories into specified grams of fat, protein and carbohydrates. For a typical 1500-calorie diet, the breakdown might read thus: carbohydrates 150 grams, protein 70 grams, and fat 70 grams. The nurse can then use the diabetic exchange lists.

If the client has been told to lose weight and no particular number of calories has been specified, the CHN can discuss the following general instructions for weight reduction. These are based on the four-group food plan, plus preparation and control of saturated fats (University of Iowa Department of Nutrition, 1973; West Virginia Medical Center Dietetic Department, 1978; Williams, 1981).

| *Foods to Use* | *Their Preparation* |
|---|---|
| A. Milk and dairy products | 1. Use low-fat or skimmed milk in place of whole milk. |
| B. Meat, poultry, fish, and eggs | 2. Luncheon meats are extremely fatty and should be avoided. Prime cuts have more marbling. Trim fat from meat before cooking. Do not bread or flour, and omit added fat in cooking. Use cooking methods that help to remove fat, such as baking, broiling, roasting, boiling, and stewing. |
| | 3. Poach or boil eggs; do not fry. If eggs are scrambled, |

add only a very little unsaturated cooking oil or
margarine. Teflon pans require no cooking oil.

C. Vegetables and fruit

4. Cook vegetables with no
added fat, salt pork, or
bacon. Omit cooking or
stewing vegetables in butter, sauces, or breading.
Do not add butter or other
fats after cooking. Eat raw
vegetables as desired.
When raw vegetables are
used as salads, use vinegar
or lemon juice as dressing
instead of French dressing,
oil-based salad dressing, or
mayonnaise.

5. Prepare potatoes baked,
boiled or mashed. Eat
skins of potatoes. Do not
fry. When preparing
mashed potatoes, use skim
milk, no butter. Omit
French fries, potato chips,
corn curls, and corn chips.

6. Use fresh fruit and fresh or
frozen juice. Fruits should
replace cake, cookies, pies,
and sweetened gelatin for
desserts. With pudding,
sherbet, and ice cream, use
small amounts, such as ½
cup.

D. Breads and cereals

7. Use no more than three (3)
slices of bread each day.
Use only ½ teaspoon of
polyunsaturated margarine
per slice. Do not use jelly,
jam, marmalade, or honey
on your bread.

8. Use skim milk on cereal, no sugar. Artificial sweeteners are permitted.

E. Miscellaneous

9. Use no more than 2 teaspoons of polyunsaturated margarine each day, or 4 teaspoons of one of the new diet margarines if it is polyunsaturated. This includes margarine used in cooking.
10. Count calories in beverages and all drinks except sugar-free beverages.
11. Alcohol tends to increase fat levels in the body, contains many calories, and has little nutritive value, so keep use to a minimum.
12. You may have unlimited amounts of the following foods and beverages: raw vegetables, decaffeinated coffee, lemon or vinegar, spices and herbs, unsweetened gelatin, and artificial sweeteners.

All persons, but particularly those with an elevated blood cholesterol and MI clients, should control cholesterol in their diets. To control intake of saturated fat, the client should follow these guidelines for the milk and meat food groups, in addition to those above (University of Iowa Department of Nutrition, 1973; West Virginia Medical Center Dietetic Department, 1978; Williams, 1981):

A. Milk and dairy products

1. Use skimmed milk cheeses. Yogurt is acceptable.

B. Meat, poultry, fish, and eggs

2. Select veal, chicken, turkey, and fish, and limit your use of beef, pork, and lamb.

3. Eat only two (2) egg yolks per week. Shell fish or organ meats such as liver or brains can be substituted occasionally for an egg yolk.

C. Miscellaneous

4. Instead of butter and hydrogenated fats, use liquid oils and soft margarine that contain polyunsaturates.

Weight control follows naturally from diet control and is accomplished with a calorie reduction diet. Obesity continues to be a risk factor for a repeat attack. It may be necessary to go to a lower-calorie diet, such as a 1200- to 1800-calorie diet, which then must be adjusted as the client continues to lose weight.

Sodium restriction is usually ordered if heart failure has complicated the MI. Booklets on sodium restriction, which can be obtained from the American Heart Association with a doctor's order, are excellent guides for both nurse and patient to follow. *The American Heart Association Cookbook* (Eshelman & Winston, 1977) is also good for patient use.

REST, EXERCISE, AND ACTIVITIES OF DAILY LIVING. Suggestions for proper rest, exercise, and daily activities have been outlined earlier. They will require adjustment as the client makes progress. Although a physical therapist does not usually visit the home, the nurse may consult with one regarding the exercise regimen. The CHN assists the client with the exercises on each home visit.

COORDINATION WITH CLINIC OR PHYSICIAN'S OFFICE. If he experiences no arrhythmias, the patient returns to see the doctor in one month. If arrhythmias return, he goes sooner, perhaps in 1 week. Later the visits are made monthly or bimonthly, decreasing to semiannually (Flink, 1977). Most visits to a busy doctor are brief, with little teaching or counseling being done. When a CHN visits the home, she should help prepare the client for his clinic visit by suggesting he write down exactly what he wants to talk to the physician about, such as the frequency with which he should take his nitroglycerin. On his first return visit there is usually adjustment in medication, diet, and/or exercise. If he has not returned to work, plans are usually made for this.

The CHN should write a brief note to the physician about the client's follow-up at home, including such items as his vital signs and the presence of dyspnea or pain, and recommending changes in his existing medical orders if these are indicated. This procedure assists the clinic in planning for the patient, and it is a readily available way to renew medical orders. It has the added advantage of providing current professional information on the day the client is seen in the clinic. The client usually delivers the form to the clinic. He can also return it to the CHN, or the clinic can mail it to the nursing agency.

RETURNING TO WORK. A gradual return to normal functioning is recommended. If the patient has been in a sedentary job, such as banking, he can return to work in 6 to 8 weeks. But if his work involves heavy labor or strain, such as mining or truck driving, retraining for another job can be done through the local department of vocational rehabilitation (Jain, 1978).

*Implementation of client care.* Implementation follows each step as outlined above in "Assessment of Patient Care." If an adjustment in the home environment is needed, such as the hiring of a temporary homemaker, the CHN may assist the family in arranging this. A telephone call may also be needed to the physician to adjust or supplement the medical orders. Diet teaching may be required on several of the CHN's visits before it is sufficiently understood by the patient.

A client's family is an important factor in his recovery. Family members must understand the essentials of his care, such as the required rest and exercise, so that they do not do too little or too much for him. A family member may be urged to quit smoking along with the patient to motivate him to stop.

Psychological or vocational counseling is often necessary during the convalescence of the MI patient. A portion of each home visit is usually spent in counseling the client and family about any psychological problems that arise. The MI may well have been caused initially by stress. In addition to his preillness stress, the client at home now worries about his prospects of getting well. He wonders whether he can return to work, how his fellow workers will regard him, whether he will have another attack, and how he can remove some of the stresses that existed before the attack. Petrowski has often cited to clients the example of Lyndon Johnson, who had a massive coronary attack in 1955 and subsequently assumed the Presidency, as encouragement to get well and return to work.

Referral to a department of vocational rehabilitation for job retraining may be required. Vocational rehabilitation services, which are available to every citizen, are supported by the Rehabilitation Services Administration in the DHHS's Office of Human Development. If an MI patient is too handicapped to return to his past employment, he can qualify for job retraining with a vocational rehabilitation office in his city or county.

And, finally, a patient's perception of his recovery is absolutely essential in planning for his return to normal living.

*Evaluation of client care.* Evaluation of the client's convalescence basically comprises evaluation of the degree of his compliance with medical and nursing orders and the rate and degree of recovery as perceived by the patient, his family, and the nurse and physician.

An innovation useful in evaluation is a written contract covering the patient's care or treatment, set up between the patient and the CHN. It includes the patient's compliance with medical and nursing orders, the patient and family's participation, and the CHN's accountability. The contract states what is expected of the CHN and the patient; it sets a time limit for actions and a termination date for the CHN's visits. It may prescribe the patient's exercises, including walking on the level and stairs, going outdoors, and aerobic exercises. It can include a possible date for return to partial or full employment or for referral to vocational rehabilitation. A copy is given to the patient, and another is kept in the patient's record (Ossler, 1976).

# References

American Association of Occupational Health Nurses. *Guide for the development of functions and responsibilities in occupational health nursing.* New York: Author, 1976.

American Medical Association. *Scope, objectives and functions of occupational health programs.* Chicago: Author, 1971.

American Nurses' Association and U.S. Department of Health, Education and Welfare. *1977 national sample survey of RNs: A report on the nurse population and factors affecting their supply.* Washington, D.C.: Authors, 1979.

Bates, B. Nursing in a health maintenance organization: Report on the Harvard Commission Health Plan. *American Journal of Public Health,* 1972, 7, 991–993.

Beeson, B., & McDermott, W. *Textbook of medicine.* Philadelphia: W. B. Saunders, 1975.

Belloc, N. B., & Breslow, L. Relationship of physical health status and health practices. *Preventive Medicine,* 1972, 1, 409–442.

Bernhardt, J. H. Anticipated benefits from an effective occupational health program. *Occupational Health Nursing,* 1976, 24, 9–14.

Bernhardt, J. H. Personal communication, March 16, 1982.

Brief, R. S. *Basic industrial hygiene.* New York: Exxon Corporation, 1975.

Cooper, K. H. *The new aerobics.* New York: Bantam, 1970.

Diekelmann, N. *Primary health care of the well adult.* New York: McGraw-Hill, 1977.

Dolinsky, E. M. Health maintenance organization and occupational medicine. *Bulletin of the New York Academy of Medicine,* 1974, *50,* 1126.

Erikson, E. *Identity: Youth and crisis.* New York: Norton, 1968.

Eshelman, R., & Winston, M. *The American Heart Association cookbook.* New York: Ballantine, 1977.

Fielding, J. E. Preventive medicine and the bottom line. *Journal of Occupational Medicine,* 1979, *21,* 79–88.

Flink, E. Personal communication, April 26, 1977.

Gentry, W. D., & Haney, T. Emotional and behavioral reaction to acute myocardial infarction. *Heart and Lung,* 1975, *4,* 738–744.

Gordon, J. B., Akman, A., & Brooks, M. L. *Industrial safety statistics—A reexamination: A critical report prepared for the Department of Labor.* New York: Praeger, 1971.

Goth, A. *Medical pharmacology: Principles and concepts.* St. Louis: C. V. Mosby, 1976.

Health Maintenance Organization Act of 1973 (PL 93-222, S. 14). Washington, D.C.: U.S. Government Printing Office, 1974.

Health Services Administration. *Vital statistics of the United States, 1968–1973* (Vol. 2, *Mortality*). Washington, D.C.: U.S. Department of Health, Education and Welfare, 1977.

Hricko, A., & Brunt, M. *Working for your life: A woman's guide to job health hazards.* Berkeley, Calif.: Labor Occupational Health Program/Health Research Group, 1976.

Jacknowitz, A. Personal communication, August 3, 1982.

Jain, A. Personal communication, January 27, 1978.

Kannel, W. B., & Dawber, T. R. Contributions to coronary risk implications for prevention and public health: The Framingham Study. *Heart and Lung,* 1972, *1,* 797.

Kannel, W. B., & Gordon, T. (Eds.). *The Framingham Study: An epidemiological investigation of cardiovascular disease* (DHEW (NIH) Publ. No. 74-599). Washington, D.C.: U.S. Department of Health, Education and Welfare, 1974.

Kannel, W. B., & Gordon, T. Recent decline in fatal heart attacks: What caused it? *Primary Cardiology,* 1978, *4,* 10–12.

Kimberly-Clark health management program aimed at prevention. *Occupational Health and Safety,* 1977, *46,* 25–27.

Lee, J. *The new nurse in industry: A guide for the newly employed occupational health nurse* (DHEW (NIOSH) Publ. No. 78-143). Cincinnati: National Institute for Occupational Safety and Health, 1978.

MacIntyre, L. J., & Haywood, L. J. Survival factors following myocardial infarction recorded by a nurse. *Heart and Lung*, 1975, 4, 23–26.

Mann, J. J., Vessey, M. P., Thorogood, M., & Doll, R. Myocardial infarction in young women, with special reference to oral contraceptive practice. *British Medical Journal*, 1975, 12, 242.

National Center for Health Statistics. *Facts of life and death*. Washington, D.C.: U.S. Department of Health, Education and Welfare, 1978. (a)

National Center for Health Statistics. *Health United States, 1978*. Washington, D.C.: U.S. Department of Health, Education and Welfare, 1978. (b)

National Center for Health Statistics. *Monthly vital statistics report* (Vol. 30, No. 12). Washington, D.C.: U.S. Department of Health and Human Services, 1982.

New Drugs—Drug News: Transdermal nitroglycerin systems. *Drug Therapy*, January 1982, pp. 35 and 39.

1975 National Conference on Preventive Medicine. *Preventive Medicine U.S.A.* New York: Prodist, 1976.

*Occupational Safety and Health Act of 1970* (PL 91-596, S. 2193). Washington, D.C.: U.S. Government Printing Office, 1971.

Oliver, M. F. Ischemic heart disease in women. *British Medical Journal*, 1974, 4, 253–259.

Ossler, C. C. *Written nurse-client contracts: Assessment of satisfaction with nursing care in a community health setting*. Unpublished master's thesis, The Catholic University of America, 1976.

Phibbs, B. *The human heart—A guide to heart disease*. St. Louis: C. V. Mosby, 1979.

Plant, J. Small firms look to hospitals for occupational services. *Hospitals*, 1978, 52, 135–137.

Ralston, G. Keeping the small plant healthy. *Ohio's Health*, 1973, 25, 9–12.

Serafini, P. Nursing assessment in industry. *American Journal of Public Health*, 1976, 66, 755–760.

Smith, D. E. *Informal discussion of work in the areas of alcohol and drug abuse in Haight-Ashbury*. Talk presented at the Alcohol and Drug Awareness Forum, Milwaukee Alcoholism Council, Milwaukee, March 19, 1981.

Stellman, J. M., & Daum, S. *Work is dangerous to your health*. New York: Random House, 1973.

Strasser, A. L. Preplacement screening: An exercise in preventive medicine. *Occupational Health and Safety*, 1979, 48, 23–24.

Thom, T. Personal communication, April 11, 1980.

Tinkham, C. W. The plant as the patient of the occupational health nurse. *Nursing Clinics of North America*, 1972, 7, 99–107.

U.S. Department of Health, Education and Welfare. *Environmental health problems*. Washington, D.C.: U.S. Government Printing Office, 1976.

University of Iowa Department of Nutrition. *Recent advances in therapeutic diets* (2nd ed.). Iowa City: The University of Iowa Press, 1973, pp. 68–76.

Weinblatt, E., Shapiro, S., & Frank, C. Prognosis of women with newly diagnosed coronary heart disease: A comparison with course of disease among men. *American Journal of Public Health*, 1973, *63*, 577–578.

West Virginia Medical Center Dietetic Department, Morgantown, West Virginia. Printed instructions for coronary patients upon discharge. Unpublished material, 1978.

Williams, S. R. Nutrition and diet therapy (4th ed.). St. Louis: C. V. Mosby, 1981.

Zeldes, G., & Verme, C. Calcium channel blockers. *Pharmacy Newsletter for Physicians*, 1982, *13*, 1–3.

# 8

# The Middle Years

*Dorothy D. Petrowski*

## Introduction

A common understanding of "middle age" is that time span between the ending of the younger adult years at about age 40 and the beginning of old age at about 65; it is the period of full maturity, and for many the peak of their working careers. This chapter sees "middle age" as those years when a person generally has reached fulfillment in major areas: human relationships, employment, avocation, community involvement, and spiritual matters. It is usually the most productive period of one's life. For example, a middle-aged worker may be selected to perform a difficult task because he has the necessary experience. Most middle-aged persons have lived enough years to understand life, but still have many years to look forward to. Some may experience a lessening of physical powers and/or the beginning of some chronic illness. There are natural stages in human development and illnesses in this age group, such as menopause and breast cancer, respectively.

Health conditions or illnesses discussed in this chapter include adult wellness and aging; diabetes; breast cancer; chronic obstructive pulmonary disease (COPD); and hypertension. There are many others, but these are selected because they usually have great impact and are often encountered by the community health nurse (CHN). All of the discussions overlap with other chapters on younger or older clients.

## Wellness and Aging in Middle Aged Adults

The period termed "the middle years" is a relatively new developmental period in America, because people are living longer. Life expectancy has increased approximately 25 years, from an average of 49 years in 1900 to an average of 73 today, and there are now over 44 million people in the United States between 44 and 64 years of age (U.S. Bureau of the Census, 1981).

## Definitions of "Wellness" and "Aging" in Middle Age

Positive health is often seen "through a glass darkly," because our eyes have been so long fixed on disease and death. Adult wellness has not been a main theme in Western society, because communicable diseases took a fearsome toll of human life until recent times. Most individuals are concerned about their unhealthy states, not their healthy state. They usually go to a physician when they are ill, and probably do not really know what a healthy state is for them. I define "adult wellness" as a state of physical, mental, emotional, social, and spiritual health that permits clients, within the limits of their abilities and disabilities, to be productive members of society and enjoy life. Dunn expresses a similar view:

> High-level wellness for the individual is defined as an integrated method of functioning which is oriented toward maximizing the potential of which the individual is capable. It requires that the individual maintain a continuum of balance and purposeful direction within the environment where he is functioning. (Dunn, 1973, p. 4)

The definition of "wellness" is intrinsically bound up with the definition of "aging." Gerontological researchers continue to study the effects of two aspects of aging on the human body. "Normal aging" or "primary aging" refers to inherited biological processes on a time continuum, which are detrimental to the body but independent of disease, trauma, or stress. "Pathological aging" or "secondary aging" refers to declines in functioning as a result of chronic illness or trauma (Elias, Elias, & Elias, 1977).

When does aging begin? How far has aging progressed when clients are between 40 and 65 years of age? Aging begins at different ages for different individuals, for a variety of reasons related to genetic endowment, environmental exposures, and life styles. Some physiological decline begins in everyone at about age 30.

## The Tasks of Middle Age

The developmental tasks of the middle years arise naturally from within the organism, from environmental forces, and above all from the demands of the individual's own values and aspirations. Both Erikson

(1968) and Havighurst (1948) emphasize the personal changes and increasingly complex human relationships this stage of life brings. Erikson (1968) refers to this stage as "generativity versus self-absorption"; one brings active concerns for self and others, younger and older, while the other brings stagnation and defeat. Middle-aged persons bridge the gap between the young generations and their aged parents; with this perspective, they can do some self-assessment. Those who practice "generativity" may regret goals not achieved or acknowledge that some things will never get done, but they can feel pride in a variety of accomplishments. A "self-absorbed" person does not necessarily view his life and accomplishments as successful, according to Erikson. Middle-aged persons do have losses—children leaving home, loss of employment, or divorce—and some may experience great difficulty in adjusting (Craig, 1980; Eklind, 1970). Many other middle-aged persons enjoy this stage and move into old age feeling fulfilled.

## Highlights of Normal Aging in the Middle Years

There is actually a dearth of research on development in the middle years. Until recently, the years between 40 and 65 were not considered marked by a process of development.

### Physical characteristics

The human body usually functions very well during the middle years. Physical vigor lasts throughout this period, unless disease takes its toll. Some changes in outward appearance are the beginning of greying and loss of hair and loss of skin elasticity, resulting in wrinkles and a redistribution of fatty tissue. Many people see beauty in hair that is greying.

Alterations in the functional ability of the sensory organs also occur in the middle years. Presbyopia occurs between ages 45 and 50, because the elasticity of the crystalline lens of the eye decreases so much that it no longer adjusts its curvature to accommodate for close-up vision. Glasses can easily correct the condition. A gradual hardening and deterioration of the auditory cells and nerves, which starts in young adulthood, continues in the middle years. Thus, one experiences some loss of auditory acuity or, more particularly, presbycusis (a loss of hearing for tones in the higher ranges). Usually these changes do not substantially affect one's work or relationships.

Other characteristics of the middle years are a lowered metabolism, general decrease in the elasticity of the lungs, and often some chronic illnesses. Metabolism slows at age 40; persons must then adjust diet and exercise to maintain normal weight. Loss of elasticity of the lung tissue can produce chronic bronchitis, but not necessarily, especially if the person has exercised and has not smoked. Knowledge about chronic illnesses helps the client care for himself in the early stages; this care often prevents later problems (Kaluger & Kaluger, 1974).

### Mental and emotional characteristics

Mental functions have usually arrived at their peak by middle age and do not weaken significantly until age 70 or later. Many cultures, in fact, look to their middle-aged populations for wisdom and experience. After 40 a person may become more anxious in a new learning situation, but once the material is learned, it is retained as well as in youth.

Personality usually does not change from the younger years. If a person has been flexible earlier in life, changes such as employment and menopause can be approached with equanimity. Persons practice Erikson's "generativity" if they adjust well to this stage. There is no question that the change from adulthood to middle age is equal in difficulty to any other period of transition in growth and development, but it is probably not a distinct midlife crisis, as first described by Jung.

### Social and vocational characteristics

Most individuals enjoy their highest social status in a community during middle age. Careers are usually at a peak of work production in stable job situations. Generally more money and more leisure time are available than earlier in life. However, loss of status in this period of life can result from losses on the job, children leaving home, and chronic illnesses that decrease socialization and consume much of a person's energies. An understanding by the client of the phenomena and associated risk factors for disease in this developmental stage can contribute to adjustment.

## Prevention of Chronic Illnesses

Wellness would be more prevalent in middle age if disease were prevented—that is, if the risk factors for chronic disease in the middle years were minimized. There are three types of prevention: primary, secondary, and tertiary.

Primary prevention occurs before the clinical phase of a disease. For example, cigarette smoking is a main risk factor for emphysema. Thus, a teenager should be encouraged not to start smoking, in order to prevent emphysema and other ill effects. For a client with newly diagnosed emphysema, smoking should be curtailed and postural drainage and breathing exercises—secondary prevention—can be taught. If the disease has progressed to a point at which the client can no longer assume daily activities, oxygen therapy and other medications may be required as *tertiary prevention* (i.e., rehabilitation). One can readily see that treatment is more costly than is prevention, especially primary prevention.

## Adjustment to Chronic Illness and Aging

About one-fourth of the diseases of the aging and aged are infectious. The remainder are chronic (i.e., with a duration of 3 months or more); many have multiple causes and numerous clinical manifestations. Chronic illnesses demand an attitude of caring as much as curing, concern with the environment of the client, and an acceptance by both client and nurse of the limitations of treatment (National Institutes of Health, 1978). An older adult may adjust to an illness, particularly a chronic one, and still maintain a normal life style.

The CHN should assist her middle-aged clients to understand and cope with the two kinds of aging mentioned earlier—normal and pathological. For example, as a result of decreased metabolism processes (a normal event), the client requires fewer calories. An adjustment in his diet should be suggested in order to prevent obesity. On the other hand, if the client has a familial tendency to essential hypertension (a pathological condition), attention to monitoring of his blood pressure is necessary.

Regimens to regulate a chronic illness may be prescribed by a physician, nurse practitioner (NP), or CHN, but clients and families make the decisions about what regimens they will follow. In order to expect compliance, health professionals must help the client and family to understand the disease, treatment, and expected outcomes, and must also understand the constraints and fears of the client and family. Factors interfering with compliance are lack of understanding, cost, discomfort, time and effort, denial, and lack of support systems. Thus, for example, with chronic bronchitis, a client may skip postural drainage until symptoms become bothersome (Strauss, 1975).

Along with the physical illnesses that affect clients in their middle years, there are mental and emotional concerns. It is thought by some that during the 40s one enters a midlife crisis or authenticity crisis.

At this time people may agonize over jobs, health, families, and unfulfilled dreams, as during adolescence. It is a time for reassessment because earlier goals may be unattainable, and there are fewer years ahead (Peplau, 1975). People discover signs of aging and may become aware of their mortality. Anxiety and depression may result. As they work through this new crisis of identity, they can move toward an exciting and adventuresome middle age, especially if supported by friends and family. If the crisis is too painful to handle and adequate coping skills and support systems are not present, functional mental illnesses may become evident. Functional mental illnesses such as depression are caused by emotional stress. Most of the functional disorders are curable (National Institutes of Health, 1978).

Mental illness due to organic causes such as cerebral arteriosclerosis or excessive alcohol intake may also affect the middle-aged with increased frequency. It is thought that about 15% of the organic mental health disorders are curable (National Institutes of Health, 1978). It should be noted that in many cases it is difficult to differentiate between organic and functional mental illnesses without a thorough assessment.

## Nursing Care for Middle-Aged Clients in Clinic, Home, Industry, and Community

The CHN teaches well or sick clients in a variety of settings about the normal aging process and adjustments to chronic illnesses, thus minimizing the ill effects of these changes. Each middle-aged person and his family should understand what to expect from normal aging and the risks associated with aging. For example, while providing home nursing care to clients with arthritis, the CHN could discuss minimizing the effects of the disease with a preventive approach such as exercising. Other clients may ask whether the CHN thinks they need bifocals, or may have numerous other concerns. Referral to nutrition classes in a clinic setting may help an obese client.

Employees at work may wish to share health concerns, such as a discussion of the Occupational Safety and Health Administration (OSHA) safety regulations for asbestos, in informal group sessions (Brown, 1975). Community groups may request that the CHN discuss normal aging with them or teach breast self-examination (BSE). A television presentation on the prevention of diabetic complications or healthy life styles would be another way to reach many persons and promote wellness.

For the well middle-aged person, it is important to discuss the developmental changes from physical, mental, emotional, social, vocational, and spiritual viewpoints. Viewing health in totality is essential to an understanding of a client's concerns, symptoms, and progress. For example, if a client is experiencing frequent exacerbations of multiple sclerosis, the CHN should review the person's health history to assess for new stressors.

In summary, the CHN's responsibilities to this age group are (1) to provide information on the processes of normal aging, wellness, and risk factors to health for middle-aged clients; and (2) to suggest, provide, and evaluate the care given to middle-aged clients with chronic illness. These responsibilities are based on a view of the client as a whole person. In addition to wellness and normal aging, several illness concerns common in middle-aged clients are discussed in detail in this chapter.

## Care of the Client with Diabetes Mellitus in the Clinic, at Home, and in Industry

### Introduction

#### Background

Diabetes has been known since about 2000 B.C.; its name is Greek for "the capacity to siphon," which aptly describes two symptoms of diabetes—polyuria and polydipsia. The symptoms or the pathology of diabetes were demonstrated in 1889 by Von Mering and Minkowski when they removed a dog's pancreas. The only major breakthrough has been the discovery of insulin in 1921 by Banting, Macleod, and Best. Oral hypoglycemic agents developed in the 1960s are not the panacea they were thought to be, because research has shown that they can produce serious cardiovascular problems (National Institute of Arthritis, Metabolism, and Digestive Diseases, 1970). The insulin implants introduced in 1981, which release insulin into the blood stream, are still in the experimental stage. A recent important event was the establishment of the National Commission on Diabetes (discussed later in this chapter), which has resulted in research and improved treatment.

#### Definition, diagnosis, and epidemiology

Diabetes is a metabolic disorder characterized by hyperglycemia, a relative or absolute insulin deficiency, and frequently accompanied by accelerated vascular disease. The oral glucose tolerance test (OGTT), although imperfect, is the method against which other diagnostic criteria are measured.

There are known to be over 4 million Americans with diabetes, and more than 6 million other cases are estimated to be undiagnosed. About 600,000 new cases are diagnosed each year, with a 50% increase in both prevalence and incidence since 1965. Although diabetes is associated with obesity, increasing age, poor economic status, and heredity, the precise extent of these factors is not known. There is a familial tendency in diabetes, and genetic factors play a part, but how diabetes is inherited is not well understood (National Commission on Diabetes, 1975).

### Morbidity, complications, and mortality

The main acute complication of diabetes is ketoacidosis or coma. Some other less acute conditions are excessive cataract formation and glaucoma, retinopathy, renal disease, and gangrene of the extremities.

Diabetes ranks as the fifth cause of death in the United States. While many persons die from diabetic complications, mostly vascular pathology, the death certificate may not state the underlying cause to be diabetes. Therefore, it is estimated that if these cases were reported accurately, diabetes might be the third leading cause of death in this country (National Commission on Diabetes, 1975).

## Care in the Clinic

Clients come to a diabetic clinic for (1) diagnosis and monitoring to control the disease with a calorie-controlled diet or with medication (insulin or the oral hypoglycemic drugs); (2) detection of complications of infection, degenerative vascular disease, and neuropathy; (3) instruction in how to care for themselves; and (4) support in dealing with symptom management, regimen compliance, and all other stresses associated with diabetes. Only aspects of screening, monitoring, and detection are discussed in this clinic section.

### Blood tests

Two different blood tests, the fasting blood sugar (FBS) count and the oral glucose tolerance test (OGTT), are used to ascertain the blood sugar level and to assist in formulating a diagnosis of diabetes. The two tests are designed to accomplish different things. Historically, the FBS test has been used as a screening test for diabetes mellitus. It is a simple test, requiring only a single early-morning blood specimen after fasting since midnight, and indicates the *probable* presence of diabetes. In the OGTT test, more than a screening is done: Glucose is given in large amounts (galactose 40 gms) to stress the mechanisms of the body that control blood sugar. It measures the ability of the pancreas to bring blood sugar down to a normal range after glucose is taken orally. It is possible that someone might have a normal FBS count and an abnormal OGTT, because the OGTT is a more sensitive test ("Ask the Doctor," 1978). The normal range for the FBS count is from 60 to 120 mg/ml. A client is considered a probable diabetic if the FBS value is greater than 130 mg per 100 ml. However, this commonly used test may miss as much as 85% of the diabetic population. An OGTT value above 140 mg percent for a client below age 50 should be considered a diagnosis of diabetes. Older clients exhibit higher normal OGTT levels (Guthrie & Guthrie, 1977; National Commission on Diabetes, 1975).

### Weight control and diet

Weight control and diet are essential for the regulation of a client with diabetes. These aspects are discussed in more detail later.

### Detection of chronic complications

Monitoring of the client's clinic care includes the detection of complications, which fall into three main categories: (1) infections, (2) degenerative vascular disease, and (3) neuropathy. Familiar examples of infections are the bladder infections of many diabetic clients, as well as greater susceptibility to minor infections, such as furuncles. Peripheral vascular disease, which can result in leg gangrene and amputation, and blindness from retinal changes are examples of degenerative vascular disease and neuropathy. Loss of sensation in the lower extremities from peripheral nerve degeneration can aggravate already existing gangrene. The list of possible complications is very lengthy. The treatment for all these conditions is basically control of the blood sugar level, which is accomplished by diet, hygiene, and insulin if required.

A discussion of the acute complications—ketoacidosis (coma) and hypoglycemia (insulin shock)—can be found in the following section.

## Care at Home: Teaching the Diabetic Client

Clients at home with diabetes are referred to a CHN, usually after a hospital discharge, for assistance in managing their disease. A newly diagnosed diabetic will require much teaching and support. A review of the information and skills required to keep well is necessary. If the client has been hospitalized because of ketoacidosis or hypoglycemia, it is imperative that the client and family receive help to understand how the crisis came about, so that they may minimize its future probability.

The CHN offers information and support, and together the CHN and the client determine the best way to manage the disease process. Diet is a primary concern, because all clients diagnosed as diabetic are prescribed a calorie-restricted diet, and many are given weight loss and exercise regimens. Diet restrictions must take into account the likes and dislikes of the client. In addition to diet facts, the CHN reviews the disease process, complications, foot care, urine testing, the medication regimen if drugs have been prescribed, and symptom control. Concerns of the client's family also need to be discussed. Other concerns include when to return to the clinic, to work, or to a resumption of the usual activities of daily living. Many middle-aged clients will want to talk about how symptoms have affected their lives physically and emotionally. The disease process may have a disrupting effect on the family.

In the protected, often rushed hospital atmosphere, the client may not have been taught enough about the disease to carry on adequate self-care at home. The stay may have been brief, or there may have been teaching in a group situation, which might not have been effective personally for this client. In the home setting, the spouse and other family members should be involved in the teaching, since the illness also affects them and their life styles. The whole family may change what they eat. Some clients live alone and need special help to understand their diet and its preparation. In teaching the diabetic client about the disease, the CHN must stress its usual manifestations and crisis complications.

### Diagnosis and disease manifestations

The anatomy and pathophysiology of the human body relative to the disease should be clarified with the client, using pictures to illustrate the discussion. The absence or decreased secretion of insulin from the Islands of Langerhans in the pancreas should be mentioned as the cause. The main factors are a genetic history of diabetes or obesity, with the diagnosis based on a positive OGTT. It is a chronic illness, with possible acute episodes such as ketoacidosis and with many complications of a chronic nature if blood glucose is not maintained at a normal level. The motivation of the client to learn about his disease and accept responsibility for self-care is of paramount importance to the wellness of the client with diabetes.

A client who has received a diagnosis of diabetes usually has concern over his lack of knowledge about the disease. He may become very fearful, anxious, and depressed about the amount of care he must provide to stay well and about the eventual outcome of the disease. The CHN can be tremendously helpful in supplying facts about diabetes that relate to his individual problems and in helping him to see that adjustment normally is a gradual one over months.

### Crisis situations

*Diabetic ketoacidosis.*   Diabetic ketoacidosis or coma, diabetic ketosis, and hyperglycemia are acute complications of diabetes mellitus. Diabetic ketosis is characterized by glucose and ketones in the blood and urine; in hyperglycemia glucose is found in the blood and urine, but ketones are absent. Both of these states resemble diabetic ketoacidosis, but are less acute (Guthrie & Guthrie, 1977).

Diabetic ketoacidosis is the most acute state of insulin deficiency and can lead to a derangement of carbohydrate, fat, and protein metabolism, dehydration, and electrolyte imbalance. These metabolic changes affect all body tissue, especially adipose, muscle, and liver tissue. Insulin stimulates hepatic conversion of fatty acids to triglycerides, and lack of it reverses the effect (i.e., triglycerides break down to fatty acids, resulting in excess ketones). Normally, insulin also facilitates muscle use of ketones (Walesky, 1978).

In ketoacidosis, ketones (beta-hydroxybutyril acid, acetoacetic acid, and acetone) are increased. Acetone imparts a distinct odor to the client's breath and urine and can be detected by the client and others. Hyperglycemia is a direct result of insulin deficiency. Other primary signs are polyuria and nocturia, with occasional bedwetting; polydipsia; dull headache; subnormal temperature at first; thready pulse; Kussmaul respirations (air hunger); lowered blood pressure; nausea and vomiting; sometimes "coffee ground" emesis, suggesting gastrointestinal bleeding; dry mucous membranes; and weakness and listlessness. These symptoms can progress to coma. The severity of symptoms is relative to the extent of the ketoacidosis. Coma due to ketoacidosis develops over a period of days and weeks, and the symptoms are present before coma ensues. This fact is important for the CHN and the client to recognize, because coma can be prevented (Slater, 1978; Walesky, 1978).

The most common cause of ketoacidosis is infection, because this increases the need for insulin. Other causes are failure to take insulin or an increased need for insulin due to surgery, trauma, or excessive food intake. Frequently, the cause is not known.

If a client is in ketoacidosis at home, the CHN should call an ambulance immediately. The client's physician should be called for insulin and other orders. The goal of treatment is immediate administration of insulin and fluids. Short-acting insulin is always used, subcutaneously and intravenously. Treatment must be accompanied by fluid replacement to combat dehydration and supply the essential electrolytes.

When it cannot be determined whether a diabetic client is semiconscious or unconscious from ketoacidosis or hypoglycemia, the client should be treated for hypoglycemia. If the cause is hypoglycemia, the positive results will be almost immediate, and such treatment will not be harmful to ketoacidosis (Slater, 1978). Coma can be caused by factors other than ketoacidosis, such as Hypersmolar (nonketonic) coma (Beeson & McDermott, 1975).

*Hypoglycemia.* Hypoglycemia or insulin shock is in some ways the opposite of ketoacidosis, because in this state the client usually has too much insulin from overdose or lack of diet control. All clients on insulin, and occasionally clients on oral hypoglycemic agents as well, are subject to episodes of hypoglycemia. In this state the client exhibits disturbances in cerebration, such as inability to perform addition and subtraction or mood swings, followed by parasympathetic signs and symptoms, such as salivation and hunger. Then sympathetic hyperactivity such as sweating, tachycardia, and anxiety can occur. The pattern varies among clients. Treatment is administration of carbohydrates, such as candy or sweetened beverages, if the client is awake (Beeson & McDermott, 1975). This should be followed by a well-balanced meal that includes protein and complex carbohydrates.

While preparing students at the University of Texas–Austin to make their first home visit, I was asked, "What do I do if I find a problem I cannot handle?" I replied, "I am only as far away as the telephone." The student who asked the question found a client home alone in a semihypoglycemic state on her *first* home visit in the course, telephoned for verification of symptoms, and then administered orange juice with a successful outcome. This was indeed a dramatic way to begin one's community health experience!

A hypoglycemic state can become severe if not treated with carbohydrates. Unconsciousness and convulsions can occur. Education of patients is most important in preventing this state. If a client has recurrent hypoglycemic attacks, the CHN may need to assess diet, exercise, and insulin dosage. Reeducation in insulin administration may rectify the problem.

Care at Home: Aspects of Nursing

*Urine tests*

Testing urine for glucose and ketones is one tool for estimating control of diabetes. Blood tests for glucose are more accurate, but are usually not feasible at home. However, British researchers recently reported two different studies showing that a blood test for glucose could be done at home for clients whose diabetes was difficult to control or in whom complications had begun. They used a finger puncture to gather the blood sample, which was spread on enzyme strips to monitor blood glucose levels. These results correlated highly with automated readings (Ryan, 1979).

The excretion of glucose depends upon the amount of glucose in the glomerulus of the kidney. When blood glucose levels are sufficiently increased, glucose is excreted in the urine. The usual nonfasting blood sugar level is 180 mg/ml. A fasting level ranges from 60 to 110 mg/ml, with a random range never exceeding 170 mg/100 ml in normal individuals, even after a great deal of sugar has been eaten. Therefore, under usual circumstances with a normal renal threshold, glucose should never appear in the urine, even postprandially. It does appear in clients with diabetes (Guthrie & Guthrie, 1977).

Some experts prefer that the urine show no glucose, and others think that a trace or one plus on a urine test is helpful in indicating that the client will not go into hypoglycemic shock. The acetone urine test determines the presence or absence of ketones. The CHN should demonstrate urine testing to the client and family, ensuring that they have the necessary equipment. With some clients, only a return demonstration or review is necessary.

In adults the most accurate urine specimen is a premeal, second-voided specimen when possible; however, this may not be necessary or feasible. A first-voided specimen, or "A specimen," is collected 1 hour to 30 minutes before a meal or at bedtime. The second-voided specimen, or "B specimen," is collected after the bladder has been emptied once, 30 minutes or less before mealtime. The reason for testing the B specimen is that there is about a 20-minute lag while urine passes from the glomeruli of the kidney to the ureters. This fact makes the B specimen preferable for testing purposes, because the A specimen may represent an overlapping of postmeal and premeal glucose values. Postmeal samples are useful for detecting intermittent glucosuria and monitoring for diabetes postcontrol. The B sample correlates more positively with blood glucose levels. Steps in collecting the B urine specimen are as follows:

1. The client voids 30 minutes to 1 hour before the urine is to be tested. This is the A specimen, the first-voided, and should be discarded.
2. The client may drink water if he has difficulty obtaining the second urine.
3. The client empties the bladder about 30 minutes after the A specimen was collected. This urine is the second-voided or B specimen, the one to be tested (Guthrie & Guthrie, 1977).

Ideally, a diabetic would collect four B specimens each day for testing. This is usually not done at home if the diabetes is controlled. Alternate testing recommendations for testing B specimens are as follows:

1. Four daily for 2 or 3 days during the week.
2. One before breakfast and at bedtime.
3. One before breakfast.

The frequency of testing depends upon the control of the diabetes. If it is controlled, the client need not test it for several weeks at a time.

Occasionally a client is requested to bring a 24-hour urine sample to the hospital clinic or laboratory for testing. The CHN should review the instructions that the client has been given. A gallon glass jar that has been washed with soap and warm water and rinsed thoroughly should be used. If the client does not have a gallon jar, he can use several small ones or obtain one from the hospital laboratory.

Written records should be kept of the urine tests for glucose and acetone (ketones) levels. The frequency of testing depends upon how well the disease is controlled. It may be done before each meal and at bedtime. The CHN assists in decisions about this record keeping. The client can take this record to his clinic appointment with the physician or NP.

### Diabetic diets

The CHN assists the diabetic client in planning a diet under a variety of circumstances. The client may be a newly diagnosed diabetic or a known diabetic who has been hospitalized. He may have seen the physician in a clinic because his diabetes needs controlled supervision for a variety of reasons. The CHN provides nursing care to newly diagnosed clients, clients with control problems, or clients with severe complications; diet planning is an important part of this care.

When a client is on a diabetic diet in the hospital, the dietary staff calculates and supervises the diet. The hospital nurse usually has very little to do with this phase of the client's hospital care. It has been my experience that most clients do not understand their diet after they return home. The prescription is often incomplete, listing only the calorie restriction and not the breakdown into the amount of carbohydrate, protein, and fat in grams. Little consideration is given in the hospital teaching to shopping and preparation of meals; these aspects are essential if the client lives alone, but they are also important to families who may be changing their dietary habits with the patient. Very often, particular likes and dislikes or cultural dietary patterns are not considered or planned for in building a dietary regime that is both safe and palatable for the client.

*Diet plans.* It is a good idea for the CHN to explain to the client that the diabetic diet is based on the four-food group plan, which is the proper basis of anyone's diet. Two special aspects of the diabetic diet are these: *Calories are controlled, and refined sugars are restricted.* The diabetic diet is similar to a weight reduction diet. Occasionally a client with diabetes is underweight and needs to increase calories.

The calorie-controlled diabetic diet can be calculated according to two methods: the Exchange List for Meal Planning or the newer Point System. The Exchange List (American Dietetic Association, 1976) has been recommended since 1950 by the American Dietetic Association and the American Diabetes Association. This plan includes six food groups. The client chooses foods from the group indicated on the meal plan. One food may be exchanged for another (e.g., cereal for bread) within the same group. Instructions for this type of planning are available from either of these associations and from commercial companies such as Eli Lilly and the Carnation Company (see Appendix 8A for addresses). The commercial literature may not reflect the latest diabetic diet revisions.

The Exchange List for Meal Planning was revised in 1976 by a joint committee from the American Dietetic and American Diabetes Associations, in cooperation with the National Institute of Arthritis, Metabolism, and Digestive Diseases. The major changes, made to emphasize low cholesterol in the diet, are these: (1) the main milk exchange is skim milk, not whole; (2) there is one group of vegetables instead of two (one exchange contains 5 gm of carbohydrate, 2 gm of protein, and only 25 calories), with starchy vegetables such as peas and navy beans moved to the bread group; (3) there are three meat groups—lean, medium-fat, and high-fat—instead of one; and (4) fat exchanges show polyunsaturated fats in bold type.

A newer type of diabetic diet plan is the Point System. As above, the carbohydrate, protein, fat and calorie composition is considered, but only two groups, calories and carbohydrates, are controlled. The client chooses any foods that give the prescribed amount of calories and carbohydrates (and protein and fat if regulated) (Guthrie & Guthrie, 1977). Although recommended dietary allowances (RDAs) are a guide for any person's nutrient requirement, the diet for the diabetic is calculated more precisely (National Research Council, 1980).

*Calculating a diabetic diet prescription.* The number of calories in the diet is based on the RDAs for age and sex, daily activity, and type of insulin. The newer recommendations from the American Dietetic and American Diabetes Associations distribute the calories as follows: 50% for carbohydrates, 20% for protein, and 30% for fat. These newer percentages reflect a decrease in fat from 35% to 30% and a 5% increase in carbohydrates, in an attempt to decrease the unsaturated fats and lessen the vascular complications of diabetic clients (Christianson, 1982). The diet prescription is calculated as follows (Stucky, 1977):

*Step 1.* Convert the client's weight from pounds to kilograms by dividing the pounds by 2.2 pounds.

$$\text{client's desirable weight} \div 2.2 = \text{kg}$$

*Step 2.*

a. Ascertain the client's daily activity level, which is based on the number of hours of vigorous activity in a 24-hour period: light work = under 1 hour; medium work = 1–3 hours; heavy work = over 3–4 hours with a pulse of 120.
b. Using the client's weight in kg (determined in Step 1), multiply that weight by the calories per kilogram. The following shows the calories per kg for different activity levels:

| | |
|---|---|
| For a bed patient | 25 cal/kg |
| Light work | 30 cal/kg |
| Medium work | 35 cal/kg |
| Heavy work | 40 cal/kg |
| Weight loss (obese) | 20–25 cal/kg |

Therefore, to determine the total calories according to weight in kg and activity level,

$$\text{kg} \times \text{cal/kg} = \text{total calories}$$

*Step 3.* To convert calories to grams, divide calories by caloric values of each of nutrients. To determine carbohydrate,

$$\text{total cal} \times 0.50 = x \div 4 = \text{gm carbohydrate}$$

To determine protein,

$$\text{total cal} \times 0.20 = x \div 4 = \text{gm protein}$$

To determine fat,

$$\text{total cal} \times 0.30 = x \div 9 = \text{gm fat}$$

For example, to calculate a diabetic diet for a female client aged 52, who weighs 128 pounds and performs at a medium activity level, the CHN should do the following:

*Step 1.* Convert 128 pounds to 58 kilograms.

*Step 2.* Multiply 35 cal by 58 kilograms of body weight to arrive at 2030 total calories in the diet.

*Step 3.*

$$2030 \times 0.50 = 1015 \div 4 = 254 \text{ grams of carbohydrate}$$

$$2030 \times 0.20 = 406 \div 4 = 102 \text{ grams of protein}$$

$$2030 \times 0.30 = 609 \div 9 = 68 \text{ grams of fat}$$

Hence, one arrives at the diet prescription of 2030 calories—250 grams of carbohydrate, 102 grams of protein, and 68 grams of fat for a 24-hour period.*

Assignment of foods on the basis of the grams of carbohydrate, protein, and fat in the diet prescription should be made from the six groups in the Exchange List or the four groups in the Point System by a nutritionist. The CHN does not have the necessary professional background for this step.

When a CHN visits a client, she should review the diet prescription, ascertain what the client actually eats, and list some special food habits. The diet prescription and the calorie allotment (broken down into percentages assigned to carbohydrate, protein, and fat) should be explained in terms of arriving at a balanced diet. A 2- or 3-day diet study or a 24-hour recall should be obtained. The CHN can facilitate this great-

---

*Adapted from "The Meal Plan" by V. Stucky, in *Nursing Management of Diabetes Mellitus*, edited by D. W. Guthrie and R. A. Guthrie. St. Louis: C. V. Mosby, 1977. Adapted with permission.

ly during the home visit by writing down what the client ate the day previous to the visit and what he has eaten that day; or she can call him prior to the home visit and ask him to list the foods. If it is to be a 2- or 3-day diet study, the client completes the remainder. Ideally, a 3-day study should include two weekdays and one weekend day. Besides the type of food, the amount (size such as 1/2 cup), method of preparation (fried), and additives (1 teaspoon of sugar to coffee) should be listed in all cases. Special food habits, such as that the client eats no fish, can be listed at the bottom of the assessment. This study is useful in later teaching.

If the client is visited over a number of months, the CHN can do a second diet study and correlate it with the first. This is to check on the client's accuracy in reporting and efforts at improving his nutrition, and it is more representative of the diet habits. If a 2- or 3-day diet study was done the first time, a 24-hour recall should be chosen for the second study, or vice versa (Christianson, 1982).

After the diet study is completed, the CHN collects it on her next visit or has the client mail it to her. The CHN can calculate the results of diet study by comparing it to the RDAs for all nutrients. However, it may be sufficient to compare it to the number of exchanges required on the Exchange List and then to make recommendations to the client on a subsequent home visit (Christianson, 1982). Cardboard food models from the National Dairy Council (see Appendix 8A for address) are good teaching aids to show portion sizes. Ideally, a family member should be involved in this instruction to help reinforce the client's learning and motivation. This family member may, in fact, be the person who does the shopping, prepares the meals, and gives psychological support to the client.

Consultation with a nutritionist is a good idea if one is available. This consultation usually takes place in an office situation in the agency, but almost never in a home visit. About once yearly, the client should return to a hospital class for a review of the diet by a nutritionist or should talk to a consulting dietitian (in person, or by telephone if outside an urban area). A class also allows for discussion of diet management techniques that clients have designed for themselves; these may be helpful to others in the class.

Just as the new food plans reflect research done on the relationship between saturated fats and vascular complications, new research suggests that high-fiber, moderately high-carbohydrate diets do lower blood sugar in diabetic clients. This type of diet appears to help control diabetes in clients on oral hypoglycemic drugs or on less than 20 units of insulin daily (Trowell, 1978). Periodic review of the diet will permit the incorporation of research findings.

*Medication*

*Insulin.*   Insulin is administered at least once daily to those individuals who are insulin-dependent. Because insulin is a protein and would be destroyed by digestive juices, it must be administered by injection, usually subcutaneously. In the hospital, some types are occasionally given intravenously.

There are several kinds of insulin available. They differ in time of action and concentration. In terms of action, there are three general types: (1) rapid-acting insulin, which includes regular (or crystalline) and semi-lente insulin (zinc suspension); (2) intermediate-acting insulin, which includes NPH (Isophane), Lente, and Globin insulin; and (3) long-acting insulin, which includes Protamine Zinc insulin (PZI) and Ultra-Lente insulin. Globin, PZI, and Ultra-Lente are used much less frequently than the other kinds. Often a short-acting and an intermediate-acting insulin are given together ("mixed" insulin regimen). Other times, two injections daily of intermediate-acting insulin are used ("split" insulin regimen). Often, other combinations are given—for example, morning and evening injections, each with short-acting and intermediate-acting insulin ("split and mixed" insulin regimen). These various combinations are used because of variations in individual response to insulin, varied life styles, and the imperfectness of insulin regimens in normalizing blood sugar (National Commission on Diabetes, 1975). Table 8-1 outlines the insulin preparations by type of action.

Approximately 99% of all insulin is administered in U-100 strength (100 units/ml) using a U-100 disposable syringe. The standardization to U-100 from U-40 and U-80 was done to eliminate dosage errors. U-100 insulin is a more concentrated insulin, which was made possible only after insulin became more perfected (Eckert, 1983). In addition to the ease of calculating U-100 insulin dosages over U-40 and U-80 dosages, there is another advantage to the newer system. Because U-100 insulin is more concentrated, the client receives less solution, resulting in less damage to tissue and a decreased chance of local infection (Anderson, 1983).

Because insulin is protein, it should be refrigerated. All vials of insulin (except regular, which is not a mixture of types) should be gently (*not* vigorously) rotated between the hands and inverted end to end several times before the dose is withdrawn.

The daily dosage is prescribed in writing or over the telephone by the physician, and the order should be renewed in writing at least every 2 to 3 months. If the client's diabetes is not well controlled, dai-

## Table 8-1
### Insulin, Classified by Type of Action

| Type of Insulin | Onset | Peak | Duration |
|---|---|---|---|
| **A. Rapid-Acting** | | | |
| 1. Regular (or Crystalline)* | 1/2-1 | 2-4 | 6-8 |
| 2. Semi-Lente (zinc)** | 1/2-1 | 2-4 | 8-10 |
| **B. Intermediate-Acting** | | | |
| 1. NPH (Isophane)* | 1-2 | 6-8 | 12-14 |
| 2. Lente** | 1-2 | 6-8 | 14-16 |
| 3. Globin | 1-2 | 6-8 | 12-14 |
| **C. Long-Acting** | | | |
| 1. Protamin Zinc Insulin (PZI)* | 4-6 | ±18 | 36-72 |
| 2. Ultra-Lente** | 4-6 | 8-12 | 24-36 |

*Note.* Adapted from information in *Nursing Management of Diabetes Mellitus*, edited by D. W. Guthrie and R. A. Guthrie. St. Louis: C. V. Mosby, 1977.
*All are cloudy except regular and globin which are clear.
**All Lente insulins contain zinc, and therefore cannot be given intravenously.

ly or weekly orders may be needed for a time. Orders may be changed, too, if the client is ill, requiring less insulin because he is not eating or exercising.

All clients on insulin are also on a prescribed calorie-controlled diet, although the converse is not true. To determine the insulin requirement, the doctor must know how much insulin the patient produces himself (diabetics have relative or absolute insulin deficiency), how much dextrose will be obtained from the diet and how this will be metabolized, and what the client's glucose tolerance level is. One unit of insulin metabolizes approximately 1.5 grams of dextrose. These facts are usually established during a hospitalization. In a home setting, the changes required in insulin dosage are determined by testing the urine for glucose and ketones four times times daily (before each meal and before bedtime).

The client usually selects either a plastic (disposable) or glass syringe calibrated to 100 units, as shown in Figure 8-1. This replaces the earlier U-40 and U-80 syringes. A blind client can obtain a special syringe called a "Truset," on which the dosage can be set with a screw.

A client learning to administer insulin can practice on an orange. The hypodermic injection should be rotated among various body sites to prevent hypertrophy (with loss of nerve endings) and atrophy (with loss of cutaneous fat). Rotation should be followed so that the same site is not used more often than once a month. The nurse must be very specific about these sites, as shown in Figure 8-2, or she can work out another plan with the client.

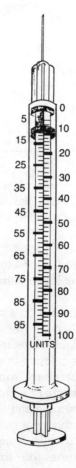

Figure 8-1.  Disposable U-100 Insulin Syringe. (Drawing by Mary Gainer.)

A CHN teaching insulin administration must consider the impact of self-injection on the client. Many may initially find the procedure scary or distasteful and may need to talk about their feelings. Others may arrange for a family member to administer insulin for a time. It is important to support the client's acquisition of independence, so patience but firmness in teaching self-injection is important.

A glass syringe can be cleaned in the home if a client prefers it to the plastic one. The syringe can be kept clean by boiling or using alcohol. In the boiling method, the syringe is taken apart and put with the needle into a strainer that fits into a pan. After they have boiled 5 minutes, the strainer is lifted out, and the water poured out. Distilled water is best, as it will not leave a deposit on the syringe and needle. In the alcohol method, a narrow-necked 4- to 6-ounce glass bottle is boiled for 5 minutes. It is filled with a new supply of 70% alcohol, and the syringe is placed in it with the needle attached. Before using, the syringe is dried by rapidly pulling the plunger back and forth. After use, the syringe and needle are rinsed out with alcohol and left in the bottle until the next use. The needle must not touch the bottom of the bottle (District of Columbia Visiting Nurse Association, 1979).

*Oral hypoglycemic agents.*   Oral hypoglycemic agents are drugs in pill form that enhance *release of insulin action* in those patients who produce some insulin on their own (the insulin-dependent, maturity-onset category). These agents have no role in the management of the juvenile diabetic.

Several such drugs are commercially available in two general categories. These are the first-generation sulfonylureas (including tolbutamide or Orinase, acetohexamide or Dymelor, tolazamide or Tolinase, and chlorpropamide or Diabinese; see Table 8-2) and the biguanides (including phenoformin or DBI or Meltrol). Five second-generation sulfonylurea compounds (Gilbenclamide, Gilbornuride, and three others) have been available in Europe for a number of years and may be released in the United States in the near future.

Although these drugs were once thought to be a major breakthrough, their role in the treatment of the client with an insulin-independent type of diabetes is controversial, in view of a study conducted by a group of 12 universities cooperating as the University Group Diabetes Program. The Food and Drug Administration has supported the findings of the Program and has required altered labeling of these agents. The study (see National Commission on Diabetes, 1975), covering clients with mild, nonsymptomatic diabetes who used fixed doses of tolbutamide and phenformin over a prolonged period, showed a statistically significantly higher death rate from cardiovascular disease

Figure 8-2. Rotation of Sites for Morning and Evening Insulin Injections. (From A. M. Fonville, "Adult Diabetes: Teaching Patients to Rotate Injection Sites," *American Journal of Nursing*, 1978, 78, 880–881. Artist: Neil O. Hardy, Medical Illustrator, Westport, Conn. Reprinted by permission.)

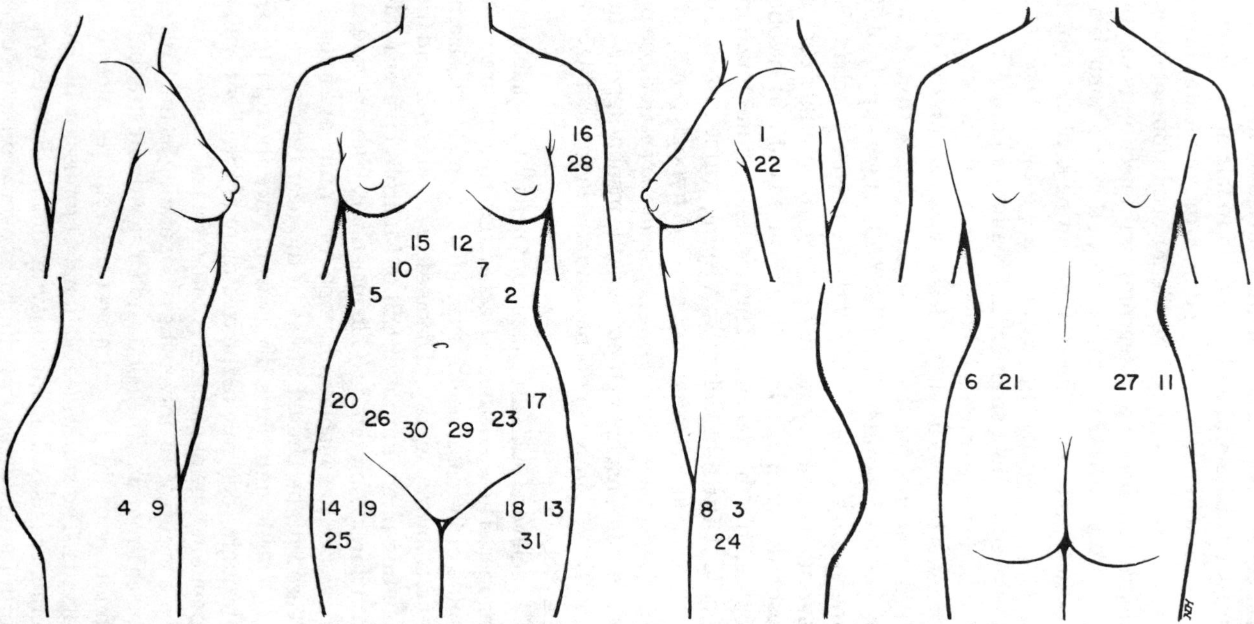

This rotation plan for insulin injection sites helps patients who take their insulin injections twice a day. The "A" sites are for morning injections,

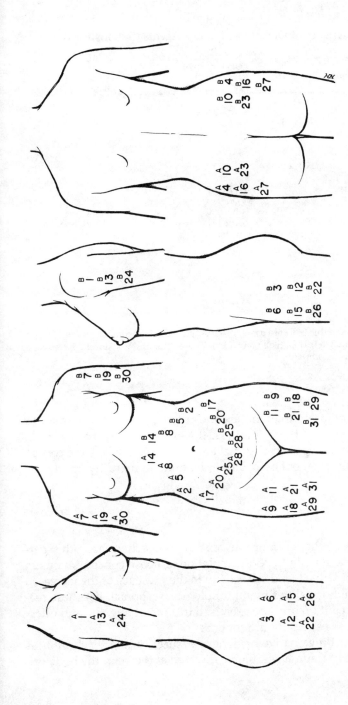

This plan, for patients on once-daily injections, avoids sites on the dominant right arm. The number of the injection site corresponds with the day of the month, which also helps the patient remember.

Table 8-2
Characteristics of Oral Hypoglycemic Agents (Sulfonylureas)

| Compound (1st generation) | Tablet size (mg) | Usual Dosage Range (mg) & Frequency | Approx. Potency Ratio (mg)* | Approx. Duration of Activity (hrs) |
|---|---|---|---|---|
| acetohexamide (Dymelor) | 250,500 | 125-1000 (single or divided) | 2.5 | 12-24 |
| chlorpropamide (Diabinese) | 100,250 | 100-500 (single, but may be divided) | 5 | up to 60 hrs |
| tolazamide (Tolinase) | 100,250, 500 | 100-1000 (single, but may be divided) | 5 | about 24 hrs |
| tolbutamide (Orinase) | 500 | 500-3000 (divided, but may be single) | 1 | 6-12 |

*Note.* The statistics in this table are drawn from A. Jacknowitz, personal communication, December 1982; and from T. G. Skillman and M. Tzagournis, *Diabetes Mellitus.* Kalamazoo, Mich.: The Upjohn Company, 1977.

*5 = strong

in the treatment group than in the control groups treated with placebo or insulin. In view of these findings, the exact role of these agents is not well defined. It appears that diet and weight control are the cornerstone of the management of insulin-independent, maturity-onset category of clients.

*Hygiene*

The diabetic client is more susceptible to infection than other persons; this is due mainly to poor circulation, glucose concentrations in the blood, poor white blood cell activity in the presence of the increased glucose, and abnormalities in immunological response. For these reasons, extreme caution must be exercised in general hygiene and infection prevention, especially in foot care.

*Foot care.* Preventative hygienic measures, primarily cleanliness and avoidance of trauma, should be directed at the skin, the body orifices, and the extremities, especially the feet. This is necessary because diabetic clients have a reduced blood supply to and reduced sensation in the feet, and they do not always feel pain when they are developing foot problems. *Foot Care for the Diabetic Patient*, a fact sheet from the National Institute of Arthritis, Metabolism, and Digestive Diseases, provides excellent recommendations (see Appendix 8B).

*Care of the skin.* Persons with diabetes are more likely than others to contract staphylococcal, beta-hemolytic streptococcal, and fungus infections. These can result in furuncles and carbuncles, necessitating an increase in insulin.

Several lesions of the skin are peculiar to people with diabetes. Diabetic dermopathy occurs from localized traumas, such as bumping into furniture. It is a hyperpigmented area on the skin, tan in color and cosmetically unattractive. Since there is no treatment for it, prevention is the answer. Clients should be instructed to arrange their furniture for ease in walking about their homes. Clothing such as boots that rub excessively in any area on the leg should not be worn.

Two other skin conditions are necrobiosis lipoidica and xanthoma diabeticorum. Although these are less common than diabetic dermopathy, they do occur—necrobiosis lipoidica as a result of trauma, and xanthoma diabeticorum from extended periods of elevated blood glucose levels (Guthrie & Guthrie, 1977).

*Body orifices.*

ORAL CAVITY. The oral cavity requires special attention because several oral problems can occur, such as pyorrhea, loose teeth, and bleeding gums. Normal daily brushing and flossing are recommended. In addition, the client with diabetes should be examined oftener by the dentist—every 3–4 months instead of only every 6 months, as is usually recommended.

VAGINA. *Candida albicans* (Monilia) is normally present in the vaginal canal and multiplies readily to pathological levels with increased concentrations of glucose in the urine. Candida can cause vulvovaginitis and severe pruritis. It can spread to the oral cavity, to the axilla, and to the skin under a pendulous breast. The best protection is prevention by keeping the blood glucose levels normal.

*Psychological aspects*

The psychological "drain" of diabetes is enormous on the client, the family, and society. The emotional problems result from the daily need to adhere to a strict diet, exercise regimen, and medication, often by injection; from frequent medical appointments; and from the threat of a variety of acute and chronic physical complications. The CHN must regularly reassure family members that their support is absolutely essential for the client. Among those areas that need careful assessment, because of their emotional significance, are the effects of diabetes on body image, normal life style, employment, and sexual functioning. It is important for the nurse to listen for concerns in these areas and be ready to explore feelings with the client, to emphasize the normality of these concerns and problems, and to help the client build coping strategies. In some cases, such as with sexual dysfunction, referral for sexual counseling or fertility counseling may be necessary.

Ketoacidosis can occur in any diabetic, and the fear of this life-threatening event (as well as of other changes, such as a leg amputation or renal failure) takes special coping stamina. The fear of a premature death can also be difficult for the client and family. Maintaining control of the metabolic condition is often contingent on satisfactory emotional response to the illness. Anger, anxiety, depression, and denial reflecting lack of adjustment may threaten the client's metabolic stability (Haukenes, 1982).

Family life can be disrupted by restrictions on the client's working potential. For example, a recent panel of federal judges upheld a 1973 ruling prohibiting insulin-dependent diabetics from obtaining licenses as commercial interstate truck drivers ("Judges uphold ban on diabetic truckers", 1979).

Traditional medical practice focuses on control of the symptoms in the individual chart. Diabetes is a complicated chronic illness that should be viewed in a family and societal context. For clients without families or for those who need support in addition to their families, a diabetic self-help group may be the answer. The CHN or the client can contact the local diabetes association for information, or the CHN may assist in organizing and leading such a group.

As the chronicity of diabetes and its ensuing complications take their toll, the medical and nursing profession have little to offer the diabetic beyond the usual regimens of diet, medication, and supportive therapy. In addition to client education in a home setting, the CHN can contribute substantially with psychological counseling. This may, in fact, be the major part of her nursing care to some clients and families.

*Referral to outside sources for assistance*

*American Diabetes Association.* The American Diabetes Association is a national, voluntary organization of both professional and lay people, with affiliates in all states and offices in many cities in the country; it promotes an understanding of diabetes, aids diabetic clients in leading a richer life, and works toward the ultimate goal of determining the cause of diabetes and a cure for it. It engages in patient, professional, and public health education and in diabetes detection, raises funds for research and disseminates findings of research, publishes a variety of literature and monthly papers, and conducts summer camps for diabetic children. Its services are available to anyone (American Diabetes Association, no date).

*Medic Alert Foundation.* The diabetic should wear a Medic Alert bracelet or necklace to identify his condition. When someone calls the telephone number on the bracelet, there are 16 operators at computers based in New York or California to answer the call. The bracelet is available from the Medic Alert Foundation, P.O. Box 1009, Turlock, California, 95380, or at a local drug store; it costs $10–$28, depending upon the metal used. In addition, the diabetic can carry a billfold card that states, "I have diabetes." They are printed by drug companies and are available from the American Diabetes Association.

Care in Industry

*Job placement*

The occupational health nurse may assist the client who has diabetes with placement in a more suitable job after his return from a hospitalization with complications from the disease. The CHN may make a referral to the nurse in industry by telephone. (Frequently the client must sign a "Release of Information Form" before there can be an exchange of information by telephone or in writing.)

*Nursing care and screening programs*

A client with diabetes may need assistance with diet and insulin administration. The occupational health nurse needs to be alert to possible physical or emotional problems indicated by failure to adhere to the medical regimen, frequent absences from the job, and/or changes in personality. Counseling to determine the source of any problems may be necessary. If there are a number of diabetics in one location, they can be taught in classes. This helps the clients to learn from each other, as well as providing peer support in coping with the rough times that may occur in a diabetic's physical, social, and emotional life.

A diabetes screening program may be instituted in industry. This would involve urine testing, FBS tests, obesity control, and education about the disease process.

## Social Support Systems

The diabetic requires the broad understanding and help of society. Physical and psychological care during repeated hospitalizations may require government support. Public education is necessary for a better understanding of diabetes as a chronic disease that is increasing in incidence and that has many complications. The CHN may be involved in presenting facts about the disease at workshops, to groups, and on television, and in developing the community's ability to provide care for clients and families affected by the disease.

There is no known cure for diabetes. The National Diabetes Data Group of the National Institute of Arthritis, Metabolism, and Digestive Disease has confirmed that there have been about 612,000 new cases of diabetes per year—an increase of more than 40% since 1965. It is not known whether prevalence has increased or whether greater awareness has led to more accurate diagnosis (Ryan, 1979).

Because of the increased incidence and absence of a cure in sight, the National Diabetes Mellitus Research and Education Act (PL 93-354), signed by President Nixon on July 23, 1974, directed the appointment of a National Commission on Diabetes to formulate a long-range plan of research and education to combat diabetes mellitus. The Commission made its report to Congress on December 10, 1975. Four major committees were established to carry out the recommendations of the Commission: Scope and Impact, Treatment, Etiology and Pathology, and Education (National Commission on Diabetes, 1975).

# Nursing Care of the Client with Breast Cancer in Home, Clinic, and Industry

## Introduction

Breast cancer is discussed in the chapter on the middle years, because most of the morbidity, treatment, rehabilitation, and mortality of breast cancer occur in this age group. The CHN sees these patients in clinics, homes, and places of employment. Regular inspection for early detection of possible breast cancer is essential. Young women should be taught to conduct BSE from adolescence onward and should continue this the rest of their lives. Breast cancer does occur in males, but it is a leading cause of death in women in the United States.

## Statistics

### Morbidity and mortality

Breast cancer is the leading site of cancer incidence and death among women, and the third leading type of all cancers in the population, with 107,000 new cases of breast cancer and 35,000 deaths from the disease expected each year. Nearly one out of every 13 American women will develop breast cancer at some time during her life, and it is the main cause of death among women aged 40–44. Every 15 minutes, one woman dies from breast cancer in the United States (American Cancer Society, 1981; Leis, 1977; National Cancer Institute, 1974).

### Risk factors

Breast cancer occurs mainly in women over 35. Risk factors, in order of importance, are these: age 50, a personal history of breast cancer in the woman herself, nipple discharge and other abnormalities, a family history of breast cancer on either side of the family, late menopause, no children, first child at age 30 or over, and early onset of menstruation (American Cancer Society, 1981).

Although breast cancer occurs only occasionally in men, the male breast should be examined for changes and nodules during a general physical examination. The male breast consists chiefly of a small nipple and areola, which top a thin disc of breast tissue that cannot be separated clinically from surrounding tissue (Bates, 1979).

### Survival rates

If lymph nodes are not involved, 85% of mastectomy clients survive 5 years or longer; otherwise, the 5-year survival rate is only 56% (American Cancer Society, 1981). Little, if anything, has been written about the quality of life in these survival years. A young epidemiological researcher at the University of Pittsburgh, Dr. Evelyn Talbott (1978), is studying the quality of life in the postmastectomy survival years.

## Prevention and Diagnosis

### Breast self-examination

Breast cancer is potentially curable if diagnosed early and treated promptly. To achieve early detection, a patient must be taught to examine her own breasts. There are several suggested methods for BSE. Both the American Cancer Society and the National Cancer Institute publish brochures on technique.

### Medical breast examination

An NP or a medical doctor should examine the breast once yearly, and should include an examination of the seven sets of lymph nodes in the axilla and upper chest. Since the lymphatics of much of the breast drain toward the axilla, axillary anatomy is included with a professional breast examination. If the nurse visualizes the axillary as a pyramidal space, the examination of the lymph nodes can be easier. The base of the triangle is formed by axillary skin, and the apex lies between the clavicle and the first rib.

### X-ray (mammography and xerography) and computerized axial tomography scans (radioisotope studies)

Breast X-rays (mammography or xerography) can detect some breast cancers in preclinical stages, 1 or 2 years before they could be palpable on a BSE. Breast X-rays offer excellent additional assistance in confirming or denying a clinical impression of whether a lesion is benign or malignant, but routine use of mammography may involve risk of radiation damage (Leis, 1977).

The computerized (trans)axial tomography (CAT) scanner, which uses radioisotopes in conjunction with computers, has been available since 1971. Using the CAT scanner, a physician or technician can accurately locate a disease process anywhere in the body, determine the nature of the process (cystic, solid, or inflammatory), and ascertain its extent, including any involvement with adjacent organs. Scans can be used in pretreatment plans and posttreatment evaluation, including detection of metastases (Watson, 1978).

The Total Mastectomy: A Newer Decision

For about 80 years the Halsted mastectomy, named for the Baltimore surgeon who devised it, was the standard procedure. It is a "radical" mastectomy, which involves removing not only the breast tissue, but also the axillary lymph nodes and the underlying chest muscles. In June of 1979, a medical conference at the National Cancer Institute (National Cancer Institute, 1979) endorsed "total" mastectomy (as opposed to radical), with axillary dissection when tumors are still small, even if the lymph nodes are cancerous. This leaves the pectoral muscles intact and does not lessen the chances of survival. The newer procedure enhances the chances of breast reconstruction. A "simple" mastectomy is the removal of the breast without lymph node dissection.

The same panel, at the urging of a member who was a breast cancer victim, was persuaded to endorse a two-step approach to surgery. This involves a diagnostic biopsy, followed by a delay of as much as a month before a mastectomy to give the woman and surgeon time to discuss alternatives. The CHN should insist that the client be informed of these new decisions (National Cancer Institute, 1979).

*Postoperative care at home*

*Care of the wound and scar.* The client who has had a mastectomy usually returns to her home in about 10 days. The CHN may visit her for several weeks or months for several reasons: to observe the wound's healing, to assist in air drying and changes of dressing, and to supervise the exercise regimen and follow-up drug and radiation therapy. Other reasons include psychological support, assistance in being fitted for a prosthesis, referral to support groups such as the Reach to Recovery Program of the American Cancer Society (Lasser, 1977), and vocational counseling. Furthermore, she must be taught to continue BSE of the remaining breast.

The wound's healing should be well begun by the time the client leaves the hospital. If a drainage tube was inserted during surgery, this site may not have healed. If the patient is obese, the original sutures may have given way. The CHN would then check the wound for evidence of infection such as redness, soreness, and swelling. Often she needs to recommend air drying to the surgical site to promote healing. This simply involves exposing the site to the air for 20 to 30 minutes two or three times a day. The patient may need to have the surgical site bathed with a mild soap and warm water before a dressing is applied. A sterile dressing is used as long as there is any opening in the incision. A clean dressing may be used until the client feels comfortable with the wound uncovered. A client should assist with the wound care in order to become accustomed to the care of her mastectomy and to adjust psychologically to it. The American Cancer Society supplies dressings free to clients at home.

In her book *First You Cry*, Betty Rollin (1976) points out the great anxiety connected with viewing the scar. The client's husband (if she is married) and close family members should look at it also, so that it does not become something disgusting to hide. Like any scar, it becomes softer, smaller, and lighter in color with age. In the first few weeks it may be very tender to touch and may even itch. A soft pad is recommended to ease the irritation from clothing. The area can be massaged lightly with hand lotion or cold cream to relieve irritation and itching. A client usually cannot lie comfortably on the affected side for long periods. Pillows placed under the abdomen relieve strain on the chest muscles and allow her to sleep on her stomach. At this time, she requires a great deal of support.

*Clothing.* When a patient feels well enough to take care of herself, she should wear comfortable clothes. At first she may want to dress in a nightgown fuller than usual to disguise the asymmetry. A robe or blouse should be opaque, should open in the front, and should have a deep armhole. Temporary bras can be furnished by the Reach to Recovery group. Tight bracelets and watchbands should not be worn on the affected arm, because they may interfere with circulation. When the client ventures out, she should carry a lightweight handbag or carry it on the unaffected side.

*Exercise regimen.* Whether the client has had a simple or a radical mastectomy, physical exercises are necessary to improve circulation and restore function to the affected chest and arm. As soon as the client returns from the recovery room, she is encouraged to flex and extend her fingers and to pronate and supinate her forearm (turning palm up and down). On the first postoperative day, she is encouraged to brush her hair and teeth, incorporating activities of daily living in her exercises. During the 7 to 10 days the patient is hospitalized, the nurse, physical therapist, and occupational therapist continue a graduated exercise regimen.

The exercises for the arm and chest continue after hospital discharge and until the prosthesis is fitted or until the client returns to her work in or outside her home. If her job is sedentary, she may want to continue some of the exercises longer. The importance of the exercises should be discussed with the client; a written contract should spell out the intent of each exercise, what joints and muscles are being exercised, a schedule, the substitution of activities of daily living to replace the exercise, and the appropriate time at which to discontinue the exercises. If the client and her family do not understand the importance of the exercises, they will probably not be done. The postmastectomy exercises to exercise pectoral and arm muscles are as follows:

1. *Moving hand up a wall.* With elbows bent at shoulder height, move hands, palms against wall at shoulder height, up wall until pull is felt in incision. Daily activities with same action are combing hair, reaching in cupboards, and cleaning mirrors.
2. *Rope or pulling.* Place rope over closet or shower rod or pulley on door. Grasp the two ends of the rope with each hand, alternately pulling up and down, until felt in incision.
3. *Arm circling.* Bend at waist and swing arms in circles clockwise and counterclockwise.
4. *Shoulder straightening.* With hands at sides, gently thrust chest forward and arms slightly backward. Repeat motion.

The specific exercises including the shoulder, elbow, wrist, and finger joints and strengthening the accompanying muscles in the arm, chest, and back on the affected side are included in the American Cancer Society's booklet, *What Is Reach to Recovery?* (Lasser, 1977), as well as in several other sources. Swimming is an excellent overall exercise for a mastectomy client, too. Bathing suits can be fitted with a prosthesis that does not react to chlorine in pools.

*Psychological counseling*

*Individual and family acceptance of loss.* Psychological counseling after the crisis of a mastectomy is essential to enable most clients to work through their feelings. Several characteristics of a crisis after primary breast cancer are important to consider. The crisis is limited usually to 4 to 6 weeks, calls up feelings of death, and is resolved sooner if the diagnosis and prognosis are discussed. Families, including husbands, vary in their ability to cope and to help the clients cope. They usually require assistance from the CHN in understanding their feelings and those of the clients. Help is needed to enable everyone involved to face the future (Klein, 1971).

The client should confront her problems and fears in open discussion with family, friends, and professionals. If she wants to cry, this should be supported. Families should be encouraged to talk to the client. The CHN should help the client and her family see that what is happening is manageable and that life will go on. Longer-term psychiatric intervention may be necessary.

Breast cancer is a multifaceted disease entity, in that it requires the surgical removal of a body part, can become a chronic illness, and is linked to female sexuality and reproduction. Inherent in the chronicity is an extended period of treatment and rehabilitation. Adjustment to the loss of a body part that is associated with physical attractiveness in a woman requires special attention. Cancer is viewed with a special dread because most of its causes are unknown, as is the outcome after surgery; the best that medicine and surgery have to offer is usually a remission of the disease (Marino, 1976). Nursing, however, can help enhance the quality of life during the remission by providing nursing measures such as special skin care and supportive therapy such as listening.

*The community health nurse's contributions.*   A CHN can counsel a postmastectomy client in her home; or, if she knows several such clients, a group can be formed for counseling and information purposes. In past years, such a group was formed by the District of Columbia Visiting Nurse Association. During the posthospital period, two to four clients met with a nurse for a few weekly sessions in the agency to ventilate their concerns about the recurrence of cancer, changes in their body image, acceptance by their husbands, prosthesis fitting, and exercise regimens.

*Prosthesis.*   Most mastectomy clients know very little about prostheses. They want to know about types of prostheses; about when and where they can be fitted; and about comfort, care, and cost. They will want to know how to adapt a bra to a prosthesis. A volunteer, a former mastectomy client, from Reach to Recovery can visit the client in the hospital or at home to discuss the purchase of a prosthesis, to describe the types of prostheses available, and to give directions for making breast forms and night bras (Lasser, 1977). In the absence of a volunteer in the community, the CHN can do this teaching and counseling. The advantage of the volunteer's visit is that she has actually had a mastectomy. However, it does not substitute for the professional nursing care the CHN can give, which includes monitoring of physical status, as well as provision of emotional support to the whole family.

Most surgeons recommend that a patient be fitted for a prosthesis about a year after surgery, because the body does not normally return to a relatively consistent shape until then. What should be worn before the prosthesis is purchased? Homemade prostheses can be fashioned from lamb's wool, cotton, sanitary napkins, bird seed, or padded bras. Inexpensive bra inserts might be all right for some clients. It is recommended that a woman eventually purchase a commercial form, because it does appear more natural.

Where should the client be fitted? Corset shops, department stores, and surgical supply stores sell prostheses. Mail order is definitely a second choice, because the fit will not be as good. Some women prefer their own bras; others prefer special mastectomy bras; and some ask a dressmaker to customize one for them.

There are several prosthesis types: silicone-gel-filled, liquid- or air-filled, weighted and unweighted foam rubber, and polyester-filled. (See Figure 8-3.) They usually come with nylon covers, are washable, and dry quickly. Most women seem to prefer the heavier silicone- or liquid-filled types, because they do not ride up. Brand names of popular forms are Yours Truly, Tru Life, Companion, Identical Form, and Jodee. Prices in 1982 ranged from $125 to $160 on the average, with customized versions costing as much as $800 and some temporary bra forms as little as $10 (American Cancer Society, Milwaukee Division, 1982).

*Breast reconstruction.* Breast reconstruction following mastectomy is being done by a few plastic surgeons. It is more feasible with the total mastectomy than with the radical, because the pectoral muscles are intact.

### Cancer as a chronic disease

*Multimodal treatment.* Chemotherapy is used as an adjunct to surgery and radiation following breast cancer. Antibiotics, hormones, and specific cancer drugs may be used, often in combination—antibiotics to control infections; hormones such as estrogen for replacement if an oophorectomy has been performed; and cancer drugs when metastases have occurred. Explanation of the treatments and their effects, skin care, bed baths, continuation of physical therapy, and psychological support are appropriate nursing interventions.

*Survival years.* Survival statistics have been discussed, but the quality of life in the survival years is another matter. After surgery, the client may resume her normal life patterns, and then after several years may become ill again if metastases increase. She may be confined to her home, at which time the CHN may be called. This may require teaching family members about narcotic administration, bed baths, and other supportive measures that any chronically or terminally ill client requires. Although the client may be chronically ill, she and her fami-

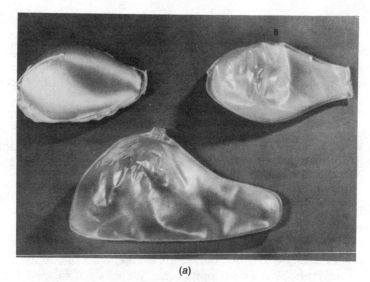

*(a)*

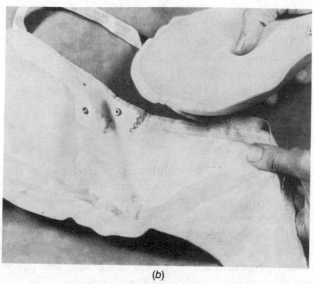

*(b)*

Figure 8-3. Types of Prostheses and Means of Securing Them: (*a*) *upper left,* foam rubber prosthesis; *upper right,* prosthesis containing fluid; *bottom,* prosthesis containing air; (*b*) inner pocket that will hold padding or prosthesis securely can be made in patient's own brassiere (note snaps that simplify removal of padding). (From B. C. Long and D. M. Molbo, ''Problems of the Breast,'' in *Medical-Surgical Nursing: Concepts and Clinical Practice* (2nd ed.), edited by W. J. Phipps, B. C. Long, and N. F. Woods. St. Louis: C. V. Mosby, 1983. Reprinted by permission of the editors and the publisher.)

ly may be assisted to design a life style for themselves that is both rewarding and enjoyable. There may be an intimacy fostered that indeed fosters growth for all involved. There is also in the healthy adjustment a hope that should not be destroyed. It is not the same as denial, but is a positive adjustment to the condition and making the most of remaining weeks, months, or years.

### Nursing care in the clinic

During the initial clinic visit, usually 3 to 4 weeks after the operation, the surgeon and nurse assess the healing process. If the wound is healed satisfactorily, the nurse helps finalize plans for obtaining a prosthesis. Arrangements for follow-up scans, radiation, or chemotherapy may be instituted, with instructions to the client as to reasons, possible side effects, and duration of treatment. Scheduling of future visits depends upon the nature of the follow-up treatment.

Usually on a subsequent visit(s) the client is referred to help groups such as Reach to Recovery to work out her feelings and seek advice. In the Oncology Clinic at West Virginia University, one of my master's students started an outpatient counseling group for mastectomy clients. Sessions were arranged on an individual basis or in groups, usually preceding a client's visit to the clinic for chemotherapy or radiation. Clients wanted to discuss prognoses and ways to alleviate discomfort, and to be reassured that they were still "whole" persons; as noted earlier, mastectomy clients suffer an identity crisis triggered by the threat of cancer to life and the loss of a significant and highly symbolic body part.

A client should be counseled about when she can resume her normal housework or career. If job retraining is required, a referral should be made to the local department of vocational rehabilitation, which assists with the plans and financing. A careful assessment is needed of what the client's current job requires and what the client can actually be expected to do, given the nature of the mastectomy.

### Occupational health

*Demonstration of breast self-examination.* Several aspects of nursing care are important in an occupational health setting. Female workers should be encouraged to perform BSEs, with a nurse in industry setting up teaching and demonstration sessions. The nurse in industry should see that the postmastectomy client knows how to perform a BSE on her remaining breast, and that she is seen regularly by her physician to check for any signs of metastases following her surgery for at least 5 years.

*Assistance with return to work.*  A client who has had a radical mastectomy may need someone to talk to about her feelings, especially if she has a different job than she had before surgery. She may also need encouragement and reassurance that she looks all right. The CHN needs to let such clients know of both the CHN's presence and her willingness to help the clients get back to normal in the work world. If job transition occurs, support is particularly important because not only has the client lost part of her body; she has also lost a job and perhaps coworkers.

## Conclusion

In conclusion, since breast cancer is at present the leading cause of death in women, research into this disease continues at an increased rate. Research suggests that there may be an environmental factor in breast cancer. At present only risk factors are known, not causes (National Cancer Program, 1976).

# Clients with Chronic Obstructive Pulmonary Disease in Home, Clinic, and Industry

## Introduction

The umbrella term "chronic obstructive pulmonary disease" (COPD), or "chronic obstructive lung disease" (COLD), is applied to a group of conditions in which the common physiological pathology is obstruction to breathing (more precisely, in the phase of expiration). The most prevalent diseases within this wide spectrum are chronic bronchitis, emphysema, and asthma. Others, less common, are cystic fibrosis, bronchiectasis, and obstruction associated with other fibrosing diseases. Chronic bronchitis and emphysema often coexist in a client, with each process contributing to airway obstruction. Only chronic bronchitis and emphysema are considered in this chapter, because they are the major manifestations of COPD in the middle years and do require home care. Asthma is the most common chronic disease in childhood and a leading cause of school absenteeism (Respiratory Diseases Task Force, 1977; Tomashefski, 1977).

Diseases: Definitions and Characteristics

*Chronic bronchitis*

Chronic bronchitis is characterized by daily coughing and expectoration of at least 2 to 3 tablespoons of sputum daily for at least 3 months of each year for 2 years or longer. It involves minor or major airways, with additional symptoms of inflammation and edema. The most characteristic pathology of chronic bronchitis is hypertrophy and hyperplasia of the submucosal mucous glands in the main bronchi with crypt formation. Unlike emphysema, which is confined to lung parenchyma, the lesions of chronic bronchitis are distributed uniformly throughout the lungs. It can occur alone (sometimes as a very disabling disease), or with emphysema or asthma, or with both (Benjamin & McCormack, 1977; Tomashefski, 1977).

*Emphysema*

The emphysemous process manifests destruction of alveolar walls, with resultant enlargement of air space and dilation of airways distal to the terminal bronchioles. The terminal bronchioles lose their supporting structure and therefore collapse prematurely. This results in decreased airway flow. Emphysema is also referred to as "small-airway disease" (Benjamin & McCormack, 1977; Duffy, 1981).

The predominant symptoms in emphysema are shortness of breath, coughing, expectoration, wheezing, and symptoms associated with recurrent respiratory infections. The major sign in earlier stages is shortness of breath. A hallmark of emphysema is decreased breath sounds. Emphysema is further characterized by hyperresonance on percussion of the chest due to lung hyperinflation and a barrel chest, another later sign. Rhonchi are expiratory in both chronic bronchitis and emphysema, and are discernible when breathing is forced (Duffy, 1981; Tomashefski, 1977).

Statistics

About 3% of the population have abnormal pulmonary functions. The incidence is approximately 30% in men and women above 35 years of age, and much higher in cigarette smokers. The prevalence of COPD can be as high as 80% in smokers in their sixth decade of life.

Morbidity is difficult to estimate, because it is not consistently reported. The 1975 mortality for COPD had increased to a rate of 19 per 100,000 and this statistic is believed to be underreported. Even if COPD is listed on the death certificate, it is listed as a cause of death in only one-third of the cases. There is a tendency to assign a death to a cardiac condition if such a condition coexists with COPD. The economic impact from COPD morbidity and mortality is about $5.7 billion. The COPD syndrome is indeed a major cause of pulmonary illness and disability, and is on the increase (Respiratory Diseases Task Force, 1977; Tomashefski, 1977).

## Etiology of Chronic Bronchitis and Emphysema

Many factors, internal and environmental, can contribute to the development of the various types of COPD. In chronic bronchitis and emphysema, cigarette smoking is the most common causative agent. Pipe and cigar smokers are at less risk than cigarette smokers are. Atmospheric pollution and occupational exposure to dusts play a much lesser role in the development of COPD than does cigarette smoking. A heredity factor does exist.

## Normal Anatomy and Physiology of the Respiratory System

The CHN should be familiar with the anatomy and physiology of the respiratory system if she is going to provide nursing care to a client with COPD. The anatomy of the respiratory system resembles an inverted tree: The right lung has three lobes, and the left two lobes, into which branch the bronchi. The right and left bronchi lead into the bronchioles, which terminate in alveoli.

During inspiration, air enters the nose or mouth and passes down through the bronchi and bronchioles, where it is dispatched to millions of alveoli or air sacs in the lungs. Oxygen passes across the walls of the alveoli into minute blood vessels. Then red blood cells distribute the oxygen to all body cells. In the reverse process, expiration, carbon dioxide is released. Inspiration takes approximately 1 second, and expiration takes 2 seconds; the total cycle comes to 3 seconds, which in turn equals 20 breaths per minute.

## History and Physical Examination of the Respiratory System by the Community Health Nurse

The CHN assesses the respiratory system, mainly to determine the current status of the client and to evaluate therapy outcomes. The history and physical examination may be done in a home or clinic setting on a form provided by the agency. The CHN should list the client's present complaints, recent hospitalization(s) if any, patterns or shortness of breath and coughing, prescribed medications and treatment, and other appropriate information required to provide adequate health and nursing care. Further examinations may help determine whether nursing care and treatment are successful or require adjustments. Subsequent examinations should probably be done routinely every 2 to 3 months when a client is confined at home, depending on the client's symptoms.

Pieces of equipment needed for the physical examination include a stethoscope, a marking pencil, and a centimeter ruler. The room should be well lighted, warm, and private. The CHN or NP utilizes inspection, palpation, percussion, and auscultation in the examination. Usually the lungs, heart, and breasts are included in a chest examination. However, this section focuses on the respiratory system of a COPD client, primarily to observe normality of breathing and detect any type of obstruction in the breathing process. The reader should refer to other physical assessment resources (books, tapes, charts, etc.) to develop skill with physical assessment of the respiratory system. The examination outlined in Table 8-3 is a guideline or a review for the CHN or NP.

## Prevention

Primary prevention can be accomplished mainly by a reduction in the amount of cigarette smoking in public; this would reduce or eliminate the smoke inhaled by nonsmokers as well as the smokers themselves. The air in a smoke-filled room is high in carbon monoxide. Carbon monoxide binds with the hemoglobin molecule and displaces oxygen, thereby decreasing the oxygen-carrying capacity of the blood to the lungs.

Secondary prevention is cessation of cigarette smoking by the individual before his disease has produced major damage. It is quite possible that small-airway disease represents an early and still reversible stage. The etiology and manifestations of chronic bronchitis and emphysema should be discussed in elementary and high schools in an attempt to discourage persons from becoming smokers. Classes to assist smokers in breaking the habit can be valuable and are often conducted by a local health department or proprietary groups.

Action on Smoking and Health is a voluntary organization formed in 1968 to protect the rights of nonsmokers, based in Washington, D.C. It has been instrumental in obtaining major nonsmoking actions, such

# Table 8-3
## Physical Examination of the Respiratory System

Examiner should request that client sit on examining table and turn his head away, so he does not cough on examiner.

| Examination Technique | Normal Finding | Probable Findings with COPD |
|---|---|---|
| **A. Posterior Chest** | | |
| Inspection thorax | symmetrical | retractions and/or bulging of intercostal spaces |
| respiratory rate and rhythm | 16-20/min, regular | rate increased, accessory muscles used, and/or body position affected |
| Palpation explore area and thoracic expansion, | symmetrical, 5-8 cm; | decreased |
| tactile fremitus | symmetrical over lungs | decreased |
| Percussion explore area and diaphragmatic excursion | resonance; N = 3-6 cm | hyperresonance; decreased |
| Auscultation breath sounds | vesicular | sounds decreased and expiration phase increased |
| adventitious sounds | none | rales, rhonchi or wheeze |
| voice sounds | normal | normal or increased |
| **B. Anterior Chest** | | |
| Inspection thorax | A-P < lateral convex | A-P diameter increased, "barrel" chest retraction, and/or bulging of intercostal spaces |
| nails | normal | clubbing |
| Palpation explore area and tactile fremitus, | symmetrical over lungs | decreased |
| trachea position | midline | may be deviated in unilateral emphysema |
| Percussion explore area | resonance | hyperresonance |
| Auscultation breath sounds | vesicular | sounds decreased, expiration phase increased |
| adventitious sounds | none | rales, rhonchi or wheeze (in asthma) |

*Note.* The CHN or NP should consult a more detailed source for problems associated with a particular COPD. I acknowledge the assistance of Joan Trekas in the preparation of this table.

as the creation of nonsmokers' sections on airlines in 1972 (Action on Smoking and Health, 1978). Nonsmoking ordinances for restaurants and Environmental Protection Agency standards for cleaner air were also enacted in the 1970s. The individual citizen can heighten awareness of nonsmokers' rights by constantly asking whether nonsmoking sections are available in public places.

## Rehabilitative Nursing Care at Home

Usually COPD is advanced and irreversible by the time a client seeks care. The overall objective clinically is to improve the client's quality of life, functional ability, and psychological well-being. The goals are to reduce the coughing, wheezing, and dyspnea, as well as infections and hospitalizations. The therapies for the COPD client include the following: (1) teaching the client about the disease process and prescribed therapies; (2) supporting the client in his decisions to follow treatment regimens; (3) urging the client to discontinue smoking; (4) contributing to bronchial hygiene through the use of respiratory therapy equipment; (5) administering pulmonary physiotherapy; (6) giving medications; (7) administering oxygen; (8) overseeing nutrition; and (9) providing humidification. These therapies differ for various clients. For example, not all clients have been smokers or require oxygen.

### Teaching about the disease process and therapies

The CHN on a home visit discusses the diagnosis with the client and family in order to increase motivation to comply with the therapies prescribed, clear up confusion, and aid the client and family in understanding that the client can reach a state of relative wellbeing. This teaching can be done with visual aids showing the anatomy and physiology of the respiratory system. *Chronic Obstructive Pulmonary Disease: A Guide for Teaching Patients* (Chicago Lung Association, 1977) is an excellent teaching aid.

The following therapies are not necessarily given in order of priority, because the client's respiratory status dictates the precise treatment intervention.

### Supporting the client in his decisions to follow treatment regimens

COPD is a chronic disease, and the client will need support and encouragement from the CHN and his family until his status is stabilized. He may need help to understand that a specific treatment will eventually relieve the condition. Sometimes a client with COPD requires more intensive counseling from a mental health or psychiatric NP.

### Discontinuance of smoking

*Any client with COPD should stop smoking!* The CHN may need to encourage him to discontinue or support him when he does. Occasionally the client is successful in stopping smoking if he joins a group that is set up for that purpose, such as the one conducted by the American Cancer Society. Many clients are too ill to leave their homes to join a group, however.

### Bronchial hygiene using bronchial therapy equipment

Bronchial hygiene can be maintained by liquefying sputum and facilitating its drainage. Aerosolized saline delivered by a nebulizer or by means of a device for intermittent positive-pressure breathing (IPPB) produces temporary relief in the hyperreactive bronchial tree. Chest physiotherapy using postural drainage, percussion and vibration, exercises, and controlled coughing are effective in increasing expectoration of mucous. In the home, supplemental liquefying assistance can be attained by use of the extra humidity in a shower. Further benefit may be gained if a bronchodilator is taken first (Golish & Ahmad, 1977).

*Aerosol therapy.* Aerosol generators or nebulizers are devices that produce aerosol vapors, which are visible as a cloud or mist. An aerosol is a suspension of particles (as medication) in a gas stream. Aerosolization takes place in the nebulizer. Aerosol generators are used to deliver aerosolized medication directly to the bronchial tree for the purpose of liquefying the secretions, so that they can be expectorated more easily. This is necessary because the airways of the client with COPD have been so damaged by the disease that the mucous secretions are not naturally removed. Also, there is an increased amount of mucous secretion. The ideal nebulizer produces a uniformly sized particle that will travel deep into the left and right bronchi, depositing very little medication on the upper airways.

There are two types of nebulizers, venturi and ultrasonic. The venturi nebulizer operates by directing a fast-moving stream of gas across one end of a tube, thus creating reduced pressure in the tube. Medication is drawn up through the tube by this reduced pressure, picked up by the rapidly moving stream of gas, directed against the wall of the nebulizer, and broken into tiny particles. An oxygen tank, a compressor (aerosol generator), or even a hand-held bulb can provide the stream of gas to produce the aerosol. The aerosol is inhaled by a deep breath or forced into the lungs by an IPPB device.

The ultrasonic nebulizer, which uses an ultrasonic beam, is more effective because the particle size is smaller and reaches deeper into the lung tissue. It is much more complicated than the venturi nebulizer and not generally used in the home. There is also a danger of inducing pulmonary edema because of the volume of liquid delivered (Duffy, 1981).

Most stable home therapy patients probably do as well with the inexpensive, low-volume, low-pressure aerosol generators as they would with the most expensive and complex IPPB units or ultrasonic nebulizers. The hand-held squeeze bulb is usually too physically tiring for the client to use and produces the least effective size of aerosol particle (Chicago Lung Association, 1977; Glover & Glover, 1978).

Specific cleaning instructions come with each aerosol device. It is important also to keep in mind the following instructions for the care of the aerosol equipment (Chicago Lung Association, 1977):

1. Rinse the medicine container (i.e., the nebulizer), and blow a little water through it after each use.
2. At the end of the day, disassemble and wash the nebulizer and tubing in a mild detergent, such as that used for washing dishes.
3. Nebulizer and tubing should be air-dried with a clean towel and covered to protect them from dust. Do not blow-dry with a hair dryer.
4. At least twice a week, the nebulizer and tubing should be soaked in a solution of 1 part white vinegar and 13 parts of water for at least an hour. Vinegar aids in dissolving and removing the medicine from the equipment. Rinse and air-dry after soaking.
5. Plastic parts deteriorate if boiled.
6. Do not try to repair the unit. Call the sales representative or the manufacturer.

*Pulmonary physiotherapy*

The purpose of pulmonary physiotherapy is bronchopulmonary drainage. Its value, and that of the bronchodilator medications, are not well established; both are viewed by some health professionals as palliative measures at present. Pulmonary physiotherapy includes (1) breathing exercises, (2) postural drainage, and (3) chest percussion and vibration. In COPD, loss of lung elasticity and the downward displacement of the diaphragm interferes with breathing; air becomes trapped in the lungs due to overdistension of the lungs. These factors, combined with damaged air passages, make respiration difficult. Oxygen can be administered after a physical therapy program.

Breathing retraining exercises, postural drainage positions, and physical exercise can improve muscle tone, lessen fatigue, and help to empty the secretions from the lungs. These new patterns take motivation and practice (Chicago Lung Association, 1977; Respiratory Diseases Task Force, 1977).

*Breathing retraining exercises.*

PURSED-LIP BREATHING.   Pursed-lip breathing is the correct breathing for the COPD client, and is done as follows:

1. The client inhales through the nose.
2. The client then exhales slowly, pursing the lips as if whistling or raising his tongue to the roof of his mouth as if forming the letter ''s.''

Pursed-lip breathing delays collapse of the airways and can to some degree improve oxygen distribution. Controlled expiration should take at least twice as long as inspiration (Chicago Lung Association, 1977; Glover & Glover, 1978).

CONTROLLED BREATHING.   In controlled breathing, the goal is to increase the client's exercise tolerance and enable him to carry out useful daily activities. The procedure is as follows (Chicago Lung Association, 1977):

1. The client lies flat on the back, with the dominant hand on the abdomen just below the sternum and the other hand on the chest.
2. With lips pursed, the client exhales, allowing the abdomen to fall. The chest is at rest during this phase.
3. The client inhales through his nose, with the abdomen rising. The chest should not move.
4. After this breathing technique has been practiced and mastered in the supine position, it should be practiced in the sitting and standing positions until it becomes habitual.

*Postural drainage.*   The client with COPD is often hampered by excess tenacious mucous. These secretions plug the airways, provide a medium for bacterial and viral infections, and restrict breathing. With proper positioning, gravity may aid emptying of the lung secretions with less expenditure of energy than is used with vigorous coughing. A physician's order is needed for postural drainage. In some instances, it is necessary to modify the treatment to accommodate the client's age or physical condition or the home setting, where a slant board and sufficient pillows may not be available.

The lungs are divided into lobes and the lobes into segments. In postural drainage, the client is strategically positioned to drain the clogged segments most effectively. Drainage of the most severely affected areas is done first. If no particular segment is ordered to be done first, drainage of the upper areas is recommended first. Ausculation of the lungs and/or a chest X-ray can establish which areas need to be drained, and can be useful also in evaluating the effectiveness of this therapy (Glover & Glover, 1978). Postural drainage is not indicated for someone with cerebral edema, unstable vital signs, or excessive secretions that could block the airways (Duffy, 1981). The postural drainage positions can be found in *Respiratory Therapy: Basics for Nursing and the Allied Health Professions*, by Glover and Glover (1978).

*Percussion and vibration.* Percussion (also called "clapping") and vibration should only be done by a CHN trained in this technique. The client is placed in the postural drainage position to assist drainage of the lungs; percussion is usually done with the client in a position favorable to drain the segment of concern. Percussion should be done on the back or anterior chest wall (rib cage) over a towel or a blanket. With her hands in a cupped position and fingers and thumbs closed, the CHN percusses the area involved by flexing and extending the wrists. The process is continued at a slow, rhythmic rate for a few minutes. Air trapped between the hand and the client's skin causes vibrations through the chest wall, loosening secretions. The percussion and ensuing vibration procedures are not done if the client has pain, a severe heart condition, a history of pathological fractures, or active tuberculosis. Percussion is not done over the kidneys or the spinal column, below the rib cage or over the breasts. Clapping over the scapula, clavicle, or sternum is ineffective (Chicago Lung Association, 1977; Glover & Glover, 1978).

*Effective coughing techniques.* Special cough techniques are an essential component of a rehabilitative program. The diaphragm is supported by placing a pillow or the client's arms against the abdomen. Secondly, when coughing, the client leans forward while pushing up on the pillow, giving support to the diaphragm (Chicago Lung Association, 1977).

*Medications for clients with COPD*

Oxygen, antibiotics, bronchodilators, mucolytics, and steroids are drugs used for the client with COPD (Bergersen, 1976; Chicago Lung Association, 1977; *Physician's Desk Reference*, 1981). Diuretics and digitalis are also ordered if the client has cor pulmonale.

*Oxygen.* Oxygen is discussed under "Oxygen Administration," below.

*Antibiotics.* Systemic antibiotics are the drugs of choice to control a pulmonary infection. A client and his family should be taught to recognize signs and symptoms of a respiratory infection, such as an elevated temperature or changes in the color of expectorated secretions, because they may be instructed by the physician to administer an antibiotic at the first notice of the illness. Antibiotics should be stored in a cool, dark place. Certain antibiotics are too toxic when administered systemically, but can be given by nebulization. These antibiotics are Neomycin and Bacitracin. Because they can cause bronchospasm, bronchodilators are administered along with them.

*Bronchodilators.* Bronchodilators are the crux of the antibronchospastic therapy and are administered locally or systematically. Metaproterenol sulfate (Alupent, Metaprel, Orciprenaline Sulfate) is an effective bronchodilator given by oral administration or inhalation. Oral bronchodilators are usually prescribed for home administration before the use of aerosols. Terbutaline sulfate (Brethine, Bricanyl), which is administered orally or subcutaneously, is an effective alternative but is slower to act. Bronkosol is the most commonly used medication for preaerosol bronchodilation, because it has a rapid action with few side effects.

*Mucolytics.* Mucolytics are enzymes that break down secretions, making them easier to expectorate. Acetylcysteine (Mucomyst, Respaire) is a local mucolytic agent.

*Steroids.* The effectiveness of the nebulized steroids has not been well established. Beclomethasone diproprionate (Vanceril Inhaler) is a relatively new metered-dose aerosol unit and inflammatory steroid.

*Oxygen administration*

The only purpose of oxygen administration is the relief of hypoxia, which occurs when insufficient oxygen is reaching the cells, interfering with metabolism. Prolonged hypoxemia can lead to right-sided heart failure. Symptoms include hypotension, cardiac arrythmias, tachypnea, dyspnea, drowsiness, headache, disorientation, nausea, and excitement. Cyanosis, a visual sign, may or may not be present, depending upon the hemoglobin status. An anemic client will not get cyanotic.

*Methods of delivery.* The method of delivery of oxygen depends upon the degree of illness. Clients with COPD require oxygen delivery with a low concentration, usually a flow rate of 2 to 3. This should not be increased, because carbon dioxide could be retained, which could stimulate respirations and thus cause hypoxia. The nasal cannula or venturi mask are the usual methods of choice for oxygen administration. Oxygen therapy is a medical intervention, and the CHN must have a physician's order to administer it.

The Oronasal venturi mask was designed principally for the COPD client (see Figure 8-4). In addition to the mask (when the concen-

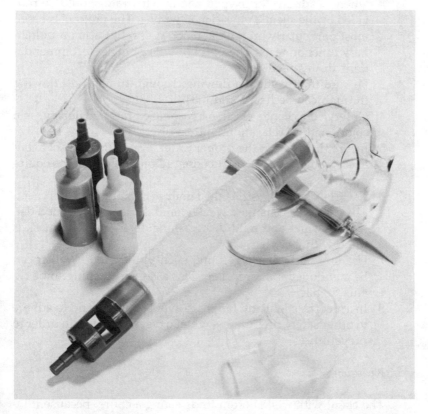

Figure 8-4. Oronasal Venturi Mask. (Photo used by permission of the Puritan-Bennett Corporation, Lenexa, Kansas.)

tration is 30% or below), it is necessary to have oxygen tubing, a tank of oxygen, and an oxygen flow regulator. If the concentration is to be above 30%, additional pieces of equipment needed are an aerosol adaptor, aerosol tubing, and compressed air.

*Oxygen administration in the home.* The client has undoubtedly had oxygen in a hospital setting prior to administration of it in the home and is familiar with certain aspects of its use. However, the method of administration may differ. Nursing care at home for the client who requires oxygen would include the following items (Duffy, 1981; Glover & Glover, 1978; Long, 1982):

1. Observe the client to determine whether oxygen therapy is necessary.
2. Adjust the flow regulator to prescribed rate. A protocol of when to administer oxygen and at what rate should be provided by the client's physician in writing. The protocol is based most particularly on arterial blood gases, but also on pulmonary function tests. The CHN or NP can make recommendations in this regard.
3. Be sure that oxygen is flowing through tubing (gas flowing through can be heard and felt).
4. Observe the client's reactions: respiration rate and quality, skin color, state of relaxation, and so on.
5. Insure that there is the proper water level in the aerosol nebulizer, if one is used. (Instructions are provided with the equipment.)
6. The CHN should instruct the family in cleaning the equipment. The cannula is changed weekly, and the mask is cleaned daily with water and mild dishwashing detergent. The mask is dried with a cloth.
7. Use of a portable oxygen unit such as the Linde Walker can be mentioned if appropriate. This assists in keeping some clients mobile.
8. Instruct the client and family to avoid smoking and to adhere to other safety precautions when oxygen is in use, in order to prevent fires.

*Nutrition*

The client with COPD often finds eating a chore, because it increases his dyspnea and coughing. Smaller and more frequent meals (five times daily) are recommended, with very little food taken after

6 P.M., so that the stomach does not become distended and impair the diaphragm movement during sleep. The diet should be high in protein and low in carbohydrates with adequate liquids, 10–12 glasses daily. Liquids help to liquefy secretions. Clients should be instructed that there is an adequate fluid intake when the urine is pale yellow in color.

### Humidification

Room humidifiers may be necessary for the client with COPD. Optimal room humidity (30–40%) is difficult to maintain, especially in the winter. Rooms with low relative humidity can make the sputum thick and difficult to raise and can increase the client's susceptibility to infection. The room humidifier should be scrubbed weekly with detergent and rinsed thoroughly (Chicago Lung Association, 1977).

Inspired gas must be humidified to protect the client's airways whenever it is administered to him. This can be done with a cool or heated humidifier or a nebulizer. A humidifier is used with a nasal cannula, nasal catheter, or oxygen mask (Glover & Glover, 1978).

## Clinic Care for the Client with Chronic Obstructive Pulmonary Disease

### Medical and nursing care

The client with COPD usually goes to the clinic to see the physician, unless he is cared for on a home care program (which provides care at home by a team of health professionals). Arterial blood gas specimens, which are usually drawn in the laboratory, are used in the clinic periodically to determine the client's oxygenation status. Also in the clinic, adjustments are made in medicines, respiratory therapy, lung physiotherapy, diet, and counseling. The CHN or NP may take the client's history, do tests of pulmonary function, teach or reinforce the teaching of the lung physiotherapy, review the diet, and listen to the client's concerns about disease and therapy. Tests of pulmonary function are done to determine the extent of changes in the disease. A spirometer is used to measure the volume of inhaled and exhaled air, which is recorded on paper and from which several tests of pulmonary function are interpreted. Referrals to organizations such as a local COPD group are often appropriate for the information and support these groups offer. Psychological counseling may be needed, because COPD is usually a long-term illness that interferes with the client's occupation, activities of daily living, sexual functioning, social activities, and body image, all of which may lead to feelings of loss and depression.

### General physical fitness

Outpatient rehabilitation should include physical exercise such as the exercise bike, walking, and occupational therapy geared to the client's tolerance. Exercise is important for *all* clients who have COPD in order to keep muscle functioning at peak efficiency within the confines of their disease. One client's exercise might be simply walking across a room three times a day, and another's might be biking (Fergus & Cordasco, 1977).

## Occupational Health: Workers with Chronic Obstructive Pulmonary Disease

### Statistics and economic impact

Approximately 400,000 workers develop occupation-related diseases, and 100,000 die annually; more than half of these deaths are probably due to diseases of the lung, including cancer. Morbidity and mortality statistics in occupational health, as noted in Chapter 7, are very likely underestimated. Another way to estimate the toll of occupational diseases is by examining their economic impact through compensation payments. By way of example, Social Security payments of $900 million were made to "black lung" victims or their widows in 1975 (Respiratory Diseases Task Force, 1977).

### Legislation

The federal government's recognition of the importance of occupational hazards in disease is reflected by the magnitude of recent legislation. The Federal Coal Mine Health and Safety Act of 1969 led to the establishment in 1973 of the Mining Enforcement and Safety Administration (MESA). The 1970 Occupational Safety and Health Act preceded the formation of the Occupational Safety and Health Administration (OSHA) and the National Institute of Occupational Safety and Health (NIOSH).

As regulatory agencies, OSHA and MESA are responsible for recommending standards for safe levels of exposure and surveillance, and for the enforcement of these in the work place. NIOSH develops statistical information about OSHA programs and criteria for standards, and provides for laboratory and technical services and personnel development to effect the changes. In the Target Health Program of OSHA, asbestos, cotton dust, and silica were among five types of materials included, with coal dust a specific concern of MESA (Respiratory Diseases Task Force, 1977).

### Nursing functions in occupational health programs: prevention and rehabilitation

Primary prevention of occupational lung disease is possible only when the causes of these diseases are understood and when harmful materials are replaced by less harmful ones or exposure is reduced to safe levels. Chemicals that are specific lung irritants, such as carbon tetrachloride and carbon disulfide (used in the manufacture of rayon), should be avoided. Nurses can inform employees about these hazardous compounds and the government health standards that have been set by OSHA. These include safe levels of exposure, information about the specific industry's current exposure levels, use of protective equipment such as masks and goggles, and the correct disposal of hazardous wastes. Work areas should be properly ventilated and lighted, and broken equipment should be repaired (Respiratory Diseases Task Force, 1977).

Preemployment and subsequent physical examinations establish whether clients have COPD and to what extent. If they have symptoms, the employees should be placed in protected situations.

## Community Health Programs

The present consideration of respiratory diseases cannot be limited to pulmonary status, but must include general health. Regular exercise, balanced nutrition, weight control, and adequate sleep are paramount to good health and good respiratory health. The Canadian government in 1974 listed five health risks or diseases, the etiology of which is often self-imposed by life style or environment. These are (1) motor vehicle accidents, (2) ischemic heart disease, (3) all other accidents, (4) respiratory disease/lung cancer, and (5) suicide, and they account for many years lost to illness and death between ages 1 and 70. Community action programs, to be effective against these conditions, must inculcate positive health values, promote health practices that improve the health status, modify life styles that are deleterious to health, and minimize or eliminate environmental health hazards such as air pollution. The CHN can teach sound health practices through radio and television discussions or in neighborhood groups. The role the school nurse plays in teaching grade-school and high-school students the hazards of smoking and in clarifying values for health attitudes in general cannot be emphasized enough (Respiratory Diseases Task Force, 1977).

Conclusion

In summary, reduction of environmental hazards to the lungs, cessation of cigarette smoking, pulmonary function tests to diagnose COPD, treatment regimens, and educational strategies are the current recommendations for decreasing the incidence of morbidity and mortality of COPD. Although there are rehabilitative measures for COPD, such as the bronchodilators, they are only marginally effective. The best method of controlling these diseases is prevention, specifically in regard to cigarette smoking. The cost to the client alone for oxygen around the clock at a low flow is in excess of $100 to $500 a month. This alone tells one that prevention is the best choice (Duffy, 1981; Respiratory Task Force, 1977).

## Middle-Aged Clients with Hypertension in Home, Clinic, and Industry

Introduction

Hypertension, popularly known as "high blood pressure," is probably the principal factor in the genesis of cardiovascular problems and a major public health problem. Hypertension accounts directly or indirectly for a substantial share of disability and death in the United States and other countries. The magnitude of the problem is highlighted by estimates that between 12 and 15% of all adults are hypertensive

Research since World War II has enhanced the understanding of high blood pressure and has advanced clinical treatment. Research on the pathogenesis of hypertension is incomplete, as is the understanding of the fundamental mechanisms that control arterial pressure in healthy and hypertensive persons. However, the advent of antihypertensive drugs in the last couple of decades and the beginning in 1972 of the federal High Blood Pressure Education Programs for communities has contributed to a very significant decline in hypertensive diseases (Hypertension Task Force, 1979a, 1979b; National Heart, Lung, and Blood Institute, 1979; Weber & Laragh, 1978).

Classsification of Hypertension

The following arbitrary classification or stratification of elevated diastolic blood pressure levels has become conventional (Joint National Committee on Detection, Evaluation, and Treatment of High Blood Pressure, 1980):

| Class | Blood Pressure (mm Hg) |
|---|---|
| Stratum I (mild) | 90–104 |
| Stratum II (moderate) | 105–114 |
| Stratum III (severe) | ≥ 115 |

Much more information about elevated diastolic pressures is available, because research has been directed primarily at them. Findings from future research will undoubtedly include recommendations for elevated systolic pressures.

Types of Hypertension and Their Causes

There are two types of hypertension, "secondary hypertension" and "essential hypertension." Secondary hypertension has a specific cause and can be identified in 5–10% of hypertensive clients (Kochar & Daniels, 1978). In essential hypertension, the specific etiological factors cannot be found. More than 90% of hypertensive clients have the essential type, also called "idiopathic" or "primary" hypertension (Hypertension Task Force, 1979a).

It is known that hypertension would not occur if mechanisms controlling blood vessel resistance were normal. Although most evidence suggests that alterations of the muscle in the walls of arterioles causes hypertension, more recent information indicates that small veins are also implicated, and that resistance changes of the vessels can be affected by increased activity in the sympathetic nervous system. Much of the research on essential hypertension is still very preliminary (Hypertension Task Force, 1979a; Kochar & Daniels, 1978).

Statistics

*Prevalence and disability*

The primary source of prevalence data on high blood pressure in the United States is the Health and Nutrition Examination Survey of the National Center for Health Statistics (1977). This survey, conducted from 1971 to 1974 on civilian, noninstitutionalized adults between 18 and 74 years of age, constitutes a national probability sample. Single blood pressure readings were taken with the subjects seated, and an extensive interview was done.

Based on projections from this national survey, nearly 60 million Americans in 1977 were estimated to be at risk for blood pressure problems, with heart attacks, strokes, or kidney failure as possible complications. Of these 60 million,

1.  About 35 million persons were estimated to have hypertension, and faced the immediate risk of one or more of the three complications listed above. Most of these warranted drug therapy. Only about 5 million of these nearly 35 million persons were taking medication and achieving control of their disease.
2.  The other 25 million persons were estimated to have borderline high blood pressure and to require monitoring. Specific drug therapy would probably not have been warranted for this group, but life style modifications would have been.

Disabled clients with hypertension and the associated problems of heart conditions and strokes number 52,000; a substantial part of this population is unable to work (Social Security Administration, 1978).

*Mortality*

Hypertension is still an element in the deaths of at least 250,000 Americans annually, but there is a decline in mortality rates for cardiovascular disease, apparently due in large part to hypertension control efforts. Although a downward trend has been observed since 1950, over one-third of the total decline has occurred since the advent of the federally supported High Blood Pressure Education Program in 1972. The death rate from stroke, for example, decreased 9% between 1965 and 1970, and 18% between 1970 and 1975. In recent years, deaths from hypertension-related diseases have continued to decline at a much faster rate than deaths from those categories of cardiovascular disease not related to hypertension. This trend holds truer for the younger age groups than for the older ones, and suggests that in the future fewer deaths will occur prematurely (Hypertension Task Force, 1979b; National Heart, Lung, and Blood Institute, 1979).

*Epidemiological factors*

Epidemiological studies have identified risk factors associated with hypertensive disease. These include obesity, physical inactivity, rapid heart rate, black or Native American origin, increasing age, use of oral contraceptives, pregnancy, family history, and high dietary salt intake. Many people in the United States gain weight and experience increased blood pressure as they age, especially in the presence of atherosclerosis. One study showed increased hypertension in physically inactive subjects. A fast heart rate may not be a cause of high blood pressure, only a symptom of its onset. At present, hypertension is the most prevalent disease among blacks in this country, and hypertension treatment is the most important factor in lengthening their life span. Oral contraceptives may increase blood pressure, and pregnancy may be complicated by hypertension. Persons who are most likely to become hypertensive are those with a family history of the disease. And, lastly, high dietary salt intake is a risk factor of great current interest (Hypertension Task Force, 1979a).

## Confirmation of Hypertension

All adults with diastolic blood pressure of 120 mm Hg or above during a routine screening should be referred to a physician for care. All persons with blood pressures of 160/96 mm Hg or above should have the elevated blood pressure rechecked within 1 month. All adults under age 50 with blood pressures between 140/90 mm Hg and 160/95 mm Hg should be checked every 6 to 12 months. Adults with a diastolic pressure of below 90 mm Hg should be advised to have their blood pressures checked routinely each year. Usually two to three readings a week apart are recommended to confirm an elevation. Routine pretreatment workup should define the severity of the blood pressure and identify risk factors (Moser & Ward, 1976).

*History*

The medical history should consist of any previous history of high blood pressure or its treatment: use of birth control pills or other hormones; stroke, cardiac, or renal disease; or a family history of hypertension, diabetes, or lipid abnormalities.

*Physical examination*

In addition to two or more blood pressure readings (one standing), the pretreatment physical by the NP or physician should include the following:

—Height and weight.

—Funduscopic examination of the eyes for hemorrhages, exudates, or papilledema—especially important in persons with diastolic blood pressures of 110 mm Hg or higher.

—Examination of the neck for thyroid enlargement, bruits, and distended veins.

—Auscultation of the lungs.

—Examination of the heart for increased rate, size, precordial heave, murmurs, arrhythmias, and gallops.

—Examination of the abdomen for bruits, large kidneys, or dilation of the aorta.

—Examination of the extremities for edema, peripheral pulses, and neurological deficits associated with stroke.

*Basic laboratory tests*

The baseline laboratory tests listed below should be obtained before initiating therapy:

—Urinalysis for glucose (dipstick), protein, and blood.

—Blood urea nitrogen, or creatinine.

—Serum potassium.

—Blood sugar.

—Serum cholesterol.

—Electrocardiogram.

Other tests that may be helpful include a chest X-ray, serum uric acid, microscopic urinalysis, and blood count ("Report of the Joint National Committee on Detection, Evaluation, and Treatment of High Blood Pressure," 1977; Joint National Committee, 1980; Moser & Ward, 1976).

## Antihypertensive Drug Therapy

Because clients must receive individualized therapy programs, some physicians classify them according to the severity of their hypertension in order to select appropriate initial antihypertensive therapy. An average group of untreated hypertensive clients will include 42% with mild, 24% with moderate, and 24% with severe hypertension; another 10% are classified as having labile hypertension (periodic elevated blood pressure).

Drug therapy for individuals with labile hypertension is highly individualized. Each patient should be thoroughly evaluated, with careful consideration of cardiovascular risk factors. If a decision is made to delay the drug therapy, the patient is monitored on a 3- to 6-month basis. Salt restriction, behavioral methods of blood pressure reduction, exercise, and weight control are helpful in controlling labile hypertension.

### The "stepped-care" approach

Antihypertensive drug therapy is begun with a small dose of medication. The dosage is gradually increased, and other drugs are added if necessary to achieve the predetermined level of blood pressure. Monitoring of the blood pressure levels and evaluation of the effects of the drug regimen are required at specified intervals. A gradual decrease in the drug dosages is desirable if levels of blood pressure are maintained. This so-called "stepped-care" antihypertensive approach resulted from a randomized controlled trial involving 10,940 persons, done in the 1970s by the National Heart, Lung, and Blood Institute ("Five-Year Findings of the Hypertension Detection and Follow-Up Program," 1979). The stepped-care approach, according to the Joint National Committee on Detection, Evaluation, and Treatment of High Blood Pressure (1980); M. S. Kochar, M.D. (1982), a hypertension specialist; and A. Jacknowitz (1982), a pharmacologist, is as follows:

*Step 1.* Start with a thiazide diuretic if blood pressure is not controlled and no external reason is found for the elevation. Alternatively, many physicians use beta-blockers and drugs from Step 2, such as clonidine (Catapres), prazosin (Minipres), captopril (Capoten), or quanabenz (Wytensen).

Step 2.   Add a sympathetic inhibiting agent—clonidine, methyldopa (Aldomet), metoprolol (Low-pressor), nadolol (Corgard), prazosin, propranolol (Inderal), rauwolfia alkaloids (Raudixin), or quanabenz. Beta-blockers—timolol (Blocadren), atenolol (Tenorin), or pindilol (Viscen)—are also used.

Step 3.   Add direct-acting vasodilators—hydralazine* (Apresoline) or minoxidil (Loniten).

Step 4.   Add or substitute for one of the above the adrenergic neuron blocker guanethidine (Ismelin), or substitute captopril.

The first step, as stated, is usually a thiazide-type diuretic or a beta-blocker. There is no demonstrable advantage of a long-acting diuretic such as chlorthalidone or a short-acting loop diuretic such as furosemide over hydrochlorothiazide in terms of antihypertensive effect. Dietary supplements are usually sufficient to prevent hypokalemia.

If the therapeutic goal is not achieved with the diuretic alone, one of the Step 2 drugs may be added. Diuretic therapy must always be continued. Whichever is chosen, it is first administered in small dosages and increased gradually until the therapeutic effect is achieved, until side effects develop, or until the maximum recommended dose is reached. Reversal of antihypertensive effects after the initial response may indicate fluid retention, requiring an increase in the dose of the diuretic. Usually there is little advantage in substituting one Step 2 drug for another, unless the patient experiences an untoward reaction.

When a third drug is needed, hydralazine or minoxidil are usually the drugs of choice in essential hypertension when sympathetic inhibitor drugs produce insufficient effects.

Addition or substitution of captopril may be necessary if the first three steps of the regimen are ineffective and the causes for unresponsiveness have been thoroughly investigated. These patients require very careful follow-up. Before proceeding to each successive step, the lack of responsiveness to the treatment should be investigated by checking (1) adherence to the drug regimen, (2) sufficiency of the current dose, (3) excessive sodium intake or weight gain, and (4) concomitant use of competing drugs (oral contraceptives, vasopressor decongestants, appetite suppressants). Drug treatment protocols do change as medical advances in hypertension therapy are made and as they are

*Some of the older drugs have more than one trade name.

adapted to individual clients (Kochar, 1982; Kochar & Daniels, 1978; "Report of the Joint National Committee," 1977).

*Untreated and noncompliant clients*

A great number of hypertensive clients are not treated or are inadequately treated because they do not avail themselves of the hypertensive screening programs or are noncompliant when given medication. Further education is needed to encourage all age groups to have blood pressure checked yearly or oftener. And clients on medication require instruction about the effects of the drugs, the necessity of taking the pills as prescribed, and the necessity of returning for blood pressure readings. The CHN can contribute significantly to these teaching programs at home, in the clinic, or in industry. In most instances, members of the client's family or someone else close to him should also be instructed by the CHN to assist the client in locating a support system.

## Dimensions of Nursing Care in Various Settings

The CHN's role in the treatment of hypertension consists primarily of detection, monitoring, teaching, and counseling. The detection is done when the CHN takes blood pressure routinely on newly admitted clients and periodically on other clients, regardless of the diagnosis.

*Home*

*Monitoring blood pressure readings.* Monitoring of clients with essential hypertension is the CHN's major contribution to their care. The CHN should take a blood pressure reading weekly or less often. These blood pressure readings should preferably be plotted on a graph on the client's record, in order to make the changes clear at a glance. The medication taken by the client can be noted on the blood pressure graph to show changes in readings related to accompanying drugs.

*Teaching: physiology of blood pressure and medications.* The parameters of teaching include discussing with clients the physiology of normal and high blood pressure. It also encompasses supervision of medications, diet, including salt intake, and weight control. Teaching the physiology of normal and high blood pressure is best done with visual aids. Supervision of medications includes reviewing the drugs with the client and explaining of their positive and negative effects; establishing whether the blood pressure is stabilizing as a result of the medications; and ascertaining client compliance. The CHN should consult the client regularly as to how he feels on the drug regimen.

*Teaching: weight control, diet, and physical activity.* Hypertension accelerates the atherosclerotic process; in turn, atherosclerosis speeds up the hypertensive cardiovascular changes and ensuing complications. Although these associations are unquestionable, the mechanisms are unknown. Cholesterol, sodium, alcohol, and caloric consumption are nutritional risks in hypertension. Obesity, defined as weight 25% over normal limits, is an independent risk factor in this disease. The Framingham Study concluded that overweight hypertensives experience heart disease and premature death at twice the rate of nonobese hypertensives (Kochar & Daniels, 1978).

Nutritional counseling for hypertensive clients should include the following four areas: salt intake modification; increased intake of potassium-rich foods with diuretic therapy; saturated fat (cholesterol) intake modification; and weight control and/or loss. A practical approach to teaching the above is to obtain a 24-hour diet recall from the client to use as a baseline. The basic four food groups of milk, meat, vegetables, and fruit should be reviewed first with posters, charts, pamphlets, and slides before the above modifications are imposed. These four modifications can be taught using a basic dietary approach (Christianson, 1982; Hypertension Task Force, 1979a; Kochar & Daniels, 1978):

A. To decrease salt or sodium chloride:
   1. Avoid overly salted foods.
   2. Cook with only small amounts of salt.
   3. Do not use the salt shaker at the table.
   4. Avoid convenience, processed, or ready-to-eat foods.
B. To decrease animal or saturated fats:
   See pp. 209–212.
C. To increase potassium:
   Have one or two fruits every morning along with the diuretic pill. Most fresh fruits and vegetables are high in potassium and should be eaten three to four times daily (diuretics deplete the body's potassium supply). Bananas, oranges, and raisins are especially high in potassium.
D. To control or lose weight:
   1. Plan meals.
      a. Three balanced meals.
      b. Only low-calorie snacks.

    c. No meals 4 hours prior to bedtime.
2. About 1–2 pounds weight loss permitted weekly.
3. Focus on control and establishing new habits.
E. Miscellaneous advice:
    1. Emphasize real taste of foods, not condiments.
    2. In a restaurant, order boiled, baked, broiled, and roasted foods without sauces and gravies.

Physical activity is recommended for all clients, but may need restrictions if the hypertension is severe.

*Counseling.* In order to counsel a client, the CHN requires a thorough understanding of hypertension as a disease, the client's specific hypertension problems (or potential problems in compliance with his medical regimen), and counseling and teaching techniques appropriate to the situation. The counseling can take place in a screening program, clinic, or industry, as well as in the home. The CHN could begin the interaction by stating that although the cause of hypertension is not known, there are methods to control the symptoms, including medication, dietary changes, and life style alterations. The CHN might then proceed by apprising the client of the risk factors listed earlier (p. 275) and ascertaining the motivation for health care and compliance with recommendations.

In addition to the physiology of the disease process, medication, diet and weight control, and physical activity, which have been discussed in this chapter, the CHN should review other factors, such as smoking, alcohol, heredity, race, stress, and relaxation. Smoking is one of the main risk factors. Drinking is another; the Kaiser-Permanente Study indicated that three or more drinks daily is a definite risk factor for hypertension, and six or more increases the risk by 50% (Klatsky, Friedman, Siegelaub, & Gérard, 1977). The chances of having hypertension are approximately two times greater if there is hypertension in one's immediate family. A greater percentage of blacks have hypertension than whites. Finally, stress as a cause of hypertension is being investigated extensively; various methods of relaxation can be taught to clients to reduce their stress, which contributes to the disease. A discussion with a client about his daily or weekly activities can be a starting point to motivate him to change his life style. For example, the nurse may suggest that the client take a daily relaxation break at work, planned recreation on the weekend, and a yearly vacation. Several counseling sessions may need to be held in order to accomplish the goals (Kochar & Daniels, 1978).

*Clinics*

The NP manages cases of stable hypertension and supports the medical regimen for cases of severe and uncontrolled hypertension. Her responsibilities can include such things as physical examinations and following the medication protocol under medical supervision. Monitoring for compliance with drug regimens and determining reasons for noncompliance are major activities for CHNs. Screening and monitoring of blood pressure can be done by CHNs with appropriate physician backup and a referral system. The clinics can be conducted in churches, stores, or other public places. The nurse also does client and family education, clinic management, and research.

*Occupational health*

The fundamental elements of a blood pressure control program at a work site are publicity, education, scheduled screenings, referral to medical care, and follow-up of clients with elevated blood pressure. Education can enhance client understanding, motivation, and compliance with treatment regimens. Screening can be done on an appointment schedule or in a mass screening annually. Screeners are often trained and supervised by the nurses. Any individual with a diastole greater than 120 mm Hg, or greater than 110 mm Hg with symptoms such as dizziness, headaches, chest pains, or shortness of breath, requires prompt referral to a physician. Follow-up is necessary to ascertain whether a client has complied with the referral and to do blood pressure rechecks and counseling at the work site (Kochar & Daniels, 1978). The CHN at the work site should communicate with the nurses who may be seeing the client at home or in another clinic situation, always with the client's knowledge.

Mass screening at the work site can be a useful way to detect hypertension. Alderman and Schoenbaum (1975) reported a research study done at Gimbel's Department Store in New York City, in which 84% of the 1850 employees were screened. Of the 186 who were diagnosed with hypertension (160/95), 65% (or 121) requested treatment. Care was provided at work with minimal financial cost or loss of work hours. Both employees and employers benefit from this type of program. If a client requires special placement at work, this must be done judiciously in order to protect him from loss of a promotion or job. A nurse can manage most facets of a hypertension control program in industry.

The Hypertension Program at the University of Wisconsin–Milwaukee Student Health Service, begun in 1976 in cooperation with the Milwaukee High Blood Pressure Program, is a model program aimed at prevention and treatment (Daniels, Kochar, Itskovitz, Hoffman, & Ettle, 1979; Hoffman, 1981; Milwaukee High Blood Pressure Program, 1977). Approximately 6600 students have been screened in this program; of these students, 17% had elevated blood pressure levels. Among these, 49% were labile, 42% were essential, 3% were secondary ("Pill"-induced) hypertensives, and 6% had subsequently normal blood pressure levels. Treatments were as follows: 75% were instructed in life style modification, 23% were treated with diuretics, and 2% were treated with propranolol. Follow-up revealed a substantial decrease in smoking and alcohol intake, diet changes, and normal blood pressure levels in 49% of the original group (i.e., the 17% with disease).

The program at the Milwaukee campus continues with a weekly blood pressure screening clinic for students, faculty, and walk-ins from the community; with mass screenings at planned intervals; and with treatment and referrals as indicated. The program at the campus site operates on the same principle as typical programs at the work site— that is, it reaches, identifies, treats, and counsels adults who have hypertension.

## Prevention of Hypertension

Addressing the known risk factors is the best form of primary prevention. The control and prevention of obesity is a formidable task. Considering the overall benefits of habits of good personal hygiene, such as physical exercise, these habits should be emphasized more. Ignorance about the basic physiological mechanism of blood pressure precludes total elimination of hypertension at present. Secondary prevention is accomplished with drug therapy for the known hypertensives, as well as dietary and life style changes (Hypertension Task Force, 1979a).

## Research Recommendations

The Hypertension Task Force has identified seven areas for research in which new knowledge is needed. These areas include (1) the role of sodium (salt) intake in the diet; (2) the relationship of the central nervous system to hypertension; (3) the role of hormones such as prostaglandins; (4) microcirculation and veins; (5) structure and function of blood vessels; (6) genetic determinants; and (7) blood pressure regulation during growth and development. If strides to conquer the "silent killer," hypertensive disease, continue at the accelerated pace begun in the 1970s, the basic aim could be realized in the 1980s. (Hypertension Task Force, 1979b).

## Appendix 8A: Addresses for Diabetic Diet Information

1. American Diabetes Association
   600 Fifth Avenue
   New York, NY 10020
   (212) 541-4310
2. American Dietetic Association
   430 N. Michigan Avenue
   Chicago, IL 60611
3. Eli Lilly & Company
   Indianapolis, IN 46206
4. Carnation Company
   Medical Dept.
   5045 Wilshire Blvd.
   Los Angeles, CA 90036
5. National Dairy Council
   Rosemont, IL 60018

## Appendix 8B

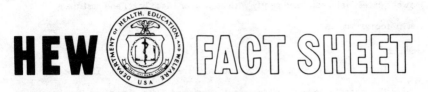

**U.S. DEPARTMENT OF HEALTH, EDUCATION, AND WELFARE**
National Institutes of Health
National Institute of Arthritis, Metabolism, and Digestive Diseases
Bethesda, Maryland 20014

### FOOT CARE FOR THE DIABETIC PATIENT

Take Care

Proper care of the feet is of utmost importance to diabetics. Since this disorder often cuts down the blood supply to the feet and also reduces sensation, diabetics do not always feel pain when they are developing foot disorders. Many major foot problems, however, can be avoided. This fact sheet is designed to help you understand the best way to care for your feet.

Corns and Calluses

Both corns and calluses are caused by the building up of hard skin at points where shoes exert pressure and friction. You may alleviate these problems by keeping them rubbed down gently and carefully with a fine emery board or pumice stone. In general, however, these lesions should be treated by a podiatrist who will also advise about improving the fit of the shoe. Be sure to consult your physician or your podiatrist.

Bathing

Bathe your feet daily in lukewarm (not hot) water, using mild soap. After a thorough rinsing, dry them gently; use a soft towel and a "blotting technique." Pay special attention to the skin between the toes. Test bath water temperature with your wrist before getting into the tub, especially if your feet are insensitive to temperature changes. If your feet are rough and dry, soak them in water

for twenty minutes, and then rub them gently with a moisture restoring cream.
(See your physician or your podiatrist about what kind to use.) If your feet
sweat excessively, rub them gently with alcohol or witch hazel and dust them
with foot powder.

Socks

Heavy cotton or wool socks (or stockings) are recommended. They should
be of the correct size and must be free of seams and darns. To ensure cleanliness,
it is important to change your socks every day. Loose woolen socks may be
worn at night to keep your feet warm.

Exercise

Walking is the best exercise for your feet. Your doctor also may advise
special exercises.

Shoes

Soft leather oxford shoes are recommended for daily wear. Shoes should
have a leather sole, a flat low heel, and should conform to the shape of your
foot. New shoes need to be worn for short periods during the first week of
wear (for example, two hours daily). Casual shoes should be worn only for short
intervals. Avoid wearing the same shoes all day long. A change at midday
is good. Do not go barefoot, especially when you cannot be sure of what is
underfoot. All shoe corrections should be done on the advice of your physician
or your podiatrist (chiropodist). If your feet swell at the end of the day, it is
a good idea to change to a more comfortable pair of shoes.

Toenails

Trim or file your toenails straight across so that they are even with the
skin on the ends of your toes. A coarse metal file with a blunt tip is a satisfactory
instrument to use. (A nail clipper also may be used.) Avoid probing with metal
tools. If you go to a foot doctor tell him you have diabetes.

Daily Inspection

Inspect your feet every day. If you notice any redness, heat, swellings, cracks in the skin, sores, or excessive of unequal buildup of calluses, consult your physician or your podiatrist.

Protect Your Feet By

Avoiding exposure of bare feet to cold, heat, and excessive sunlight.

Wearing shoes and socks whenever you can.

Some Don'ts

Don't apply a hot water bottle, a heating pad, or hot water to your feet.

Don't wear cut-out shoes or sandals.

Don't apply strong antiseptics or chemicals to your feet.

Don't wear bedroom slippers for work.

Don't go walking on a foot which has any ulcer or infection.

Always see your physician and your podiatrist at regular intervals. It is essential that you keep your diabetes under good control to ensure good foot care.

Discuss all foot problems with your physician or podiatrist promptly.

### ###

October 1978

# References

Action on Smoking and Health. *ASH: History of the war against smoking, 1964–1978* (pamphlet). Washington, D.C.: Author, 1978.

Alderman, M. H., & Schoenbaum, E. E. Detection and treatment of hypertension. *New England Journal of Medicine*, 1975, *293*, 65–68.

American Cancer Society. *1982 cancer facts and figures.* New York: Author, 1981.

American Cancer Society, Milwaukee Division. *Suppliers of protheses and bras for the mastectomy patient.* Milwaukee: Author, 1982. (Mimeographed)

American Diabetes Association. *Cure* (pamphlet). Milwaukee: Author (Wisconsin Affiliate), no date.

American Dietetic Association. Exchange list for meal planning. Chicago: Author, 1976.

Anderson, M. Personal communication, May 25, 1983.

Ask the doctor: Diabetes tests are compared, *Milwaukee Journal*, August 11, 1978, p. 9.

Bates, R. *A guide to physical assessment*. Philadelphia: J. B. Lippincott, 1979.

Beeson, P. B., & McDermott, W. (Eds.). *Textbook of medicine*. Philadelphia: W. B. Saunders, 1975.

Benjamin, S. P., & McCormack, J. Structural abnormalities in COPD. *Postgraduate Medicine*, 1977, *62*, 101–102.

Bergersen, S. *Pharmacology in nursing* (13th ed.). St. Louis: C. V. Mosby, 1976.

Brown, M. J. L. The quality of the work environment. *American Journal of Nursing*, 1975, *75*, 1755–1760.

Chicago Lung Association. *Chronic obstructive pulmonary disease: A guide for teaching patients* (booklet). Chicago: Author, 1977.

Christianson, M. A. Personal communications, February 16 and 25, 1982, and March 14, 1982.

Craig, G. J. *Human development* (2nd ed.). Englewood Cliffs, N.J.: Prentice-Hall, 1980.

Daniels, L. M., Kochar, M. S., Itskovitz, H. D., Hoffman, W. K., & Ettle, S. N. Hypertension control on an urban campus. *Journal of the American School Health Association*, 1979, *27*, 234–238.

District of Columbia Visiting Nurse Association. Untitled mimeograph, January 1, 1979.

Duffy, D. Personal communication, March 1, 1981.

Dunn, H. L. *High-level wellness*. Arlington, Va.: Bealty, 1973.

Eckert, M. Personal communication, May 18, 1983.

Eklind, D. Erik Erikson's eight ages of man. *New York Times Magazine*, April 5, 1970, 111.

Elias, M. F., Elias, P. K., & Elias, J. W. *Basic processes in adult developmental psychology*. St. Louis: C. V. Mosby, 1977.

Erikson, E. H. *Identity: Youth and crisis*. New York: Norton, 1968.

Fergus, L. C., & Cordasco, E. M. Pulmonary rehabilitation of the patient with COPD. *Postgraduate Medicine*, 1977, *62*, 143.

Five-year findings of the Hypertension Detection and Follow-Up Program. *Journal of the American Medical Association*, 1979, *242*, 2562–2577.

Glover, D. W., & Glover, M. M. *Respiratory therapy: Basics for nursing and the allied health professions*. St. Louis: C. V. Mosby, 1978.

Golish, J. A., & Ahmad, M. Management of COPD: A physiologic approach. *Postgraduate Medicine*, 1977, *62*,133.

Guthrie, D. W., & Guthrie, R. A. (Eds.). *Nursing management of diabetes mellitus*. St. Louis: C. V. Mosby, 1977.

Haukenes, E. Personal communication, February 14, 1982.

Havighurst, R. J. *Developmental tests and education* (3rd ed.). New York: David McKay, 1948.

Hoffman, W. K. Personal communication, September 27, 1981.

Hypertension Task Force. *Report of the Hypertension Task Force* (Vol. 1, *General summary and recommendations*) (DHEW Publ. No. (NIH) 79-1623). Washington, D.C.: U.S. Department of Health, Education and Welfare, 1979. (a)

Hypertension Task Force. *Report of the Hypertension Task Force* (Vol. 2, *Scientific summary and recommendations*) (DHEW Publ. No. (NIH) 79-1624). Washington, D.C.: U.S. Department of Health, Education and Welfare, 1979. (b)

Jacknowitz, A. Personal communication, December 1982.

Joint National Committee on Detection, Evaluation, and Treatment of High Blood Pressure. *Report of the Joint National Committee on Detection, Evaluation, and Treatment of High Blood Pressure* (DHEW Publ. No. (NIH) 80-1060). Washington, D.C.: U.S. Department of Health, Education and Welfare, 1980.

Judges uphold ban on diabetic truckers, *Milwaukee Journal*, February 27, 1979, pp. 1–2.

Kaluger, G., & Kaluger, M. M. *Human development: The span of life*. St. Louis: C. V. Mosby, 1974.

Klatsky, A. L., Friedman, G. D., Siegelaub, M. S., & Gérard, M. J. Alcohol consumption and blood pressure: Kaiser-Permanente multiphasic health examination data. *New England Journal of Medicine*, 1977, *296*, 1194–1200.

Klein, R. *A crisis to grow on: Rehabilitation of the breast cancer patient*. New York: American Cancer Society, 1971.

Kochar, M. S. Personal communication, November 30, 1982.

Kochar, M. S., & Daniels, L. M. *Hypertension control for nurses and other health professionals*. St. Louis: C. V. Mosby, 1978.

Lasser, T. *What is Reach to Recovery?* (pamphlet). New York: American Cancer Society, 1977.

Leis, H. P. The diagnosis of breast cancer. *CA: A Cancer Journal of Clinicians*, 1977, *27*, 209.

Long, C. Personal communication, February 14, 1982.

Marino, L. B. Cancer patients: Your special role. *Nursing 76*, 1976, *6*, 26–29.

Milwaukee High Blood Pressure Program. *Milwaukee Life Saving Program: Outstanding in the United States, 1974–1977* (pamphlet). Milwaukee: Author, 1977.

Moser, M., & Ward, G. Guidelines for hypertension control. *Primary Cardiology,* 1976, *237,* 20–21.

National Cancer Institute. *Progress against cancer of the breast* (DHEW Publ. No. (NIH) 75-328). Washington, D.C.: U.S. Department of Health, Education and Welfare, 1974.

National Cancer Institute. *The Treatment of primary breast cancer: Management of local disease* (NIH Consensus Development Conference Summary, Vol. 2, No. 5). Washington, D.C.: U.S. Department of Health, Education and Welfare, 1979.

National Cancer Program. *Report to the Director, National Institute of Health.* Washington, D.C.: U.S. Department of Health, Education and Welfare, 1976.

National Center for Health Statistics. *Health and Nutrition and Nutrition Examination Survey (HANES) 1971–1974: Blood pressure levels of persons 6–74 years, United States 1971–1974* (DHEW Publ. No. 203, Series 11, Vital and Health Statistics). Washington, D.C.: U.S. Department of Health, Education and Welfare, 1977.

National Commission on Diabetes. *Report of the National Commission on Diabetes to the Congress of the United States* (Vol. 3, Parts 1 and 4) (DHEW Publ. No. (NIH) 77-1024). Washington, D.C.: U.S. Department of Health, Education and Welfare, 1975.

National Heart, Lung, and Blood Institute. *Blood pressure statistics in the United States.* Unpublished mimeograph, 1979.

National Institute of Arthritis, Metabolism, and Digestive Diseases. *Summary of results of the University Group Diabetes Study of the oral drugs and tolbutamide.* Washington, D.C.: U.S. Department of Health, Education and Welfare, 1970.

National Institute of Arthritis, Metabolism, and Digestive Diseases. *Foot care of the diabetic patient* (pamphlet). Washington, D.C.: U.S. Department of Health, Education and Welfare, 1978.

National Institutes of Health. *Changes—research on aging and the aged* (DHEW Publ. No. 78-85). Washington, D.C.: U.S. Department of Health, Education and Welfare, 1978.

National Research Council (Food and Nutrition Board, Committee on Dietary Allowances). *Recommended dietary allowances* (9th ed.). Washington, D.C.: Author, 1980.

Peplau, H. E. Mid-life crises. *American Journal of Nursing,* 1975, *75,* 1761–1765.

*Physician's desk reference* (35th ed.). Oradell, N.J.: Medical Economics, 1981.

Respiratory Diseases Task Force. *Respiratory Diseases Task Force report on prevention, control, education* (DHEW Publ. No. 78-1248). Washington, D.C.: U.S. Department of Health, Education and Welfare, 1977.

Report of the Joint National Committee on Detection, Evaluation, and Treatment of High Blood Pressure: A cooperative study. *Journal of the American Medical Association*, 1977, *237*, 255–258.

Rollin, B. *First you cry*. Philadelphia: J. B. Lippincott, 1976.

Ryan, A. J. Editorial: Diabetes and therapeutic self-control. *Postgraduate Medicine*, 1979, *65*, 23–24.

Slater, N. L. Adult diabetes—insulin reactions versus ketoacidosis: Guidelines for diagnosis and intervention. *American Journal of Nursing*, 1978, *78*, 876–877.

Social Security Administration. *1972 survey of disabled and nondisabled adults: Chronic disease, injury, and work disability*. 1978.

Strauss, A. L. *Chronic illness and the quality of life*. St. Louis: C. V. Mosby, 1975.

Stucky, V. The meal plan. In D. W. Guthrie & R. A. Guthrie (Eds.), *Nursing management of diabetes mellitus*. St. Louis: C. V. Mosby, 1977.

Talbott, E. Personal communication, March 13, 1978.

Tomashefski, J. Definition, differentiation, and classification of COPD. *Postgraduate Medicine*, 1977, *62*, 89.

Trowell, H. Diabetes mellitus and dietary fiber of starchy foods. *Journal of Clinical Nutrition*, 1978, *31*, S3–S11.

U.S. Bureau of the Census. *Statistical abstract of the United States, 1981* (102nd ed.). Washington, D.C.: U.S. Department of Commerce, 1981.

Walesky, M. E. Adult diabetes—diabetic ketoacidosis. *American Journal of Nursing*, 1978, *78*, 873.

Watson, R. C. CT scan, its use and abuse. *CA: A Cancer Journal of Clinicians*, 1978, *28*, 100–103.

Weber, M., & Laragh, J. H. A cardiovascular basis for the treatment of essential hypertension. *Bulletin of the New York Academy of Medicine*, 1978, *54*, 931.

# 9

# The Elderly at Home, in Clinics, and in Nursing Homes

*Dorothy D. Petrowski and Phyllis Tyzenhouse*

## Introduction

The United States is no longer a nation of young people. The 24 million Americans aged 65 and older comprise 11% of the population, and the proportion is expected to reach 18% by 2030. Between 1960 and 1970, the greatest growth rate of any population group was among those aged 75 and over—36%, compared to a growth of 11% in the group aged 65 to 74 (O. W. Anderson, 1976).

As the elderly population grows, chronic health problems will increase, especially those common to people over age 75. Several prevalent social trends have forced families and community agencies to provide alternatives to institutionalization of the elderly and total care by families. These trends include the tendency for children to live apart from older relatives; the shrinking size of households, with decreased availability of relatives to provide social, psychological, economic, and physical support; and the increasing number of families with two or more generations of people over 65. If these trends continue, community health nurses (CHNs) will become increasingly involved in the care of the elderly at home and in community settings, and they will need to increase their knowledge and skills in gerontological nursing.

292

# Health Characteristics
# of Senior Citizens

## Definitions According to Age

It is not possible to generalize about the characteristics of the elderly, for several reasons. First, there is a lack of agreement about who is "old," and "old age" spans a period of at least 40 years. The 1965 World Health Organization Seminar on Aging in Kiev defined persons between the ages of 45 and 59 as "middle-aged"; those 60 to 74 as "elderly"; those 75 to 89 as "aged" or "old"; and those 90 or older as "very old" (W. F. Anderson, 1967). More recently, Neugarten and Havighurst (1976) considered older people in distinct groups: the "young-old," who are aged 55 to 75, and the "old-old," those aged 75 and above. Using this definition to view the older population as being divided into a younger, generally healthy, and active group and an older, more physically limited group is helpful in working with and planning for them.

## Vast Variability in Aging

A second deterrent to generalization is the fact that each person has his own pattern and rate of aging. It is possible to be chronologically old and psychologically young, and the biological effects of aging on various organs are not uniform. One's eyes may be keen and unimpaired, while the joints are worn and stiff. Aging is not synonymous with sickness and infirmity, although the numbers of persons affected with one or more chronic diseases increase with age. According to figures cited by Carpenter, McArthur, and Higgins (1974), almost 27% of the elderly have one or more chronic diseases; 20% have two or more; and 31% have three or more. However, these people may or may not be functionally impaired; in fact, 53% of persons over 65 have no activity limitation at all due to chronic disease (U.S. Department of Health, Education and Welfare, 1978).

A great challenge to nurses is to keep the functionally able older group as independent and healthy as possible for as long as possible. Or, as Selye says, "The most important thing is not just to add years to life, but to add life to the years" (quoted by Wixen, 1978).

## A Healthy and Successful Older Person

The elderly person is in the stage of life when his major efforts as an individual are almost finished, and there is time to reflect, enjoy grandchildren, travel, read, and so on. The psychosocial dimension of "integrity or despair" means that the elderly person either looks back with satisfaction on his life or sees it as a series of missed opportunities (Eklind, 1970; Erikson, 1968). Optimal growth and adaptation can occur all along the life cycle, if the individual's strengths and potentials are recognized and encouraged by the environment in which he lives (Butler & Lewis, 1977).

The many elderly people who are free of physical affliction are quite able to perform physical and mental activities. The CHN should foster this state of well-being by encouraging them to keep active. Even if the CHN has been called to a home to see a sick family member, she should also focus on the well elderly persons in the home.

The problem of determining health among the elderly is compounded by the difficulty in distinguishing between normal physiological changes and pathological processes. One can gauge health by using a combination of physical measures, such as blood pressure and visual acuity; behavioral measures, such as functional adequacy and role competence; mental and psychological measures; and ratings of health by the individual and significant others.

Health may also be defined by identifying indicators of physical and mental health, such as satisfaction with one's life, competence in self-maintenance, ability to adapt to physical and social losses, accurate perception of reality, and capacity to interact with others. Typically, the individual who is able to meet basic needs, enjoy social interaction, and set goals for himself is generally a healthy person, even though his strength and organ function may be reduced. Cape (1978) has described a healthy person as one who enjoys the sense of well-being while it lasts, and rides out stresses with determination and confidence. He believes that physical and mental assaults such as an infection or the loss of a loved one can tilt the scales of health toward morbidity, but a strong ego structure can counterbalance some of the downward tilt.

Health in the older population is delicately balanced and influenced by a combination of forces. CHNs can improve their elderly clients' health by addressing environmental, social, psychological, and physical determinants of health. They can address the living standards of the well elderly by suggesting ways to make living space safe; by encouraging visits to senior centers for socialization, engagement in hobbies, the practice of normal nutrition, and appropriate physical exercises; and by emphasizing the necessity for medical checkups.

## Health Goals for Elderly Citizens

In 1979, the United States Department of Health, Education and Welfare published a landmark document, *Healthy People: The Surgeon General's Report on Health Promotion and Disease Prevention* (Richmond, 1979); this report reviewed the present state of the health of Americans, past accomplishments that contributed to improved health, and goals for the future. In his introductory remarks, then Secretary of Health, Education and Welfare Califano pointed out that the leading causes of death in 1900 were influenza, pneumonia, diphtheria, tuberculosis, and gastrointestinal infections, claiming 580 lives out of every 100,000. Today, only 1% of all deaths before age 75 are due to infection. The efforts that led to the control of infectious diseases have been termed ''the first public health revolution.''

Health professionals can be proud of these achievements, but most are now preparing for the second revolution, involving primarily health promotion and prevention of chronic diseases. Heart disease, cancer, and stroke, which are influenced by environmental and behavioral factors, now cause most deaths among older adults. Smoking, overeating, lack of exercise, and failure to wear seat belts are examples of behaviors that contribute to the leading causes of death. Informed and motivated individuals can control these risk factors or behaviors for disease. The second revolution will need to be waged by the public, the consumer, rather than by the health care system. CHNs can play a major role in promoting the second revolution by learning the leading causes of disease and death in each major population group, the risk factors for these diseases, and strategies for motivating and enabling clients to reduce their risk factors. They must make a greater effort to seek out the elderly whose health needs are more likely to be unmet: those with existing impairments, the poor, the nonwhite, the rural aged, and those who live alone. Many old people are unaware that their problems are correctable and that help is available.

The Surgeon General's goal for older Americans in 1979 was to improve health and quality of life for them, and by 1990 to reduce the average annual number of days of restricted activity attributable to acute and chronic conditions by 20%, or to fewer than 30 days per year (Richmond, 1979). Although most chronic diseases have long latent periods, and the ideal time to initiate prevention is during early life, it is possible to reduce disease and loss of function at any age.

Improving the health of older people would not only increase their life expectancy, but also their independence and satisfactions; it would reduce the need for medical care and institutionalization. Older people require almost 30% of the total health expenditure in the United States. In 1977, the annual per capita health expenditure for the elderly, $1745, was nearly triple the amount spent for persons aged 19 to 64, and nearly seven times greater than for persons under 19. (See Table 9-1.)

The cost of hospital care for persons aged 65 and over expanded from $5 million in 1968 to $18 million in 1977. Not all of these expenses are reimbursed by Medicare or other insurance resources, and the out-of-pocket cost for each older person averaged $613 in 1977 (Gibson & Fisher, 1979). Considering the low average income of old people, it is small wonder that many of them scrimp on necessities in order to pay for medicine and medical care, and delay seeking care until their problems become serious. Obviously, the best method of reducing the need for elaborate care is prevention.

## Major Health Problems of the Elderly

The major causes of death among persons aged 65 and over continue to be heart disease, cancer, and stroke, followed by influenza and pneumonia, arteriosclerosis, diabetes mellitus, accidents, chronic respiratory disease, cirrhosis of the liver, and kidney diseases (U.S. Bureau of the Census, 1979). Other chronic diseases that do not necessarily contribute to death also affect the lives of the elderly. The prevalence of certain chronic diseases in persons 65 years of age and older offers clues as to which groups should be screened for these diseases. Much of this screening could be done by CHNs. In order of prevalence, the diseases are arthritis, hearing and vision impairments, hypertension, heart conditions, diabetes, back problems, abdominal hernias, chronic bronchitis and asthma, and ulcers. By way of example, 380 in every 1000 elderly persons are afflicted with arthritis (more females), and 29 in 1000 suffers from ulcers (more males) (U.S. Department of Health, Education and Welfare, 1976).

The 1975 Health Interview Survey, from which these figures are drawn, was far from inclusive because the list of diseases did not include conditions such as periodontal disease, which is present in about

Table 9-1
Per Capita Health Care Expenditures for Three Age Groups, 1977

|  | All Ages | Under 19 | 19–64 | 65+ |
|---|---|---|---|---|
| Total, in millions of dollars | 646 | 253 | 661 | 1,745 |
| Hospital care | 297 | 89 | 325 | 769 |
| Physicians' services | 146 | 70 | 159 | 302 |
| Other professional services | 15 | 4 | 17 | 35 |
| Drugs and drug sundries | 57 | 33 | 58 | 121 |
| Nursing home care | 57 | 5 | 14 | 446 |

*Note.* Adapted from R. M. Gibson and C. R. Fisher, "Age Difference in Health Care Spending, Fiscal Year 1977," *Social Security Bulletin,* January 1979, p. 5.

95% of the elderly (Ebersole & Hess, 1981). These authors have also found that a significant number of nursing home residents have hemorrhoids and varicose veins, which seriously detract from enjoyment of life. Although these and other diseases and physical limitations could be readily detected and treated, less than half of those over 65 reported that they had had preventive care examinations in the past 2 years (U.S. Department of Health, Education and Welfare, 1976). Of this group, 48% reported having had an eye examination during this period; 30% of the women had had a Pap smear; and 37% had had a breast examination; 37% of the group had had an electrocardiogram; and 34% had had a glaucoma test. The figures for the rural aged, the nonwhite, and those with low incomes were even lower, indicating that outreach programs are needed to improve the availability of health care for these older Americans.

## Care of the Elderly at Home

### Living Arrangements for the Elderly

In 1978, 63% of older Americans lived in family settings, and only 6% were institutionalized. Nearly one-third of the older population lived alone in 1978, and about 2% lived with nonrelatives (U.S. Bureau of the Census, 1979). The majority of the old people living alone are women, because older women outlive older men, and older men are more likely to be married. As spouses and companions die or become residents of nursing homes, the number of senior citizens who live alone increases in the upper age groups. CHNs will thus be working with mainly female elderly clients in their homes or in institutions. It is essential to assess the suitability of a client's residence; the following outline for assessing a residence may be useful:

A. General adequacy of environment
    1. State of repair
    2. Cleanliness and freedom from pests
    3. Source of heat, water, electricity, waste disposal
    4. Toilet and washing facilities
    5. Home furnishings
    6. Food preparations and storage area
    7. Recreational area (yard, porch, etc.)
B. Safety features
    1. Personal security
    2. Police and fire protection
    3. Smoke detector or similar device
    4. Telephone or communication system
    5. Availability of emergency medical aid
    6. Safe area for outdoor exercise
    7. Freedom from barriers and source of potential injury (waxed floors, small rugs, electrical hazards, loose stairs, etc.)
    8. Contact with others (family members, friendly visitors, etc.)
C. Availability of supplies and services
    1. Food
    2. Clothing
    3. Household items (soap, linens, etc.)
    4. Banking
    5. Transportation
    6. Recreation (newspaper, radio, library, companionship at a community center or elsewhere)
    7. Religious services (if desired)
    8. Neighbors

The CHN should respect the uniqueness of each client's residence, should compliment the client on positive aspects of his home, and should discuss inadequacies such as unsafe areas with the client and any family members.

Health and Social Assessments

*Purpose and uses of health assessments for the elderly*

In addition to assessing the adequacy of the residence, the CHN assesses the elderly client in the home to determine the characteristics of his health—physical, social, and psychological functioning and sources of support. These data are used to evaluate the client's skills and potential for living in familiar surroundings, and to assist him in maintaining optimal health.

The CHN who visits the client's home takes comprehensive health assessments: the client's and family's health history, a social/ interpersonal history, and a physical examination that includes an assessment of mental status. The activities of daily living or functioning that the client can still perform are also assessed. The health and social data can be collected using a general outline or a special form. Both methods have advantages, and samples of each are shown in the next section or can be found in Appendixes, A–C at the back of the book.

*Types of Health Assessments*

*The client's and family's health history.* It is a good investment of the CHN's time to elicit a comprehensive health history, not only because it provides insight into present health problems, but also because it suggests areas that require further exploration. It should be done simultaneously with the Mental Status Questionnaire or the Face-Hand Test, which are discussed in the next few pages.

Data about the client's family are used to assess his degree of risk or predisposition to diseases that may prevail in the family, such as coronary heart disease, diabetes, or cancer. The pedigree or genogram is an effective way to represent this information. General guidelines for recording the client's health and family history are shown at the end of this volume in Appendix A.

*Social/interpersonal health history.* Obtaining a social history from the client can yield important information about the client's values, strengths, habits, health practices, and potential problems. It is helpful to interview the client together with a relative or friend, because the second person can sometimes supply details not immediately recalled by the client. Clients are often able to provide additional information if questions are rephrased or repeated during follow-up visits. It takes longer to interview older people because they need time to organize their thoughts and to recall dormant information. It is sometimes wise to pursue a topic initiated by the client; cutting off a discussion that the nurse considers digressive may cause the loss of valuable information. On the other hand, some older people ramble when they are unable to recall answers to questions. Clues to selecting appropriate communication techniques can be derived from a mental functioning checklist, such as the one described below under "Mental Status Assessment." A brief guideline for social assessment can be found in Appendix B.

*Physical examination.* The physical assessment of senior citizens is best accomplished in an unhurried manner and need not be completed during one visit. The sequence depends on the nurse's objectives, and may not follow a standard head-to-toe routine. Before beginning, it is helpful to discuss the purpose and extent of the planned examination, and to instruct the client and family about their roles. The CHN might plan to assist with the bath or demonstrate an affective technique to a family member, and might incorporate these with the assessment. Many older people tire easily, and the stimulation of interacting with a relative stranger may be tiring if the examination is lengthy. Instructions may need to be repeated, or even written, and the nurse should ask for feedback to insure that the client and family understand what is expected. A suggested form for recording the physical examination can be found at the end of this volume in Appendix C.

*Mental status assessment.* Assessment of mental status in a psychosocial assessment can be done with a standard questionnaire, such as the one designed by Kahn, Goldfarb, Pollack, and Peck (Goldfarb, 1974). This questionnaire and scale for scoring the degree of mental impairment (seen in Table 9-2) has been found to be a valid and reliable indicator of mental impairment when correlated with psychiatrists' and psychologists' clinical impressions of the individual's mental state. If the client makes fewer than three errors but seems to have intellectual difficulties, the problem may be due to poor concentration or lack of motivation.

Another relatively simple test for detecting and measuring brain syndrome is the Face-Hand Test developed by Goldfarb (1974). This test is based on the premise that the failure of an individual to report the sensation of touch on the back of his hand is associated with the loss of cortical neuronal function. The client is seated comfortably, hands resting on his knees, facing the nurse. The client's cheek and hand are lightly touched or brushed with a cotton ball; simultaneously, the client is asked to report where he was touched, according to the scheme described:

1. Right cheek–left hand
2. Left cheek–right hand
3. Right cheek–right hand
4. Left cheek–left hand
5. Right cheek–left cheek
6. Right hand–left hand
7. Right cheek–left hand
8. Left cheek–right hand
9. Right cheek–right hand
10. Left cheek–left hand*

Table 9-2
Mental Status Questionnaire

1. Where are we now?

2. Where is this place located?

3. What is today's date? (day of month)

4. What month is it?

5. What year is it?

6. How old are you?

7. What is your birthday?

8. What year were you born?

9. Who is the President of the United States?

10. Who was President before him?

| Number of Errors | Presumed Mental Status |
|---|---|
| 0–2 | slight impairment |
| 3–5 | mild to moderate impairment |
| 6–8 | moderate to severe impairment |
| 9–10 | severe impairment |

The test is repeated with the eyes closed and open, although Goldfarb (1974) has found little difference in the two approaches. Failure to report touch or incorrect reporting of the location is considered indicative of brain impairment. Additional sources of rating scales and techniques for assessing the elderly may be found in Appendix 9A.

   *Assessment of client's activities of daily living or functioning.* It is helpful for the CHN and family to know what daily activities the client can perform, and thus how the client functions. Then the client, family, and CHN can decide together how much functioning or potential functioning the client retains and how much assistance is required. This information is useful whether the client is well or ill, and whether he is in his home or in a nursing home. Guidelines for the assessment of an elderly client's activities of daily living or functioning are as follows:

A. *Assess client's eating habits:*
   1. Motivation to obtain optimal diet
   2. Problems in obtaining, storing, and preparing food
   3. 1- or 3-day food record, including fluid intake
   4. Enjoyment of food; effects of food
   5. Ability to feed himself
B. *Evaluate client's activity patterns:*
   1. Normal and occasional daily activities, and satisfaction with this pattern
   2. Usual form(s) of exercise, amount, and effect
   3. Sleep/rest patterns and factors promoting and detracting from sleep
   4. Hobbies, recreational activities
C. *Check client's elimination pattern:*
   1. Problems associated with elimination
   2. 3-day record
D. *Observe client's personal care:*
   1. Ability to bathe and groom self, comb hair
   2. Ability to get in and out of bed
   3. Ability to go to the toilet
   4. Ability to dress and undress, tie shoes
E. *Assess client's mobility:*
   1. Ability to walk about the room, walk outside, and walk stairs
   2. Ability to drive a car or use public transportation
F. *Evaluate client's household tasks:*
   1. Ability to shop for food and other items
   2. Ability to keep the kitchen clean, dust the house, vacuum or mop floors, make a bed

   3. Ability to pick up mail, mail letters
   4. Ability to perform seasonal tasks—rake leaves, wash windows, put in screens, and shovel snow
G. *Observe client's communication:*
   1. Ability to read and write
   2. Ability to understand the spoken word
   3. Ability to use the telephone
H. *Observe client's socialization:*
   1. Ability to negotiate in society
   2. Ability to give and receive friendship and love
   3. Ability to feel self-worth
I. *Review client's finances:*
   1. Ability to manage spending money—bank money, write checks, tally account, and pay bills on time
   2. Ability to plan and follow a budget
   3. Ability to complete tax forms on time

It is extremely helpful to know the level of a client's daily functioning in relation to certain diseases such as cerebral vascular accidents (CVAs), which are discussed later in this chapter.

## Care of the Senior Citizen in the Nursing Home

### Criteria for Admission to a Nursing Home

The methods for assessing older people in nursing homes are similar to those used in the home, although an additional assessment tool might be useful in planning for nursing staff assignments. This tool, ''Functional Classification for Institutional Clients'' (see Figure 9-1), can also be used to indicate the client's progress or regression over time, or to evaluate the effectiveness of nursing intervention. If these scores are kept for a group of older people in several wards or units, they provide documentation for reallocation of staff members or requests for additional staff members.

In some nursing homes, the client may be considered a permanent resident, and the institution becomes home. If the client is mobile, has intact social skills, enjoys crafts and other activities, and has adapted successfully, he will have established a new network of friends and may have a support system within this new environment that must be

|  | Score 0-5* |
|---|---|
| 1. Capable of unlimited mobility and unsupervised activity<br><br>   a.  ambulatory:  able to travel about safely and independently<br><br>   b.  free of physical conditions requiring supervision | |
| 2. Capable of moderate mobility:  minimal supervision<br><br>   a.  physical condition may require infrequent supervision<br><br>   b.  may have mild chronic illness or disability | |
| 3. Limited mobility:  independent for personal care<br><br>   a.  dependent on others for some personal services<br><br>   b.  usually needs assistance outside (walking aid or escort)<br><br>   c.  may require periodic health supervision<br><br>   d.  may have moderately severe chronic illness or disability | |
| 4. Mobility limited to indoors:  requires personal care<br><br>   a.  needs nursing supervision<br><br>   b.  requires protective environment | |
| 5. Severe chronic illness or disability<br><br>   a.  confined to own rooms<br><br>   b.  requires constant supervision<br><br>   c.  needs assistance with activities of daily living | |
| 6. Bedfast<br><br>   a.  requires intensive nursing care | |

*5 is a high or desirable score        TOTAL

Figure 9-1.  Functional Classification for Institutional Clients.

304

taken into consideration, along with relatives and friends who live in the community. Thus, he no longer lives alone and now has ready access to friends and care providers, though he may still require encouragement from the nurse to continue his interests. On the other hand, the mentally or physically impaired client may be relatively isolated in his bed or room, and the nurse may be challenged to fill the role of friends and/or to create opportunities for the client to interact with others. It may be necessary to plan a program of mental or physical restoration to increase the individual's level of social functioning.

If the client has been isolated for a long time, former social skills may be rusty from disuse and must be relearned. Much encouragement and positive reinforcement of successes are needed to build such client's self-esteem and reestablish their independence, making it possible for many to return to the community.

## The Community Health Nurse's Role in a Nursing Home

The CHN's role is to assist in the improvement of care for the clients and to provide education to the staff. On occasion, the CHN may be invited to a nursing home on a consultative basis to provide inservice education for the staff in specific areas. Suggested areas are wellness and aging; care of a client with a colostomy or following a CVA (as discussed in the last half of this chapter); or dying and death (as discussed in Chapter 10). The CHN may also assist in the inspection of a nursing home with a sanitarian from a health department.

# Significant Developmental Changes and Health Problems of the Elderly

A client may have some problems that, while not necessarily life-threatening, are of concern to the nurse because they contribute to social withdrawal and therefore interfere with enjoyment of life.

## Incontinence

Loss of either bowel or bladder control, or the fear that one may lose control, is a powerful deterrent to social interaction. No one knows how many older people remain at home for this reason. In fact, current prevalence figures for incontinence among the elderly are scarce. The National Center for Health Statistics (1965) reported that in 1963 13% of older men and 20% of older women residing in nursing homes had some form of incontinence. No figures for incontinence among senior citizens living in the community are available, but prevalence can possibly be inferred from the older data. Milne, Williamson, Maule, & Wallace (1972) do address the problem of incontinence in the elderly.

The main causes of incontinence in women are loss of muscle tone in the perineal muscles, the cystocele and the rectocele. Men and women with spastic colons or diverticulosis often have a sudden urge to defecate, and may soil themselves before reaching a toilet. Diuretic medication for hypertension requires frequent trips to the bathroom. Sometimes diuretics are ordered in unnecessarily high doses, despite the fact that older people usually need smaller doses than younger people and should be given the smallest possible dose that accomplishes the purpose. They should be taken at a time when the planned effect, urination, can be done in a convenient place. The nurse can act as a client advocate, if necessary, to bring this to the physician's attention. In men, hyperplasia of the prostate will stimulate the urge to void.

When a client reports incontinence, the nurse should establish, if possible, the client's pattern of elimination and intake. Perhaps the client can be motivated to go to the toilet at regular intervals, regardless of whether or not he feels an urge to void, in order to establish a regular pattern. Some points for assessment of incontinence are as follows:

1. *History.* The CHN should determine patterns of voiding and defecation, past and present; fluid intake pattern; medications; history of infection or trauma; sources of stress or anxiety.
2. *Structure.* The CHN should examine for abnormality, including cystocele, rectocele, relaxed pelvic floor, vaginitis, enlarged prostate, and fecal impaction.
3. *Associated factors.* Mobility problems may prevent reaching the bathroom on time; cerebral deterioration and certain medications may dull the client's awareness of a full bladder or contribute to retention and overflow.

Incontinence and bladder retraining programs are discussed further in the section on CVAs, later in this chapter.

## Hearing Loss

Problems of hearing loss tend to decrease the elderly person's capacity to enjoy social activities, group dining, and theatrical presentations. It is frustrating to miss the punch line of jokes or to produce laughter when one responds inappropriately to misinterpreted conversation. Embarrassing experiences can cause the older person to dread interaction with others. Hearing may be adequate when the client is speaking with one person in a quiet room, but if there is competition with traffic, music, multiple conversations, or other background sounds, the older person may be unable to screen out the interference and comprehend the speech.

Decreased auditory perception is not always due to physiological or pathological changes. Sometimes the removal of accumulated cerumen will produce a dramatic improvement in hearing. So-called hearing loss in the aging may be partly due to decreased ability to process essential information because of central nervous system deficiency, rather than due to physiological changes (Bergman, 1971). Hearing decline often begins abruptly at about age 40, accelerating rapidly thereafter, so that by age 65 about 50% of the population suffer from reduced hearing acuity. In spite of this, only 15% of the elderly report having had a hearing test within a 4-year period.

Properly fitted hearing aids amplify sounds, but they have the disadvantage of accentuating some unwanted sounds and distorting certain musical tones. Hearing aids require a period of adaptation for some people, like bifocals, and cannot be expected to replace natural hearing.

## Visual Changes and Impairments

The eyes serve most people well through early middle age, but by the fifth decade, age-related changes begin to alter visual perception. Although most older people need glasses, approximately 80% have fair to adequate vision to age 90 and beyond. Many may have the use of only one eye, but this is true also for younger persons (Butler & Lewis, 1977). Only about 9% of Americans aged 65 and over in 1974 had visual impairments that caused limitations in their daily activities (National Center for Health Statistics, 1974). Visual acuity loss begins at about age 40 and increases, so that more than 75% of the over-65 population have some decreased vision (U.S. Bureau of the Census, 1977).

Combined biological, physical, and genetic factors contribute to the eventual decline in vision. As the individual grows older, decreased pupil size, loss of transparency and increased thickness of the lens, and thickening of the capsule allow less light to reach the retina. A 65-year-old needs about twice as much light as a 20-year-old, in order to compensate for a decreased pupil size. This reduced retinal illumination can be partially corrected by providing more light for the elderly as they perform daily tasks and engage in recreational activities. The CHN's application of knowledge about developmental eye changes should encourage the use of night lights, adequate lights in stairways and corridors, better light than candlelight at mealtime, and the placement of switches so that lamps can be turned on before the elderly enter rooms.

The accommodative power of the lens begins to decrease at age 40, causing presbyopia. Presbyopia does not affect the nervous tissue of the eye, but it diminishes the ability to focus sharply on objects closer than 3 feet. The stiffening of collagen fibers decreases the ability of the lens to shorten and focus on objects close at hand. The individual compensates by holding reading material farther away from the eyes. Reading glasses or bifocals can correct the eyes' loss of accommodation, even though the physical changes in the optic lens are irreversible. Use of large print and large letters on nurses' name tags are appreciated by older clients with presbyopia.

Another developmental problem, changes in color vision, begins to occur after age 20. With increasing age, the lens tends to pick up more of the yellow-orange range of colors. Blues and violets are filtered out, and are thus more difficult to differentiate than are colors at the red end of the visible spectrum. This has practical implications for elderly persons on medications. If a client codes pills by color and takes two purple ones instead of blue ones, the results could be drastic (Steinberg, 1976). The CHN should help the client by teaching him to feel the shapes of pills, to place certain ones in specific containers, or to label containers in large print.

Several serious visual eye impairments (cataracts, glaucoma, and detached retinas) occur in the population aged 65 and over at the rate of 37.2 per 1000 for males, and 49.6 per 1000 for females. Figures are higher for the poor, the nonwhite, and the poorly educated (National Center for Health Statistics, 1981). A cataract develops when the fibers of the lens become dense and less able to transmit light. The anterior chamber of the eye becomes shallower, decreasing the angle between the root of the iris and the corneo-scleral posterior surface (Cape, 1978). These changes render the eye more sensitive to glare, reduce the amount of transmitted light, and decrease the ability to focus. Usually cataracts are bilateral and are treated surgically if there are no contraindications.

Only about 3% of adults over age 50 develop glaucoma (caused by the obstruction of intraocular pressure), but adults over 40 should be screened yearly for it. *Glaucoma is a preventable disease!* The nurse practitioner (NP) can assess the size of the anterior chamber by shining a penlight obliquely on the temporal side of the eye at the corneo-scleral border to screen grossly for glaucoma. The NP will see a shallow anterior chamber if glaucoma is present. A definitive diagnosis should be made by an ophthalmologist with tonometry. The CHN should encourage yearly screening for glaucoma.

Retinal detachment occurs when a separation of the two primitive layers of the retina occurs due to accumulation of fluid between them, or when both retinal layers separate from the choroid because of a tumor growth. Most often, there is no apparent cause. As the detachment extends and becomes complete, blindness occurs. The client should be referred for immediate surgery (Phipps, Long, & Woods, 1979).

The most serious of all the eye problems, and the least treatable, is macular degeneration. Over 50% of persons over age 70 show some loss of central-field vision, which interferes with the reading of fine print and threading needles. People with this problem often read by holding objects to one side and read with their peripheral receptors. Use of a magnifying device may offer some benefit.

Not all visual-field loss in older people is confined to the central area; many have lateral-field deficits. These people are at risk of injury in traffic and tend to bump into furniture or door frames. Nursing assessments should include visual-field testing to gain information for planning nursing care and client teaching.

In addition to the developmental changes in the eye that occur naturally with aging, harmful effects are caused by disease, drugs, diet, metabolic shifts, radiant energy, and other environmental factors. The retina and the rods and cones are composed of postmitotic cells that do not regenerate, so damage is irreversible. A CHN working in a school should teach students about eye anatomy and physiology, developmental changes in the lens, and eye care in order to prevent or lessen eye problems later. Adequate illumination, regular eye examinations, and use of eye drops only when prescribed are some important items that should be stressed for any age group. The problem of assisting the visually impaired elderly is compounded when multiple vision problems coexist. Nurses who are mindful of the common eye changes and diseases will be better equipped to plan safe environments for elderly clients and to help them to a fuller enjoyment of their varied pursuits.

Falling

Falling occurs more often among the elderly and takes place at home more frequently than elsewhere. A 1974 study of emergency room visits for falls in a metropolitan area of Washington State reported that 56% of the falls occurred at home, and that 44% of all nonindustrial falls were experienced by persons over 60 years of age ("Injuries Due to Falls—Washington," 1978). The frequency of falls was 407 per 100,000 for persons 60 and over, compared to 173 per 100,000 for persons aged 40 to 59.

The tendency to fall or the dread of falling causes some of the elderly to remain at home. They associate falls with injury, loss of precious mobility, prolonged confinement, and possibly death or disability. There is often an associated loss of confidence in their ability to remain upright (Cape, 1978). The CHN can use confidence-building strategies, such as supervised practice with a cane or walker in a client's own neighborhood; these may overcome the reluctance to venture out. Such strategies may be the only feasible intervention, if the cause of falling cannot be determined or corrected. There are many reasons for falls: neurological or cardiovascular deficits, general debility, and so on.

Reducing the physiological problems that interfere with enjoyment of social activities contributes to the quality of life of senior citizens, increases their independence and mobility, and prevents further declines in health. Everyone benefits from increasing the activity of senior citizens: The elderly feel more useful and need fewer helping services, and society gains from the contributions of a growing segment of the population.

## Nursing Care of the Elderly in Clinics

In some areas, geriatric clinics are available to the elderly; or similar services may be provided in conjunction with day care centers, group meals, or senior citizens' residences. These clients are likely to be ambulatory, but they may be functioning with a variety of social, psychological, economic, and health problems that need to be uncovered.

At times, clients present themselves at clinics with innocuous complaints but have other problems as well, and a skillful nurse can discover them through careful history taking and assessment. A client may ask the nurse to take his blood pressure, but may have problems of dizziness or falling that require investigation. No complaint should be regarded as too minor to pursue; the client may be testing the nurse's skill or interest, or he may hesitate to divulge other concerns at that time.

## Major Nursing Care Tasks with the Elderly

Care of the client with a colostomy or a CVA is discussed in detail in the remainder of this chapter, because these are major ailments among the elderly that the CHN encounters frequently and that demand much of her time and attention.

Nursing Care of a Client with a Colostomy
at Home, in the Clinic, and in the Hospice

### Introduction

The typical elderly client with a permanent colostomy has a diagnosis of carcinoma, and the CHN provides the bulk of his professional care after hospital discharge. A colostomy is performed when some portion of the colon, rectum, or anus becomes nonfunctional as a result of disease or trauma. Cancers of the colon and rectum are the most prevalent internal cancers in this country; about 114,000 cases are diagnosed yearly, with approximately 55,000 deaths. They occur almost equally in both sexes. When this type of cancer is diagnosed at a very early stage, the prognosis is good, but the majority of clients are diagnosed and operated on late in the disease (American Cancer Society, 1981a, 1981b).

### Risk factors and prevention

The major risk factors for colon and rectal cancer are these: (1) personal history of rectal polyps, (2) familial history of rectal polyps, (3) chronic ulcerative colitis, (4) blood in the stools, (5) diverticulitis, and (6) age over 40 (American Cancer Society, 1981a).

The American Cancer Society recommends the following: "All persons 40 and over should have a digital rectal examination annually; at age 50, a stool guaiac slide test should be added on an annual basis and sigmoidoscopy every three to five years after two initial negative sigmoidoscopies a year apart" (American Cancer Society, 1980, p. 17). The Society further recommends that persons at risk should receive more frequent and intensive examinations beginning at an earlier age. Such persons include those with prior colon cancer or a history of polyps, family history of colorectal cancer, ulcerative colitis, or Gardner's syndrome. Some physicians do order barium X-rays of the colon or fiberoptic colonoscopy in addition to the procedures above to aid further in detecting colon and rectal cancers, especially if the guaiac is positive. Therefore, CHNs can contribute to a lower mortality rate by stressing the importance of the screening tests, especially for persons age 40 and over. An explanation of the tests may be required.

### Medical treatment

*Surgery and colostomy.* Surgery is almost invariably the treatment of choice for cancer of the rectum. The type of surgery depends upon the anatomical position and extent of the carcinoma. A colostomy is a surgical creation of a new opening, or "stoma," of the colon onto the body surface. In England, it is also referred to as an "artificial anus."

Colostomies are temporary or permanent, single- or double-barreled, and can be done on any of the three colon sections (descending, transverse, or ascending). A permanent colostomy is created when the colon becomes nonfunctional as a result of disease. Temporary colostomies are done to divert the fecal stream from an area of inflammation or around an operative area. When only one loop of intestine is opened onto the abdominal surface (i.e., there is only one stoma), the client has a single-barreled colostomy. In a double-barreled colostomy, both loops, distal and proximal, appear on the abdomen. (See Figure 9-2.)

A single-barreled colostomy is permanent, and usually the distal bowel is removed. A double-barreled colostomy may be permanent or may be closed later, depending upon the disease present. A temporary colostomy is usually done in the upper portion of the descending or transverse colon, whereas a permanent one is done in the lower portion of the descending or the sigmoid colon (Luckman & Sorenson, 1980; O'Connor, 1980).

If the colostomy operation is performed on a client who has a diseased section of the descending colon, especially the sigmoid, the surgeon usually removes the rectum and the diseased portion of the large intestines. During surgery, the stoma is formed by bringing one end of the incised intestine up through a small abdominal incision. The intestine may be folded back like a cuff, supported slightly above the abdominal wall, and sutured into place (Phipps et al., 1979).

In some instances when the abdomen is opened, a diseased part is found in the transverse colon. The surgeon then removes the diseased section and brings both ends out through the abdominal wall, creating two stomas. This double-barreled colostomy operation is done usually when there is a chance for revision in about 6 months. A loop colostomy is a special type of double-barreled colostomy that is usually performed for diverticular disease. The two stomas are later connected behind the abdominal wall, so that the client can eliminate through the rectum again.

Postoperative care for the single-barreled and double-barreled colostomy is the same, because usually only the functioning part of the colon is irrigated. It is recommended that transverse or ascending colostomies not be irrigated. The reason is that only the descending and sigmoid colostomies can be trained to have a set pattern of elimination. Colostomies in the other locations have a semiliquid stool that cannot be regulated to a schedule. The CHN should ask the physician or the

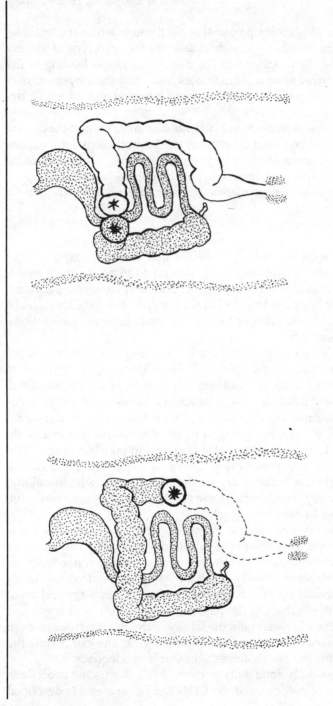

Figure 9-2. Location of Stomas for (*left*) Left-Sided (Single-Barreled) and (*right*) Right-Sided (Double-Barreled) Colostomies. (From E. Lennenberg and A. N. Mendelssohn, *Colostomies: A Guide.* Los Angeles: United Ostomy Association, 1974. Reprinted by permission.)

hospital nurse which is the proximal barrel through which the fecal material will drain, in order to be able to describe the exact type of surgery performed and the prognosis to the client. The stoma leading to the rectum is inactive. Mucus accumulates in it, and the physician may order a periodic flushing out of it to avoid infection and odor (O'Connor, 1980).

*Radiation and chemotherapy.*    Clients who have inoperable disease may be treated with radiation therapy or chemotherapy (still experimental) for palliation of the presenting symptoms, which are rectal bleeding, discharge, tenesmus, and pain. Preoperative radiotherapy is done sometimes as well (American Cancer Society, 1981b).

### Physical care at home

A client with a colostomy is discharged from the hospital about 10 to 14 days after the operation. At this time, he needs much assistance with his physical care and psychological acceptance of the surgery. The colostomy has been irrigated in the hospital, but the client may be very anxious at home because he and his family have the responsibility for doing this now.

The CHN can assist the client by discussing with him and his family the care that will be needed. Table 9-3 lists suggested areas to cover during the weeks or months in which the CHN visits the client. The CHN should follow the client for about 3 months after hospital discharge. At this time, the client is usually ready to resume normal activities, possibly including going to work. If the client is very elderly and weakened, this period of CHN supervision may last longer. The CHN should always strongly urge the client to perform his own irrigation, and self-care is necessary for the many clients who live alone. However, a family member may have to take over colostomy care if the client is unable to care for himself.

*Self-care of the colostomy site: irrigation.*    The most immediate physical nursing care is irrigation of the colostomy. The family may not have all the necessary equipment for an irrigation when the nurse visits, so she should instruct the family in what to purchase and where. Ideally, the CHN should visit the home before hospital discharge and assist the family with purchasing the necessary equipment, which is listed in Table 9-4. The CHN can help the family with this by telephone even before she makes a home visit. On the first visit, she can review the equipment with the family to see whether it is adequate.

The irrigation is done daily or every 2 or 3 days. One procedure for irrigating a colostomy that the CHN can recommend is described

Table 9-3
Guidelines for Colostomy Nursing Care

| Human dimension | Care required |
| --- | --- |
| Physical care | - teach self-care of the colostomy site<br>irrigation<br>care of stoma and surrounding skin<br>- special problems<br>diarrhea and constipation<br>diet<br>    bland or regular with individual modifications to produce a soft stool<br>    avoidance of gas producing vegetables<br>    sufficient fluids |
| Psychological Care | - adjustment to diagnosis of cancer<br>- adjustment to caring for the colostomy<br>- encourage client to discuss his concerns<br>- involve family members (if they are available) |
| Social Assistance | - eliminate social isolation by encouraging client to resume normal activities and visit with friends<br>- assist client in returning to work if of working age |

in Table 9-5. At first the irrigation may tire the client, and he may want to lie down for a while after it. This is an ideal time to use a clamped irrigating sleeve to collect any remaining stool before the bag is put in place. The CHN may use the services of an enterostomal therapist to assist with the care (O'Connor, 1980).

*Self-care of the colostomy site: the stoma and surrounding skin.* Strictures of the stoma occur in some persons. To avoid a stricture, the client is instructed to insert a gloved finger coated with K-Y jelly into the opening to stretch it; this can be painful. Vaseline should be avoided because it promotes a stricture. The passage of irrigating equipment or the stool is sufficient in most persons to keep the stoma patent. Am-

Table 9-4
Equipment for a Colostomy Irrigation

---

- Can or bag with tubing (enema cans work well)

- Cone or latex catheter No. 18 to 28 to attach to tubing

- K-Y or another water-soluble lubricant

- Irrigating sleeve

- Belt to affix irrigating sleeve

- Small piece of plastic (or cleaner's bag) to keep
  client or bed dry during irrigation (optional)

- Bath towel (to cover lap during irrigation and later
  to dry skin)

- Tissues

- Several disposable colostomy bags

- Amphogel (or another antacid not in an oil base) to
  put on stoma and surrounding skin if it becomes irritated (optional)

---

*Note.* We acknowledge the assistance of B. O'Connor in the preparation of this table.

phogel, or some other antacid not in an oil base, can be put on the stoma and surrounding skin if they become irritated. Air drying can also be suggested.

*Special problems: diarrhea and constipation.* Diarrhea occurs in persons with colostomies as it does with anyone else. If nonprescription medication and/or a diet change does not stop the loose stools, a client with diarrhea should contact the physician. Constipation can also be troublesome; usually the physician orders a stool softener, or very occasionally a small amount (5 to 10 ml) of mineral oil, to relieve the situation. If it persists, the diet probably requires more roughage.

Diet is a very important factor in the regulation of a colostomy. The client should try to establish a diet that aids in the production of a soft stool. This requires a lot of experimentation with a bland or regular diet. Excessive roughage may produce too loose a stool. Foods that are gas-producing, such as cabbage, baked beans, or Brussels sprouts, should be kept to a minimum if flatus is a problem. However, no food is contraindicated. Adequate hydration is necessary to produce a soft stool.

### Psychological care at home

Many clients become depressed when a cancer is diagnosed. This is compounded in a client with a rectal or colon cancer who must have a colostomy. A colostomy seems overwhelming because it evokes concern over inability to care for it properly, and there is direct handling of fecal material. The client worries that his partner and family will not accept him, that he will not be acceptable as a sexual partner again, and that he is undesirable in other ways. The sudden change associated with a colostomy also results in feelings of being out of control. Loss of ability to care for one's own elimination is a subject of embarrass-

Table 9-5
Colostomy Irrigation Procedure

Equipment

Irrigating bag or can with 500 to 1000cc of warm tap water

Catheter lubricated with K-Y jelly

Irrigating sleeve

Small piece of plastic

Turkish towel and tissues

Procedure: in bathroom sitting on a straight chair or toilet

1. Remove air from tubing.

2. Remove appliance or dressing and clean around stoma with a tissue.

3. Insert cone 2 to 3 inches or a catheter 3 to 6 inches (absolute maximum) into stoma and allow solution to flow in slowly.

4. If fecal material is slow to be returned, move catheter back and forth a bit, and have client change position (lean forward and move from side to side).

5. After irrigating, clean stoma and apply bag.

6. If skin around stoma is irritated, have patient air dry area for 20 minutes twice daily. Apply antacid and dry with hair dryer at cool setting.

ment for those in our culture. Nursing and family support are necessary to reduce loss of self-esteem.

The CHN usually sees the client frequently in his first 3 months after surgery; during her visits, she can assist him in working through some of his negative feelings. A counseling session is appropriate at the time the CHN first visits the home to supervise the irrigation. It is recommended that the CHN initiate a discussion about concerns surrounding the diagnosis of cancer and colostomy care on her visits if the client does not mention these first. The CHN should, of course, establish the client's prognosis with the physician to insure that she is presenting correct facts. Whatever the facts, however, she must deal with the client's perception of his own prognosis. He should be told that it takes a few months to establish an elimination routine after surgery. Once this routine is regulated, the client usually relaxes. The CHN should involve the family as much as possible and ask them to encourage the client, but it frequently happens that elderly clients live alone.

*Social assistance*

The CHN should help reduce social isolation by encouraging the client to resume normal activities and visits with friends. He will worry that he will not be able to control passing flatus and stools, or that there will be an odor. He will be concerned that the stools may leak around the bag. The CHN should reassure him that with time he will be able to set a controllable pattern of elimination. He will also have learned to omit certain bothersome foods. Petrowski encouraged a client to purchase a colostomy bag decorated with daisies; this helped her morale and enabled her to get up enough courage to go out of her home. Only a few elderly clients still go to work; the CHN should assist the client and family to ascertain if and when this is still possible.

*Clinic care*

The client who has had a colostomy returns to his surgeon 4 to 6 weeks after surgery. On the first visit, the doctor checks to see that the site is healed and that there is no infection, and checks the stoma to see whether it is patent. He further notes whether the client has regular bowel movements, knows how to perform the irrigation (one is usually ordered), and understands his diet. His conversation with the client helps determine whether his mental status is satisfactory.

On subsequent visits, a scan may be done to detect metastases.

After a number of months or a year, the client may be referred to a family practice physician for follow-up, and a family NP may also assist with the client's follow-up.

### Hospice care

A client with a colostomy whose cancer is far advanced may be admitted to a hospice. St. Christopher's Hospice in England was begun in 1967 for persons dying of cancer. A CHN should discuss advantages of hospice care and hospice availability in the community with the client and family as one alternative type of care to her visits. There the client can receive professional nursing care around the clock, while the family can visit at almost any time. Hospice care for the terminally ill is discussed in more detail in Chapter 10 (McCorkle, 1978).

### Community outreach

The American Cancer Society assists the client and public in several ways: It provides advice about colostomy care, makes referrals for professional help and volunteer visitation, sponsors the Ileostomy and Colostomy Associations, and supplies free lay and professional literature. The volunteers in the visitation program are recovered ostomy clients who visit recent colostomy patients, either in the hospital or at home, to assist in recovery by answering questions from first-hand experience; they are living examples that rehabilitation is possible. They distribute *Care of Your Colostomy*, a very useful pamphlet that the CHN can use with her clients. In some areas, the American Cancer Society trains enterostomal therapists who work with clients in homes and clinics. The Society also presents programs on cancer prevention at health fairs and on television and subsidizes cancer research.

Several self-help groups are available for cancer clients, such as Make Today Count, Living With Cancer (which grew out of Make Today Count), and various ostomy clubs (Dodd & Schell, 1978). Orville Kelly, a cancer victim, started Make Today Count as one of the first cancer groups in 1967. Peers are good therapists for one another because they can disclose problems related directly to this disease, can create empathy, and can support each other's efforts and activities. Information about groups can be obtained from the local American Cancer Society office or from the United Ostomy Association, 2001 W. Beverly Blvd., Los Angeles, CA 90057. If a CHN talks to a group, she may want to use some of the audiovisual aids listed in Appendix 9B.

Clients With Cerebral Vascular Accidents
at Home, in the Nursing Home, and in the Community

*Introduction*

CVAs are a health problem of major magnitude, as demonstrated
by the statistics cited below. "Cerebral vascular disease" is a broad term
including all types of occlusive or stenosing diseases and aneurysms
of the cerebral blood vessels. Cerebral vascular disease may lead to
strokes through two general mechanisms, those producing intravascu-
lar compromise (thrombosis and embolism) or extravascular hemorrhage
(hypertensive cerebral hemorrhage) (Melvin, 1980; Sahs, Hartman, &
Aronson, 1976). About 75% of all strokes are caused by infarctions, and
25% are caused by hemorrhage (15% by intracerebral and 10% by subarachnoid hemorrhage) (Sahs et al., 1976).

Cerebral infarction is death of neurons by ischemia, which may
be caused by any of the above mechanisms. If the ischemia lasts more
than 10 to 15 minutes, there is discernible neurological deficit (Beeson
& McDermott, 1975). Intracranial hemorrhage is usually caused by ruptured arteries, although veins may bleed as well. Arterial aneurysms
and hypertensive vascular disease are common causes of intracranial
hemorrhage. The most common cause of subarachnoid hemorrhage is
a ruptured berry aneurysm (Beeson & McDermott, 1975).

A CHN should be familiar with the prevention of CVAs and with
the treatment and rehabilitation of clients with CVAs. Frequently a CHN
assumes responsibility for care of the client with a CVA after hospital
discharge, in order to assist with the nonacute treatment and rehabilitation phases.

*Statistics*

CVAs rank third among the causes of death in the United States,
exceeded only by heart disease and cancer. In 1976, about 500,000
Americans were stricken (the incidence), and 188,623 died (National
Institutes of Health, 1979). Based on estimates, about 2500 persons experience a stroke yearly in a population of 1 million (incidence rate).
Of these, for the United States as a whole, the mortality rate is 1020
per 1 million (Sahs et al., 1976). The prevalence rate is approximately
12,500 per 1 million persons, as seen in Table 9-6. Of these, about 5000
require special services, and 1250 require institutional care (Sahs et al.,
1976). There are about 2.5 million stroke survivors (prevalence) in the
country.

Table 9-6

Estimated Incidence and Prevalence of Stroke

| Age group | Estimated Incidence of Stroke | | |
|---|---|---|---|
| | Standard million population | Estimated incidence per 1,000 | Expected new cases per year |
| 0–34* | 582,083 | 0.00 | 0 |
| 35–44 | 113,561 | 0.25 | 28 |
| 45–54 | 114,206 | 1.00 | 114 |
| 55–64 | 91,464 | 3.50 | 320 |
| 65–74 | 61,155 | 9.00 | 550 |
| 75-plus | 37,531 | 30.00 | 1,126 |
| Total | 1,000,000 | | 2,138 |

| Age group | Estimated Prevalence of Stroke | | |
|---|---|---|---|
| | Standard million population | Estimated prevalence per 1,000 | Expected total cases in community |
| 0–34* | 582,083 | 0 | 0 |
| 35–44 | 113,561 | 0 | 0 |
| 45–54 | 114,206 | 20 | 2,284 |
| 55–64 | 91,464 | 35 | 3,101 |
| 65–74 | 61,155 | 60 | 3,669 |
| 75-plus | 37,531 | 95 | 3,565 |
| Total | 1,000,000 | | 12,619 |

*Note.* From A. L. Sahs, E. C. Hartman, & S. M. Aronson, *Guidelines for Stroke Care* (DHEW Publ. No. (HRA) 76-14017). Washington, D.C.: U.S. Department of Health, Education and Welfare, 1976.

*Frequency of stroke in the 0–34 age group is so low that "estimated incidence" and "expected new cases" are considered 0 for the purposes of calculation.

In planning community health services, the morbidity and disability problems can be viewed as follows: Among 100 persons who have suffered strokes, 10 will be virtually unimpaired, 40 will have only mild disabilities, 40 will require special care, and 10 will require institutional care. Therefore, about 40% of 1 million survivors of strokes (those disabled persons requiring special care) could be potential clients of the CHN. Many of the 10% requiring institutional care are admitted to a nursing home directly from a hospital or later when their families can no longer care for them (National Institutes of Health, 1979).

There is a ray of hope in the survival statistics. In the past decade, the total of stroke deaths has been decreasing—from 214,313 in 1973 to 181,580 in 1977. This is generally attributed to better treatment for transient ischemic attacks (TIAs), so-called "little strokes"; improved control of hypertension (the presumptive cause of stroke); and better quality of care for stroke victims (National Institutes of Health, 1979). Also, many Americans seem to be taking better care of their health than previously.

### Epidemiology: the risk factors

The four main risks or predisposing factors in stroke are these: (1) hypertension over 140/90; (2) TIAs—the rate of stroke is highest in the first year after a TIA; (3) cardiac disorders such as embolic cerebral infarction; and (4) advancing age. Other risk factors of somewhat lesser importance include race, evidence of generalized arteriosclerosis, a family history of strokes, physical inactivity, cigarette smoking, obesity, anemia, syphilis, elevated serum glucose, use of oral contraceptives, and elevated cholesterol level. Nonwhites have higher incidence, prevalence, and mortality rates (Sahs et al., 1976) Kasman (1979) lists atherosclerosis as the most common cause of stroke and includes pregnancy, drugs (amphetamines), and trauma among the risk factors.

### Transient ischemic attacks

A client with an impending stroke often has prior warning in the form of one or a series of TIAs. These are transient losses of central nervous system function, which can reverse completely. About 60% of clients whose strokes are caused by an infarction report TIAs before the onset, but such "small strokes" are uncommon in clients with hemorrhagic strokes. After a TIA, neurological functions can resolve completely within 2 to 15 minutes, or the loss can last up to a day or two. Among clients who suffer TIAs, about one-third stop having them altogether for no known reason; one-third continue to have these attacks without progressing to completed strokes; and one-third will suffer completed strokes. When a completed stroke does occur, it is often within 2 months to 1 year after a TIA. The CHN should encourage a client who has had a TIA to see his physician, because drug therapy or surgery may prevent a major stroke (Kasman, 1979; Melvin, 1980; Sahs et al., 1976).

### Clinical manifestations of cerebral vascular accidents

Clients who suffer CVAs usually have hemiparesis, aphasia, dysarthria, apraxia, and bladder and bowel incontinence. Visual problems such as hemianopsia, dysphagia, emotional lability, perceptual problems, and mental impairment are often associated with it as well.

*Hemiparesis.* Body alignment on the side affected by a stroke is altered in these ways: (1) the arm is adducted and internally rotated (closer to the body than normal); (2) the elbow and wrist are flexed (bent upon themselves) and the forearm is pronated; (3) the leg is rotated externally at the hip joint (rolled away from the body—an opposite position from the unaffected leg), (4) the knee is flexed; and (5) the foot is plantar-flexed at the ankle joint (foot drop).

*Aphasia and other speech and language problems.*

ETIOLOGY, DEFINITIONS, AND CHARACTERISTICS. Speech and language problems result from the embolitic, thrombotic, or hemorrhagic lesions in the brain following a CVA. Clients requiring speech and language therapy usually have a CVA etiology of embolus or thrombosis, since victims of extravascular cerebral hemorrhage usually do not live.

Basically, there are three ways in which speech or language can be affected in these clients, depending upon which brain area is damaged: aphasia, dysarthria, and apraxia. "Aphasia" is a disturbance of language; the client may no longer be able to comprehend and/or express previously acquired patterns of language. The set of symptoms varies, depending upon where in the vascular distribution the occlusion or vessel break occurs. The most frequently occurring vascular lesions producing aphasia occur in the middle left cerebral artery and its branches. "Dysarthria" is an interference in the ability to execute the motor skills necessary to produce speech. This is always due to paralysis of the speech musculature or muscle incoordination. "Apraxias" are stroke-caused disturbances in the cognitive ability to plan the motor sequence necessary for speech formation. For example, even though the client has no paralysis of the lips or tongue, he may not be able to speak.

In addition to these three disturbances, interference with left-hemisphere functioning produces deficiencies in writing and calculation, as well as "agnosia" (inability to recognize a stimulus, such as not knowing that the color of a certain dress is red or that an object is a pen). Damage to the right hemisphere results in deficiencies in nonverbal ideation. If a client is right-handed and suffers right-hemisphere damage, he is not likely to have any aphasic symptoms, but may have dysarthria. A client who is right- or left-handed and sustains left-hemisphere damage is likely to show aphasia (Titkofsky, 1980).

CATEGORIES OF APHASIA. Aphasia is the main speech problem the CHN encounters when caring for CVA clients. The three main categories of aphasia are Werniche's (formerly called "posterior"), Broca's ("anterior"), and global. They result from lesions located in different parts of the brain. Each type results in specific speech and language characteristics as shown in Table 9-7. For example, a client with Werniche's aphasia speaks fluently, but comprehends poorly—the reverse of Broca's aphasia. Other less frequently occurring types of aphasia are also shown in Table 9-7 (Watson, 1975).

*Incontinence of bladder and bowels.* Most stroke victims have urinary incontinence (McDowell, 1976). During the acute phase of the stroke, a client may require an indwelling catheter to prevent distention of a flaccid bladder. As consciousness returns, bladder tone often returns. Some hemiplegic clients develop bladder control only after they learn to walk independently. Urinary incontinence that persists after independent walking usually indicates either a urinary tract disorder or bilateral pyramidal tract disease (Sahs et al., 1976).

Bowel incontinence correlates closely with the severity of the brain damage and usually indicates bilateral cortical injury or brain stem dysfunction. Most clients regain bowel function within a few days following the onset of the stroke. If the bowel incontinence persists 3 to 4 weeks following a stroke, rehabilitation is more difficult to achieve (Sahs et al., 1976).

*Visual problems: hemianopsia.* The degree of visual loss is generally proportionate to the total stroke damage (Boroch, 1976). Hemianopsia (loss of the same half of the field of vision in each eye) can result from a CVA. Homonymous hemianopsia is the loss of vision in the temporal visual field of one eye and the nasal vision field of the other (e.g., interference in the right hemisphere of the brain can result in vision loss in the nasal field of the right eye and the temporal field of the left). Because the left field of vision is affected, the defect is termed "left homonymous hemianopsia." A left-hemisphere lesion produces opposite symptoms (J. Johnson & Cryan, 1979; Wallagen, 1979).

*Dysphagia.* Dysphagia (difficult swallowing) occurs in some clients after a CVA if the ninth cranial nerve is damaged. The ninth cranial nerve, the glossopharyngeal, lies in the medulla. If the motor portion is damaged in a CVA, a decreased gag reflex, due to deviation of the uvula and dysphagia, can result. Trauma to the sensory portion of this nerve affects taste (Boroch, 1976).

*Emotional lability and mental impairment.* The emotional and mental changes that a person suffers after a stroke range from mild to severe. Many clients return to appropriate emotional response and full mental capacity, while others have persisting changes in personality and cognition.

Emotional reactions include anxiety, anger, crying, depression, perceptual and thinking disturbances, distortion of body image, denial, and regression. Anxiety, which is common in stroke victims, can reach

## Table 9-7
### Characteristics of Common Aphasic Disorders

| Type of Aphasia | Spontaneous speech | Characteristics Comprehension | Naming | Repetition |
|---|---|---|---|---|
| Werniche's aphasia (Posterior) | fluent | poor | poor | poor |
| Broca's aphasia (Anterior) | nonfluent | good | poor | poor |
| Global | nonfluent | poor | poor | poor |
| Conduction | fluent | good | good | poor |
| Anomic | fluent | good | poor | good |
| Isolated speech area | fluent only in repeating | poor | poor | good |
| Transcortical motor | nonfluent | good | poor | good |
| Transcortical sensory | fluent | poor | poor | good |

*Note.* Adapted from R. T. Watson, "How to Examine the Patient with Aphasia," *Geriatrics,* 1975, *30,* 76. Reprinted with permission of *Geriatrics.*

panic levels. Anger is aggravated by frustrations stemming from disability or dependency, and is often directed toward a family member; anger directed inward can result in such severe depression that it interferes with rehabilitation or results in suicide. Perceptual disturbances in which the client has difficulty organizing environmental stimuli, either psychological or physical, can occur. Stroke clients often suffer from altered concepts of themselves and their bodies; they also can suffer from denial of the illness and the disabled body part ("anosognosia"), or the inability to acknowledge the future in terms of their disability. It is not uncommon for some to regress to childlike ways.

In addition to the emotional problems, some clients display generalized mental impairments different from aphasia, including deficits in their capacity for attention, retention, abstraction, and generalization. Thinking disturbances can result in the tendency to shift from one aspect of a situation to another, inability to account for thoughts and actions, and withdrawal from reality (Sahs & Hartman, 1976). Such problems usually necessitate a fairly long rehabilitation at home.

*Nursing care at home*

The length of hospitalization for a CVA depends on the severity of the stroke, the amount of perceptual and sensory damage, other medical diagnoses, and the client's age. The hospital stay usually ranges from 34 to 48 days (5 to 7 weeks). The client most often returns to his home for a prolonged rehabilitation after hospitalization, and it is then that the involvement of the CHN begins (McDowell, 1976).

Along with a history and assessment on the first visit to the client, the CHN should also analyze the levels of rehabilitation to be worked through in order to establish realistic therapy goals and to encourage the client and family. These graded levels of rehabilitation are as follows: (1) the client is unable to ambulate and requires assistance with personal care; (2) the client performs his own personal care, but needs help to get out of bed; (3) the client moves about with mechanical aids; and (4) the client resumes "normal" activity for his age and condition.

The levels often change as the client progresses, but setting levels early gives the CHN, client, and family baselines on which to plan care. Some clients will never resume "normal" activity. Discussing the client's potential assists the caregivers in motivating the client appropriately, in planning the care, and in relieving anxiety and depression in both the client and themselves when efforts fall short of expectations.

The nursing care is guided by the physiological, psychological, social, and spiritual concerns associated with the CVA. (See Table 9-8).

## Table 9-8
## Guidelines for CVA Nursing Care

| Human dimension | Problem | Nursing care |
|---|---|---|
| Physiological | Hemiparesis | Physical therapy<br>- positioning<br>- exercises for range of motion (ROM) and strengthening<br>Adaptive equipment<br>Progressive mobility<br>- wheelchairs<br>Ambulation and mechanical aids<br>Refer to occupational therapy<br>- encouraging activities of daily living |
| | Decubiti | Prevention by repositioning, frequent turning, and proper fitting of braces<br>Treatment if decubiti develops<br>Air drying of decubitis ulcers, medications, cushions, air mattresses |
| | Incontinence - bladder and bowel | Care of indwelling catheter or bladder retraining program<br><br>Diet with roughage and ade-adequate fluids |
| | Aphasia | Refer client to speech therapy<br>CHN encourages speech sounds |
| Psychological (and Cognitive) | Emotional instability<br>Mental impairment<br>Self-image problems | Counseling by CHN<br>Involvement of family<br>Provide facts about the disease process<br>Referral to mental health nurse or psychologist<br>Occupational therapy |
| Social | Discharge planning<br>Assistance with family problems<br>Reintegration into social structure | Return to normal living<br>Socialization<br>Referral for vocational rehabilitation |
| Spiritual | Thoughts about being useless, death, and meaning of life | Counseling by CHN<br>Referral to clergy |

*Physiological care at home.*   Physiological care is the first priority for clients who have suffered a CVA. On the CHN's first home visit, she evaluates the status of the hemiparesis and makes plans with the client and family to continue a physical therapy program.

One of the most serious problems related to the pathophysiology is the hemiparesis itself. Physical restoration includes positioning, exercises for range of motion (ROM) and strengthening, progressive mobility training, and ambulation with or without mechanical aids.

POSITIONING UPPER AND LOWER EXTREMITIES AND TURNING.   Proper positioning of the paralyzed extremities is most important and will save weeks and months of physical therapy. The CHN should start positioning as soon as the client is put to bed. A bed board may be needed under the mattress to give the body firm support. The objectives of positioning are to prevent contracture, relieve pressure, and prevent edema (which occurs quickly with these clients). One should be alert to evidence of edema, because it can destroy functioning. For example, if edema is present in an extremity for about 21 days, fibrosis develops, making the hand or foot less workable. Proper positioning also decreases the chances of decubitus ulcers.

Positioning is divided into two parts: positioning of upper and of lower extremities. The upper extremity is positioned in order to prevent the following: a contracture of the shoulder, the holding of the arm close to the chest, and the inward rotation of the arm, all of which are tendencies with these clients. Enough pillows are used to keep the arm well away from the chest, so that each distal joint is positioned higher than the preceding proximal one. In other words, the wrist joint should be higher than the elbow, and the fingers should be higher than the wrists. A number of small pediatric pillows should be used instead of a few large adult ones. As the client progresses and ambulates, the arm is often placed in a sling. Wheelchair arm trays also provide support for the affected arm.

The lower extremity, without positioning, usually falls into outward rotation with a foot drop. This is not the time for a neatly made and tightly boxed bed. The covers should be loose without putting weight on the toes. Sandbags are positioned at the thigh, on the lateral aspect of the lower leg, and on the medial aspect of the foot, in order to keep the lower extremity in a neutral position, preventing rotation. A trochanter roll can be used instead of the sandbags; this trochanter roll (made of a towel, bath blanket, or sheet) should extend from the crest of the ilium to the midthigh, as the hip joint lies between these two points. Other sandbags or a foot board may be used to keep the foot at a right angle to the leg to prevent foot drop. Use of a short leg brace to align the extremity is discussed later in this chapter.

Turning is closely associated with positioning. The CHN should turn the client or help him turn every 2 hours, when he is awake or not engaged in other activity. When the client is turned on his unaffected side, the affected arm and leg should be supported on pillows above cardiac level. The affected knee and elbow may both be bent, with the wrist slightly extended and the foot at a right angle to the leg. He should not lie on the affected side for any length of time; the CHN should change his positions often, even if only slightly. The government booklet *Strike Back at Stroke* (U.S. Public Health Service, 1971) has excellent drawings of positioning.

EXERCISES FOR RANGE OF MOTION AND STRENGTHENING. Exercises for range of motion (ROM) are the passive or active movement of a body joint through its normal positions. The caregiver can start exercises 2–3 days after the onset of a CVA if the cause is thrombosis or embolism, and 6–7 days if the CVA has been caused by hemorrhage. With other causes, exercises can be started after the vital signs have stabilized. However, most clients have already begun their physical therapy when the CHN enters the picture. The purposes of exercises are (1) to maintain and build muscle strength, (2) to maintain joint function, (3) to prevent deformity, (4) to stimulate circulation, and (5) to build endurance. The exercises themselves are divided into those for the upper extremity and those for the lower extremity:

A. Upper extremity
  1. Shoulder
     a. Flexion and extension
     b. Hyperextension
     c. Abduction and adduction
     d. Horizontal abduction and adduction
     e. Internal rotation (upper arm forming right angle with lower arm and fingers toward toes) and external rotation (fingers toward head)
  2. Forearm
     a. Supination and pronation
     b. Elbow
     c. Flexion and extension
     d. Ulnar and radial deviation
  3. Fingers
     a. Flexion and extension (each finger and/or together)

   b. Abduction and adduction
   c. Thumb opposition
B. Lower extremity
   1. Hip—same as shoulder, except no horizontal abduction and adduction
   2. Knee—same as elbow
   3. Ankle—dorsi and plantar flexion; inversion and eversion
   4. Toes—flexion and extension; abduction and adduction

The exercises can be done passively by the CHN, a family member, or the client himself (if he can exercise his affected extremity with his unaffected one). They can be done actively when a client can take the affected joint through its ROM without help. Resistance can be added to an active exercise by putting weight on the extremity; this is done to strengthen certain muscle groups. For example, the client has to exert more physical effort to extend his leg if a sandbag has been placed on the foot.

The CHN starts teaching the family the exercises almost as soon as she does them for the client. It the client does not exercise his unaffected extremity, the nurse should stress that it is critically important that this be done. In the hospital, exercises are probably done once or twice daily at first, going through each motion one to three times. This schedule is increased until the exercises are repeated five, and then 10 times each and done two to three times a day (Costello, 1980).

A list of ROM exercises (diagrammed with stick men to increase the client's understanding), with the suggested frequency for performance of each one, is placed in the client's record and given to the client. This list of exercises is updated as the client, family, CHN, physical therapist, and/or physician sees a need. This updating is usually done by the physical therapist or physician during a home visit or clinic visit, or by telephone.

Throughout the course of rehabilitation, these exercises should be incorporated into the client's activities of daily living. The same muscles and joints exercised in the formal exercise program can be used in daily activities. For example, when the client is eating a meal or combing his hair, most of the motions of the hand and arm are involved. These are grasp, flexion and extension of the wrist, pronation and supination of the forearm, flexion and extension of the elbow, and some flexion, abduction, and internal and external rotation of the upper arm at the shoulder joint. However, if the client manages to eat with only grasp, supination and pronation, and flexion and extension of the elbow, adaptive equipment may be a good idea.

ADAPTIVE EQUIPMENT.   Adaptive equipment is used to aid a client in performing a function that he cannot perform for himself, or that he can perform more easily if the equipment is used. Information about adaptive equipment can be obtained from any rehabilitation center or hospital supply store. Some of the aids are manufactured especially for the handicapped (long-handled combs), some are ordinary items from general stores (soap on a rope), and others can be made by the family (small brushes with suction cups; such brushes can be made stationary for client use). Adaptive equipment is used on a selective basis. It can increase the client's physical exercise in a pleasant way and make living more comfortable. A few examples of adaptive equipment for a client who is recovering from a CVA are these:

Toothbrush with a long, built-up handle (an electric toothbrush is good, too)

Small nail brush with hooked end

Brush with suction cups

Long-handled bath brush

Shower hose

Soap in net bag or a rope

Soap mitt

Bathtub seat

Long-handled comb

Stocking with dressing stick that fits into stocking

Pulley for exercising

Swedish "pincher" to grab items out of reach

Adapted pencil for a paralyzed hand

Playing card holder

The client's motivation to feed himself, comb his hair, or play cards is increased if he comes to realize that these are pleasant ways to exercise naturally and to speed recovery. Thus, the client should be encouraged to do things for himself as soon as possible, and activities of daily living should be substituted for exercise as soon as possible.

There are numerous other ways to aid handicapped persons with improvised or specially constructed equipment. Benches or chairs in the bathtub are useful, as are plastic patches on the bottom of the tub. Grab bars to provide safety and support can be installed in hallways and at various locations near the tub and toilet. A raised toilet seat is essential if the client uses a wheelchair and transfers to the toilet from it. The CHN can inform clients that these items are available.

PROGRESSIVE MOBILITY TRAINING; WHEELCHAIRS; TRANSFERS OUT OF BED. A wheelchair enables a client to be mobile, thus increasing his daily activities immensely. There are a variety of wheelchairs, and the CHN should instruct the client about the choices available, including the importance of getting one that has locking wheels. A prescription for a wheelchair made out by a physical therapist or nurse trained in physical rehabilitation will insure that the client is provided the correct one for his needs.

The client confined to a wheelchair must be transferred from bed to wheelchair, and vice versa. This is accomplished more easily if the nurse and client plan the procedure, and if the nurse teaches the client to help himself as much as possible with his unaffected side.

AMBULATION AND MECHANICAL AIDS. Another level of independence in the rehabilitation of the CVA client is ambulation, accomplished at first with mechanical aids—a wheelchair, a short or long leg brace on the affected side, walkers, crutches, Lofstrand crutches, and canes. A prescription is required for any leg brace, and it is also a good idea to have one for the other mechanical aids in order to insure correct choice and third-party payment. Braces are used to protect weakened muscles of the affected leg, to counteract plantar flexion, and to enable the client to walk (Kasman, 1979). They should be lightweight, cosmetically agreeable, and as comfortable as possible, or they may not be worn. The CHN should insure that the braces do not cause pressure sores. She should instruct the client and family in the following procedures for brace care: (1) open, clean, and oil locks weekly; (2) clean plastic or leather with lukewarm water, and leather with saddle soap when necessary; (3) check braces periodically for worn parts and for readjustment of the fit; and (4) place braces on a table or floor in good alignment when not in use.

Some clients progress to walkers, others to crutches or canes. When the client can bear some weight on his affected side, he can use a crutch or cane. One Lofstrand crutch or a quad cane held on the side of the uninvolved extremity are the methods of choice (Costello, 1980). These aids can be rented or purchased with Medicare funds. The rubber tips of any of these aids should be cleaned periodically with soap and water to insure a proper grip on the floor.

PHYSICAL AND OCCUPATIONAL THERAPISTS. Most community health agencies employ one or more full-time physical therapists who assist in the assessment of clients with CVAs. The physical therapist plans the rehabilitation program with the physician, CHN, client, and family. The period immediately after hospital discharge is a critical time for the family, so a CHN usually visits three to five times weekly at first. The CHN continues to visit the client and conducts the exercise program, with periodic collaboration (about once a month) with the physical therapist (Sebern, 1980).

Occupational therapists are often employed part-time by a community health agency. A CHN can refer a client to them to assist in the transition from a program of exercise to activities of daily living.

CARE FOR DECUBITUS ULCERS.. It is necessary for the CHN to understand what a decubitus ulcer is and what causes it in order to prevent its occurrence. The actual cause is sustained pressure on an area, for as short a time as 2 hours. When the blood circulation to an area is diminished or stopped, the exchange of nourishment and wastes between cells and capillaries is disrupted, leading to death of cellular tissue and necrosis. Pressure causes ischemia and a pale appearance of the skin. The ischemic area is subject to breakdown. When the pressure is removed, the body's reaction is to supply nutrients and oxygen and to remove waste products from the cells as quickly as possible. This accounts for the reddened skin appearance and local skin warmth immediately after pressure is removed.

Prevention of these ulcers is much easier than treatment is. To prevent bed sores from developing, the CHN should assess the status of the client, including (1) general condition, (2) mental state, (3) activity level, (4) mobility in bed or wheelchair, (5) incontinence, and (6) availability of a family member to reposition the client. Particular attention to all of these areas is required if there is likely to be a problem with bed sores.

In accordance with this assessment by the CHN, suggested specific measures to prevent bed sores are as follows:

Change the client's position every 2 hours during daytime hours.

Check equipment (braces, crutches, and drainage tubing) for sources of pressure.

Observe meticulous skin care, including cleansing of the perineum and buttocks.

Pat the client's heels and elbows with suitable materials and his back with sheepskin.

Massage susceptible areas to increase circulation at time of repositioning.

Provide a diet rich in protein and Vitamin C.

Insure adequate hydration (up to about 2500 cc daily).

Teach the client and family about the routines. They may need to be written down.

An air mattress or a polyurethane foam cushion, 4 inches thick, should be recommended if the client is confined to bed.

These pressure sores may, however, develop when a client is in bed or a chair and the position is not changed for a few hours, especially over bony prominences, as seen in Figure 9-3. Very dry or wet skin increases the chances for skin breakdowns; pathogenic organisms can enter these sites. Thus bladder incontinency or a dripping catheter is a definite threat. Increased edema is also a threat, because it interferes with cell-capillary exchanges (Gruis & Innes, 1976).

Treatment of any ulcers that may develop includes changing the client's position, cleaning the site with soap and water, massaging, applying antibiotic ointment or other medication as prescribed, and alternating air drying and use of a dressing. It is necessary to contact the physician to report the status of the ulcer and request specific orders, because the particular medication used varies.

CATHETER CARE.  Many clients at home have an indwelling catheter, which needs daily care. Instructions as listed in Figure 9-4, should be discussed with the client and family. Further instructions appear in Chapter 10.

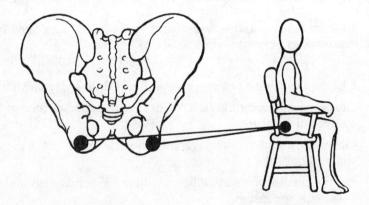

Figure 9-3.  Pressure Points (Ischial Tuberosities) When Client Is Sitting in a Wheelchair or Chair. (Drawing by Mary Gainer.)

BOWEL RETRAINING. Regular bowel habits are ideally regulated by general physical exercise and a diet with sufficient bulk and roughage. Stewed fruit, prune juice, raw vegetables and fruit, whole-grain cereals, and hot liquids are simple dietary measures that stimulate bowel movements. Adequate fluids are also indicated to prevent constipation.

Medical measures include stool softeners, suppositories, laxatives, and enemas. The CHN should determine the client's bowel habits prior to the stroke and should help the family set a regular schedule for evacuation. It may be necessary to check for impactions by digital examination in some clients. Enemas are not recommended on a regular basis, because they can stretch the bowel beyond its normal capacity. The CHN should be sure to teach the bowel retraining program to the family (Sahs & Hartman, 1976).

APHASIA: THE COMMUNITY HEALTH NURSE'S INTERVENTION. The majority of aphasic clients will not regain communicative function at their pre-stroke level; however, there can be significant reduction of their communicative impairments with speech therapy. Any client with aphasia should be referred to a speech therapist. The chance for maximum spontaneous recovery will be greater if speech therapy is begun during the first 2 months after the stroke. The CHN should do the following:

1. Observe and report findings to the doctor or speech therapist to aid in diagnosis and treatment.
2. Determine details of the client's personal background, job, hobbies, religion, and so forth, in order to provide more motivation for the client to speak.
3. Reinforce lessons administered by the speech therapist. The CHN can envelop the client in speech sounds as she performs other duties for the client. Meaningful, functional vocabulary can be reinforced. Collaboration with the speech therapist at periodic intervals is essential for assessment of the client's status and for the therapist to encourage the client, family, and CHN in achieving maximum rehabilitation results (R. Johnson, 1980).
4. Treat the client as an intelligent adult. Do not shout at him, and do not converse too rapidly or too slowly. Most clients will want to know if a response was inappropriate, so that they can modify their mistakes. The atmosphere should be relaxed and permissive if speech therapy is to be effective (Sahs & Hartman, 1976).
5. Discuss aphasia with the family. The family can be *immensely* helpful in stimulating speech patterns. The pamphlet *Aphasia*

## GUIDELINES:

1. It is important to drink fluids (at least 10 (ten) 8 ounce glasses per day) so the catheter will drain well.
2. Check amount and contents of urine: clear, light yellow color; an adequate amount is ¾ of what you take in.
3. Check tubing and bag: unkinked and below the level of the bladder—tubing taped to the thigh to prevent pulling on catheter.

## CLEANING

1. *Men:* Clean penis daily with soap and water and dry.
2. *Women:* Clean meatus daily with soap and water and dry.
3. Tubing and Bag; (also leg bag if used)
   a. Cleanse daily.
   b. Protect ends of catheter and tubing with a plug kept in alcohol in a sterile jar.
   c. Wipe ends of connecting points with alcohol before reconnecting. See Diagram #1.

### DIAGRAM #1

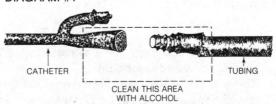

CATHETER                    TUBING

CLEAN THIS AREA
WITH ALCOHOL

   d. Clean used bag and tubing with soap and water, rinse, remove air bubbles. To remove air bubbles from tubing—attach water filled 50 cc. syringe to tubing and flush tubing with water.
   e. Place 1 cup vinegar into the bag through the long tubing (a meat baster or syringe works well for this) and clamp off the long tubing. Place ¼ to ½ cup in leg bag. Leave the vinegar in the bag until you are ready to use the bag again—no longer than 24 hours. Then empty the vinegar into the toilet.

Figure 9-4. General Instructions for Patients with Catheters. (From Visiting Nurse Association of Milwaukee, *General Instructions for Patients with Catheters* (pamphlet). Milwaukee: Author, 1978. Copyright 1978 by Visiting Nurse Association of Milwaukee. Reprinted by permission in its entirety.)

Figure 9-4. *Continued*

---

## PROCEDURE FOR CATHETER IRRIGATION

1. Position patient on back.
2. Remove bulb, syringe and glass from pot (holding syringe by end opposite tip).
3. Do not touch tip of syringe or inside of syringe or glass.
4. Squeeze water from bulb firmly into syringe.
5. Put syringe into glass.
6. Pour 3 to 4 ounces of irrigating solution into glass.
7. Place container for irrigation returns at the end of the catheter. See Diagram #1.

8. Disconnect catheter from tubing and cover end of tubing with cap from alcohol container.
9. Draw up 1 to 2 ounces of solution into syringe.
10. Insert tip of syringe into catheter.
11. Press gently on bulb to assist solution in running in.
12. Disconnect the syringe from the catheter and lower the end of the catheter to below the level of the bladder and allow the solution to drain into the container. If the solution does not return, do not add more.
13. Repeat steps 9–12 three to four times or until solution returns clear.
14. Wipe end of catheter and tubing with alcohol wipe and re-connect.
15. Discard unused solution from glass and the irrigation returns from the container.
16. Wash equipment with soap and water.

---

    *and the Family* (American Heart Association, 1977) can be very useful.

6. A major activity of the Easter Seal Society is speech rehabilitation; thus, an aphasic client can be referred to the Society for speech therapy. Vocational rehabilitation could be used for job retraining, but only if the client has some kind of work potential.

*Psychological care at home.* Physical rehabilitation can be carried out more effectively if caregivers understand some of the psychological problems the CVA client experiences. A stroke affects a particular human being with a particular personality, goals, values, and ways of coping with stressful situations. Each of us has a characteristic way of responding to anything that threatens to interfere with the usual tenor of our lives. We may minimize, rationalize, or deny the existence of the threat. Some patients initially have a great problem accepting the paralyzed hand they see as their own; others might seek a solution to this stress through a heightened dependency status. The patient needs help to maintain his sense of well-being. The altered way in which he perceives himself may lead to disorientation and mood swings— common sequelae of this disease. Many of these symptoms have an organic basis in a client who has had a CVA; he is also coping with multiple losses and grieving.

A person with severe brain damage as a result of a CVA has difficulty in abstract thought, while a client who has suffered a very mild stroke can remain quite insightful. Hence, proper nursing management rests in considerable measure on the nurse's ability to understand and interpret the nature of the client's struggle with his illness, in accordance with the extent of brain damage that has occurred. A client can be brought back to his former self through the continued stimulation of old memories and patterns and the formation of new ones with the help of those around him (Wolanin, 1964).

Working with a client with a CVA can be taxing for the family and the CHN, because the client needs assistance and encouragement to perform activities in his own imperfect way, relearning rather than learning for the first time. The CHN and the family must make a great effort to deal patiently with irrational behavior or inappropriate responses. They should not see the client as a pathetic, hopeless, confused "old person," but as a human being attempting to come to terms with an overwhelmingly stressful event.

Interpretation of these psychological problems to the family should enable them to assist in a practical way in the client's care. He should be helped to keep in contact with the world as he knows it. Not only should he be visited, but later in the course of his recovery he should visit people and places, attend parties, and go to shops. He should take part in the family activities and decisions and be made to feel that he remains an important part of the family life. Occupational therapy may also help. Understanding of his sometimes irrational behavior and guidance back into a normal social setting will help the client regain a proper image of himself. The CHN may suggest that the client could benefit from the services of a mental health or psychiatric NP or a psychologist. Many clients cannot afford long-term psychological counseling, or they may not accept it. However, a few may require intensive therapy from a psychiatrist, and the CHN can assist with the referral.

*Social assistance at home.* A main social concern is that a client with a CVA who has been living alone may no longer be able to do so, and he may have to consider available alternatives. For the 10% of CVA clients who are seriously affected, nursing home care may be the only answer.

It is extremely important that these clients maintain contact with family and friends, in order to increase their chances of a return to a normal life. They usually need assistance with ambulation and speech to be able to function at an optimal level again. A few younger clients may require referral to vocational rehabilitation.

*Spiritual care.* The client may fear death as a result of his experience with a CVA, or may continue to feel worthless and depressed. The client often reflects on the meaning of his life at this time. Reminiscing can and should be allowed, in order to assist the client to regain a positive self-image and feelings of self-worth. The CHN may need to refer the client to his spiritual advisor; such a referral is a very individual matter. If a client and his minister, priest, or rabbi have had a good rapport before the stroke, the clergyman may be an appropriate person for counseling.

### Clinic care

A client who has had a CVA should return to see a physician within the first 2 months after hospital discharge. The purposes of the appointment are to review and make recommendations for the following: (1) physical therapy regimen; (2) speech therapy referral, if indicated; (3) diet; (4) medicine; (5) incontinence retraining; (6) blood pressure reading; and (7) evaluation of mental health status.

A physical therapy regimen includes examination of the status of the client's hemiparesis, use of extremities, and ambulation. Usually the CHN who has cared for the client at home requests changes in his exercise program and mechanical aids at this time; for example, he may be ready to move from a wheelchair to crutches or a walker. The physician notes progress or lack of it during the examination. It is difficult to weigh a client who has a hemiparesis. However, if the client is overweight, the doctor may order a calorie reduction diet, limiting intake to approximately 1200–1500 calories daily. If the CHN has requested a bladder retraining program because one was not instituted in the hospital, and the physician considers this feasible, he will write an order for it. Blood pressure readings are routinely made, because hypertension is a risk factor in many CVAs.

An NP may examine a CVA victim in a clinic setting, where she will do the physical examination and make recommendations. Or the NP and doctor may alternate seeing the client on his visits to the clinic.

### Nursing home care

It is noted earlier in this chapter that 10% of clients with CVAs are so disabled that they require assistance for the remainder of their lives. Some of these are cared for at home, and others in nursing homes.

*Economic concerns and eligibility.* The selection of nursing home care frequently depends upon the client's and/or family's ability to pay or eligibility for residence in a publicly financed home. Financial assistance can be sought through Medicare and Medicaid funds. Other factors affecting choice of a nursing home include location, type of care needed, and religion of the client. The role of the CHN or the NP in a nursing home is usually consultative. A CHN may be invited to teach in-service classes about stroke care to staff in a nursing home.

*Bladder retraining program.* Incontinence of bladder and bowels can be a problem for the client who has had a CVA. Bladder retraining is recommended for CVA clients in a nursing home. It can also be done in a client's home if a person trained in catheter technique is present constantly until training is established.

General considerations for a bladder training program are varied. Four conditions are necessary: knowledge of the urinary tract, the client's participation, a nursing assessment, and a training plan with a physician's approval. Past habits and analysis of the pattern of incontinence are valuable. A 72-hour record showing when the client is dry and when wet, as well as the amount of urine, is helpful. Frequent voiding of small amounts might suggest insufficient fluids, bladder infection, or retention with overflow; continuous dribbling could mean retention with overflow or lack of sphincter control.

Training can be started as soon as exercises are started, or any time thereafter. As muscle tone improves in the larger muscles of the body, muscle tone of the sphincter and muscles used for micturation and defecation also improve. Thus, increasing physical activity within limits is very important. Many clients gain control by boosting their fluid intake. The intake should be about 2000 cc to 2500 cc daily, more if the weather is hot. Dressing in street clothes is also an incentive to become continent. Success depends upon the client's mental as well as physical state. The client must be told to expect occasional accidents.

An assessment of the client's ability to sit up (in bed and on a commode or toilet), stand, and walk is essential. Position is important for elimination. A client will be more successful in a semisquatting position. A toilet that provides maximum privacy is the best place; then the commode at the bedside; and, as a last resort, the bedpan. If the patient must use the bedpan, his trunk should be elevated so that he is as near a crouching position as possible. Adaptive equipment may be helpful for the toilet or commode, such as an elevated toilet seat for the patient who has poor flexion of hips or knees. Most clients needing retraining have an indwelling catheter; therefore, the nurse supervising retraining should heed certain recommendations (Melvin, 1980; Sebern, 1980; Wunch, 1980):

1. A physician's order is necessary for bladder retraining.
2. A urine specimen should be sent to a laboratory for culture to determine sensitivity. If an infection is present, antibiotics are ordered for 10 to 14 days. The type of antibiotic depends upon the results of the urine culture and sensitivity. Bactrim is often ordered.
3. Forty-eight hours after the first administration of the antibiotics, remove the catheter; increase fluids to 2500 cc/day.
4. The client should be encouraged to void every 4 hours. If the client voids within 8 hours, catheterize for residual urine. If the client does not void within 8 hours, he should be catheterized. He should still attempt voiding every 4 hours. If he requires catheterization after a 24-hour period, the indwelling catheter should be reinserted.
5. The client should then be checked by a physician prior to reinstitution of the retraining program for other problems, such as an enlarged prostate in males or a stricture of the sphincter. A retraining program is not reinstituted until the problem is corrected.
6. When the program is restarted, follow the plan as outlined. Also, teach the client trigger techniques to assist him to void. Trigger points (as inner or outer thighs) are sensory reflexes causing the bladder to contract. Bowel movements trigger the bladder to empty.
7. Compliment the client and family on any success with the program.

*Community programs*

Some clients recover enough physical and cognitive potential to join a stroke club and attend its meetings with their families. The American Heart Association will assist with the sponsorship if one does not exist in the client's community. One such club was jointly sponsored in 1975 by the Association and the Veterans Administration Medical Center in Butler, Pennsylvania. At the monthly meetings, such topics as drug versus nondrug therapy for anxiety in patients and families; depression; psychology of chronic disability; handling difficult spouses; and changing life styles in families as a result of chronic illness have been discussed. In the chronic phase, the families need more information about what to expect (such as the altered behavior and emotions of the client), as well as help in solving these problems (McCormick & Williams, 1979).

### Current research

Much of the current research is directed toward prevention of CVAs, especially TIAs; research is also under way to establish the relationship of CVAs to atherosclerosis or arteriosclerosis, the effects of high blood pressure, the rate of strokes in women compared to men, and the effects of "good living" (i.e., reducing stress and exercising) (Ancowitz, 1979). The effects of antiplatelet-aggregation drugs, including aspirin, are being studied by scientists supported by the National Institutes of Health. The National Institute of Neurological and Communicative Disorders and Stroke (NINCDS) is cooperating with the World Health Organization in a high-priority study of strokes (National Institutes of Health, 1979).

The course of rehabilitation for a CVA client is long and weary, and calls for much resourcefulness and creativity on the part of the client, family and CHN. Much of the CHN's work is to encourage the client and family.

## Appendix 9A: Rating Scales and Procedures for Assessing the Elderly

Bell, R., & Hall, R. C. W. The Mental Status Examination. *American Family Physician*, 1977, *16*, 145–152.

Lawton, M. P. Functional assessment of elderly people. In V. M. Brantl & M. R. Brown (Eds.), *Readings in gerontology*. St. Louis: C. V. Mosby, 1973.

Grauer, H., & Birnbom, F. A geriatric functional rating scale to determine the need for institutional care. *Journal of the American Geriatrics Society*, 1975, *28*, 472–476.

Katz, S., Ford, A. B., Moskowitz, R. W., Jackson, B. A., & Jaffe, M. W. "Studies of illness in the aged: The Index of ADL. A standardized measure of biological and psychological function. *Journal of the American Medical Association,* 1963, *185,* 914–919.

Mahoney, F. I., & Barthel, D. W. Functional evaluation: The Barthel Index. *Maryland State Medical Journal,* 1965, *14*(2), 61–65.

## Appendix 9B: Audiovisual Aids for Colostomy Care

1. *Learning About Your Colostomy* (#666); *Colostomy Care at Home* (#667) (Filmstrips) Available from the Trainex Corporation, Box 116, Garden Grove, LA 92642.
2. *Colostomy* (Flipchart with an instructor's guide) Available from Robert T. Brady, Bowie, MD 20715.
3. *Types of Surgery and Appliances; Pre- and Post-Operative Concerns; Education and Discharge Planning* (Film or videocassette in three parts) Available from Greater Cleveland Hospital Association, Room 200, 1021 Euclid Avenue, Cleveland, OH 44117. Attn: Education Department.

## References

American Cancer Society. *ACS report on the cancer-related checkup.* New York: Author, 1980.

American Cancer Society. *Cancer facts and figures 1982.* New York: Author, 1981. (a)

American Cancer Society. *A cancer source book for nurses.* New York: Author, 1981. (b)

American Heart Association. *Aphasia and the family.* Dallas: Author, 1977.

Ancowitz, A. *What you should know about stroke prevention* (DHEW Publ. No. (NIH) 79-1909). Washington, D.C.: U.S. Department of Health, Education and Welfare, 1979.

Anderson, O. W. Reflections on the sick aged and helping systems. In B. L. Neugarten & R. J. Havighurst (Eds.), *Social policy, social ethics, and the aging society.* Washington, D.C.: National Science Foundation, 1976.

Anderson, W. F. Practical management of the elderly. *Proceedings of the Royal Society of Medicine,* 1967, *60,* 1227–1235.

Beeson, P. B., & McDermott, W. *Textbook of medicine.* Philadelphia: W. B. Saunders, 1975.

Bergman, M. Hearing and aging. *Audiology,* 1971, *10,* 164–171.

Boroch, R. M. *Elements of rehabilitation in nursing: An introduction*. St. Louis: C. V. Mosby, 1976.

Butler, R. N., & Lewis, M. I. *Aging and mental health: Positive psychosocial approaches* (2nd ed.). St. Louis: C. V. Mosby, 1977.

Cape, R. *Aging: Its complex management*. New York: Harper & Row, 1978.

Carpenter, J. O., McArthur, R. F., & Higgins, I. T. The aged: Health, illness, disability, and use of medical services. In C. L. Erhardt (Ed.), *Mortality and morbidity in the United States*. Cambridge, Mass.: Harvard University Press, 1974.

Costello, M. Personal communication, April 16, 1980.

Dodd, M., & Schell, P. Oncologic self-help groups. In C. J. Kellogg & B. P. Sullivan (Eds.), *Current perspectives in oncologic nursing* (Vol. 2). St. Louis: C. V. Mosby, 1978.

Ebersole, P., & Hess, P. *Toward healthy aging: Human needs and nursing response*. St. Lous: C. V. Mosby, 1981.

Eklind, D. Erik Erikson's eight ages of man. *New York Times Magazine*, April 5, 1970, pp. 25–114.

Erikson, E. *Identity: Youth and crisis*. New York: Norton, 1968.

Gibson, R. M., & Fisher, C. R. Age difference in health care spending, fiscal year 1977. *Social Security Bulletin*, January 1979, pp. 13–16.

Goldfarb, A. I. *Aging and organic brain syndrome*. Fort Washington, Pa.: McNeil Laboratories, 1974.

Gruis, M. L., & Innes, B. Assessment essential to prevent pressure sores. *American Journal of Nursing*, 1976, *76*, 1762–1764.

Injuries due to falls—Washington. *Morbidity and Mortality Weekly Reports*, June 9, 1978, pp. 192–194.

Johnson, J., & Cryan, M. Homonymous hemianopsia: Assessment and nursing management. *American Journal of Nursing*, 1979, *79*, 2131–2134.

Johnson, R. Personal communication, April 1980.

Kasman, M. Stroke: Update on diagnostic and treatment strategies. *Modern Medicine*, March 1979, pp. 15–30, 32–41.

Luckman, J., & Sorenson, K. *Medical-surgical nursing: A psychophysiologic approach*. Philadelphia: W. B. Saunders, 1980.

McCorkle, R. Hospices: A British reality and an American dream. In C. J. Kellogg & B. P. Sullivan (Eds.), *Current perspectives in oncologic nursing* (Vol. 2). St. Louis: C. V. Mosby, 1978.

McCormick, G. P., & Williams, M. Stroke: The double crisis. *American Journal of Nursing*, 1979, *79*, 1410–1411.

McDowell, R. N. Rehabilitating patients with strokes. *Postgraduate Medicine*, 1976, *59*, 148.

Melvin, J. L. Personal communication, May 12, 1980.

Milne, J. S., Williamson, J., Maule, M. M., & Wallace, E. T. Urinary symptoms in older people. *Modern Geriatrics*, 1972, 2, 198.

National Center for Health Statistics. *Characteristics of residents in institutions for the aged and chronically ill, United States, April–June 1963* (DHEW Publication Series 12, No. 2). Washington, D.C.: U.S. Department of Health, Education, and Welfare, 1965.

National Center for Health Statistics. *Limitations of activity due to chronic conditions* (DHEW Publication Series 10, No. 111). Washington, D.C.: U.S. Department of Health, Education and Welfare, 1974.

National Center for Health Statistics. *Prevalence of Selected Impairments, United States, 1977* (DHHS Publ. No. (PHS) 81-1562). Washington, D.C.: U.S. Department of Health and Human Services, 1981.

National Institutes of Health. *The NINCDS Stroke Research Program* (DHEW Publ. No. (NIH) 79-1618). Washington, D.C.: U.S. Department of Health, Education and Welfare, 1979.

Neugarten, B. L., & Havighurst, R. J. (Eds.). *Social policy, social ethics, and the aging society.* Washington, D.C.: National Science Foundation, 1976.

O'Connor, B. J. Personal communication, May 7, 1980.

Phipps, W. J., Long, B. C., & Woods, N. F. (Eds.) *Medical-surgical nursing: Concepts and clinical practice.* St. Louis: C. V. Mosby, 1979.

Richmond, J. B. *Healthy people: The Surgeon General's report on health promotion and disease prevention* (DHEW Publ. No. 79-55071). Washington, D.C.: U.S. Department of Health, Education and Welfare, 1979.

Sahs, A. L., & Hartman, E. C. (Eds.). *Fundamentals of stroke care* (DHEW Publ. No. (HRA) 76-14106). Washington, D.C.: U.S. Department of Health, Education and Welfare, 1976.

Sahs, A. L., Hartman, E. C., & Aronson, S. M. (Eds.). *Guidelines for stroke care* (DHEW Publ. No. (HRA) 76-14017). Washington, D.C.: U.S. Department of Health, Education and Welfare, 1976.

Sebern, M. Personal communication, June 1980.

Steinberg, F. U. (Ed.). *Cowdry's: The care of the geriatric patient.* St. Louis: C. V. Mosby, 1976.

Titkofsky, R. Personal communication, May 15, 1980.

U.S. Bureau of the Census. *Social indicators, 1976.* Washington, D.C.: U.S. Department of Commerce, 1977.

U.S. Bureau of the Census. *Social and economic characteristics of the older population, 1978* (Publ. No. P-23, No. 85). Washington, D.C.: U.S. Department of Commerce, 1979.

U.S. Department of Health, Education and Welfare. *Aged patients in long-term care* (Publ. No. (ADM) 76-154). Washington, D.C.: Author, 1973.

U.S. Department of Health, Education and Welfare. Health Interview Survey: Vital and health statistics. In *Health United States, 1975* (DHEW Publ. No. (HRA) 76-1232). Washington, D.C.: Author, 1976.

U.S. Department of Health, Education and Welfare. *Current estimates from the Health Interview Survey: United States, 1977* (DHEW Publication Series 10, No. 126). Washington, D.C.: Author, 1978.

Wallagen, M. I. The split brain: Implications for care and rehabilitation. *American Journal of Nursing*, 1979, 79, 2122.

Watson, R. T. How to examine the patient with aphasia. *Geriatrics*, 1975, 30, 73-77.

Wixen, J. Lesson in living. *Modern Maturity*, October–November 1978, pp. 8–10.

Wolanin, M. O. They called the patient repulsive. *American Journal of Nursing*, 1964, 64, 73-77.

Wunch, K. Personal communication, May 1980.

# 10

# Dying at Home, in a Nursing Home, or in a Hospice

*Helen L. Swain*
*and Dorothy D. Petrowski*

## Introduction

Terminal illness, dying, death, and grief are natural processes, but they require the support of excellent nursing care. Such nursing care demands sensitive awareness of oneself and one's personal attitudes, superstitions, fears, and desires concerning death. As persons who fear the water cannot learn to swim, nurses cannot learn to help if they fear the very situation in which the help is needed. Personal attitudes are often reflections of group values and our society in general; they can be changed.

## Attitudes and Trends Regarding Death

### 20th-Century America and the Change from Dying at Home to Dying in a Hospital

In the early part of this century, death was more commonly expected, and it frequently occurred at home. Childbirth was a common cause of death, infant mortality was high, and communicable disease was rampant. In fact, it would have been unusual to find a young family unaffected by the death of at least one of its members.

347

Children in the early 1900s had experience with dying parents or siblings, and assisted with care of the dying and funeral preparations at home. The circumstances may have seemed unkind or unpleasant, but they were real and natural. But today, the majority of our people have not had the same experiences with death. Death is more of a stranger and concomitantly more frightening.

While in the first quarter of the century it was uncommon for people to enter a hospital when they were ill or dying, it gradually became more and more common. Today, an estimated 80% of our population die in institutions—hospitals, nursing homes, and hospices; this is almost a total reversal of the earlier pattern.

Dying in an institution may not be inherently bad, but it poses quite a different situation for family members than does dying at home. By its very nature, an institution can be alienating, impersonal, and fear-provoking. Families may feel they need to give up their functions involving physical care and support. Children are protected from the reality of dying. Death is taken away from the family and becomes the province of the professional.

*Factors influencing trends*

Nuclear families, increased mobility, and biomedical technological advances are among some of the reasons why death has shifted from home and family to the institution and professionals. Family members are often not within helping distance of each other. Present life styles make it difficult, if not insurmountable, for people to care for dying family members by themselves in their own homes. The alternative is for the dying to be cared for by professionals in an institutional setting. Though few would complain about these advances, they have created the belief that, given enough time and resources, every malady can be eradicated.

*Societal and professional attitudes toward death*

Because persons often are ill-equipped emotionally and intellectually to handle the death of family members, the care of the terminally ill or dying person is relinquished to professionals. Professionals, however, may also find themselves afraid to deal with death, because as members of society they share societal attitudes. Furthermore, they are taught the values of the health care professions, which primarily emphasize cure. Professionals value their curative efforts and consider themselves successful when clients return to wellness.

These values explain why few nurses choose to work with terminally ill persons. The professional emphasis on success and wellness, and the societal attitudes of denial and fear about death, make it difficult for a nurse to provide essential care to a dying person and his family. Feelings of helplessness, vulnerability, and loss of control over events are evoked in the helping person. This is particularly true in an acute care setting, which strongly emphasizes a return to wellness. Perhaps it is due to the inability of institutional staffs to provide the kind of care and caring essential to the well-being of the dying person that the trend toward returning to nonacute care settings has evolved.

Recent Trend back to Nonacute Care Settings for the Dying

*Nursing homes*

Nursing homes offering skilled or nonskilled care of the dying have been rapidly increasing since World War II. Families faced with long-term care of dying relatives may find that the nursing home offers the quality of care they seek and are unable to provide. High-quality nursing homes offer a sheltered environment, a degree of autonomy and dignity, continuous professional services and a more home-like environment than a hospital. Nevertheless, many nursing homes transport clients back to the hospital when death appears imminent. The role of the community health nurse (CHN) in a nursing home has been discussed in Chapter 9.

*The hospice movement*

To meet the needs of persons facing death, a recent phenomenon has developed in the United States in the past decade—the hospice movement, which started in England about 1950 (Saunders, 1976). Most individuals in hospices have terminal cancer. The central theme of the hospice concept is care rather than cure; since terminally ill persons cannot be cured, it is logical that they be cared for compassionately. The hospice movement emphasizes helping the dying person and his family maintain dignity and humanity while the patient receives sophisticated medical and nursing care, and helping them to live while the patient advances through the dying process (Cohen, 1979; Zorza & Zorza, 1978). Identifiable elements of any hospice program are as follows (Cohen, 1979; Milwaukee Hospice, 1979):

1. Inpatient or home care around the clock to dying persons, with medical direction and nursing services.
2. Supplemental social work, chaplaincy, and other health care personnel services.
3. Use of volunteers to assist families and cut costs.
4. Expertise in control of physical, psychological, social, and spiritual symptoms.
5. Treatment of client and family as the unit of care.
6. Home care in collaboration with hospital backup.
7. Bereavement follow-up services.

The philosophy of hospice care can be implemented in a variety of settings. Models include home care with institutional backup, a hospital-based program, or a free-standing hospice. The CHN would be most often involved in the home care hospice program, in which nursing care would be similar to that outlined in this chapter for care of a dying person at home.

### The client's home

Many people still prefer to spend their remaining days in their own homes, although they may not realize what a difficult decision this can be until actually faced with it. Dying at home, in contrast to sudden death at home, is not a one-person act, and the option to die at home should be discussed long before death is imminent. Family and friends must be considered; physical care arrangements and household accommodations must be made; and, most important, the physical and psychological demands placed on the people involved must be considered. When feasible, dying at home can be a satisfying experience for the client, and a growth experience for the entire family. It is never, however, without liabilities, concerns, and doubts. It requires effort, coordination, and extensive mutual support among all involved, including professionals and, most specifically, the CHN (Whilsmith, 1978).

For those who so choose, the home offers the benefits of a familiar environment and the proximity of loved ones. Today's concept of home care for the dying is seen as an extension of hospital services, or as a function of community health services. In either case it is most often the CHN, working with other members of the health care team, who supplies ongoing intimate support for the client and significant others during the dying process.

Preparation for Care of the Dying Needed
by the Community Health Nurse

The CHN needs formal and continuing education about the process of dying to enable her to provide objective and empathetic nursing care to a terminally ill person. She must be prepared to serve the whole person from a base consisting of knowledge of the specific terminal illness, knowledge of the individual's ways of coping with the sickness and impending death, and awareness of her own feelings about death. These ideas are further developed later in this chapter.

## Nursing Care of the Terminally Ill or Dying Person and His Family

### Definition of "Terminal Illness"

A "terminally ill" client is one who is nearing death from an illness that is progressing and unrelenting and that cannot be arrested in the present state of knowledge or ignorance (Beeson & McDermott, 1975). Closely related to terminal illness is "dying," which is a drawing to the end and a declining of all body processes. Although "terminal illness" and "dying" are often thought to be synonymous, the terms do denote different states of living. "Terminal illness" connotes a state of living with a diagnosed disease, usually with chronicity of at least 3 months' duration, whereas "dying" describes the final stage of living, regardless of the presence or absence of diagnosed disease. For example, the victim of an automobile accident or a very aged person with no diagnosed disease may be dying without being considered "terminally ill."

There is one other aspect to the definition of "terminal illness." Although a client may have been told that she "may not survive more than 2 years after a mastectomy," she is not considered "terminally ill" until she exhibits physical symptoms of her diagnosed illness and needs care that she cannot provide herself (i.e., has a self-care deficit).

Most dying clients of a CHN, in the home or in a nursing home or hospice, have been diagnosed with a terminal illness such as cancer, diabetic complications, or congestive heart failure.

### Physical Care

Dying at home can be a difficult ordeal if planning has been inadequate. Skilled nursing intervention can help prepare the client and family and can provide a unique support system and liaison with other support systems. (Throughout this chapter, the term "family" is used to designate all of the client's significant others.)

The CHN can help the family make the home as comfortable an environment as possible. Special equipment such as hospital beds and wheelchairs can be purchased, rented, or borrowed from organizations such as the American Cancer Society or the Multiple Sclerosis Society. Families can use their creative abilities to improvise equipment and supplies. These efforts should be encouraged and supported by the CHN. A homemade over-the-bed tray or table may not be quite as efficient as one that is purchased or rented, but the caring that is shared will usually far outweigh a minor inefficiency. The nurse should keep in mind that most decisions should be made by the client and family.

The family should be prepared for predictable events in the advance of the disease process. The CHN may need to educate the family about the particular disease process. Martinson (1976) provided an example of such preparation in her work with leukemic children who were cared for at home. She found that if families were prepared for the possibility of hemorrhage with a supply of clean towels, they had more time and energy for other important issues, such as airway maintenance and psychological support. Written prescriptions are obtained from the physician at the outset and reviewed with the client and family for adequacy at periodic intervals. The CHN should also establish what the physician has told the client about his diagnosis and prognosis, and should proceed accordingly. Most clients want to know if they are going to die. One of the most common fears is dying alone (Benton, 1978). Open discussions with the client and family throughout the dying process will provide the CHN with cues to changing physical and psychological needs. Curative interventions are considered inappropriate for those who elect palliative care. The basic physical needs of nutrition, warmth, positioning and skin care, toileting, bathing, and airway maintenance, along with pain control, should be considered as the primary areas of concern.

*Nutrition*

Since the goal of care is comfort, it is important to supply the client with palatable nourishment and adequate amounts of food and fluid to maintain his fluid balance. Families should be encouraged to prepare foods that have previously been a part of the diet in the home. Favorite foods will often help to stimulate the appetite of the dying person. Although highly seasoned spaghetti and meatballs may not seem to be the most appropriate choice of food, more is accomplished from both a nutritional and a psychological standpoint if they are tolerated and enjoyed by the client than if other foods are refused. Alcoholic beverages in moderation may also be used to stimulate appetite. If it has been customary to have wine with the evening meal, it should be offered. Small amounts of alcohol usually do not interfere with the medication regimen, and consultation with a pharmacist on this matter can clarify questions regarding interactions. If the client tolerates a diet similar to that of other members of the family, time and energy are conserved. Finally, small touches to make the food attractive should not be overlooked; for example, a neighbor might deliver a miniature flower arrangement every few days to place on the client's tray.

The CHN must also consider the client's diagnosis and physical status. The person dying of cancer who also has a cardiovascular disorder may require dietary salt restriction and extra sources of potassium to maintain his electrolyte balance; this in turn promotes comfort.

Another area of concern is decreasing appetite, due to the inability of a debilitated person to digest and utilize large amounts of food at one time. The CHN should alert the family that the client may refuse a full meal, because he has a physiological need for smaller and possibly more frequent servings. Palatable high-nutrient liquids can often be alternated with small servings of solid food. This may provide the additional time necessary for digestion and absorption of the solid foods. Commercial protein supplements or dry nonfat milk can be added to cream soups and beverages to increase their nutrient value. Extra calories may forestall unwanted weight loss.

As the client's physical condition deteriorates, the nurse should encourage family members to offer small amounts of fluid frequently. It is appropriate to demonstrate the use of a straw to siphon small amounts of liquid into the client's mouth, as well as the use of eye droppers and small syringes, with plastic tubing added to the ends, for offering fluids. A child's training cup sometimes works well. It is at this point that alternative methods of oral hygiene should also be discussed. Swabbing the mouth with a mixture of lemon juice and glycerine thins the mucus that is frequently present in the oral cavity.

It is important for the CHN to teach the family about safety measures in administering oral fluids to ill persons. The client's head should be elevated to prevent aspiration as fluids are given. It may be necessary to teach family members to observe for swallowing difficulties and never to force fluids on unconscious or semiconscious persons. Occasionally, intravenous feedings are administered by the CHN in the home if ordered by the physician.

### Warmth

Providing warmth for the dying client may well be the easiest physical need to meet, especially if the client is able to describe sensations of warm and cold. Several suggestions might be appropriate, depending upon the individual's overall physiological status. A thermal or electric blanket may provide adequate warmth without the burden of the excessive weight of a number of blankets. The family might also be helped to understand that as the client's circulatory status declines, he may complain of feeling cold even when the other family members are comfortable. If the client's body temperature is elevated (over 99.6°F), the CHN should alert the family to increase fluid intake and adjust the environment appropriately.

### Positioning and skin care

Proper positioning is essential to the client's comfort and well-being. If the family members understand the value of repositioning, they will be motivated to carry out the task consistently. The CHN can support the family's efforts while offering such ideas as the use of extra pillows for added support. The nurse can also easily demonstrate how quickly pressure over a bony prominence can cause "redness" by applying pressure to her own wrist or elbow for a short time, thus helping the family to understand the potential for skin breakdown and the need for proper positioning to prevent decubiti.

Although prevention and treatment of decubitus ulcers are discussed in Chapter 9, a few points should be emphasized in treatment of the dying person. Using a turning sheet to move the client can prevent trauma to skin from pressure. Suggestions about the use of small sheepskins, pieces of soft flannel, or soft crushed wool to prevent skin irritation should be shared with those caring for the client. The perineal area may need to be washed more frequently than usual to decrease skin breakdown from urine. Pressure sores develop more easily when a client suffers extensive weight loss. Some families may have initiated other creative methods of maintaining skin integrity, and the CHN should recognize and encourage these efforts. She and the family should continually be mindful that the best intervention is prevention.

## Toileting

While the client remains ambulatory and continent, toileting may pose no problem. However, the nurse should be alert to changes in bowel and bladder function that may result from inactivity, decreased intake, increased debilitation, or specific disease processes. If the client is immobile, the nurse can suggest the use of such equipment as bedpans, urinals, catheters, retaining bags, and diapers as a last resort.

Decreased food and fluid intake plus decreased mobility are the prime causative factors of fecal impaction. The family should be encouraged to keep an accurate record of the client's bowel activity and taught how to check for and remove a low fecal impaction if it becomes necessary. Other measures include added liquids, prune juice or prunes, and roughage in the diet. The physician may order a stool softener, suppositories, laxatives, or an enema.

If the client becomes incontinent, the physician may prescribe an indwelling catheter. The smallest size catheter that works should be selected, because it lessens trauma to the urethral orifice. At least one family member should learn about catheter care and handling of equipment such as drainage bags or leg urinals. Catheters should be irrigated daily with sterile water or another solution; the sterile water can be prepared by boiling for 10 minutes and then cooling it. A kitchen baster is ideal for irrigating the tubing. The drainage tubing and bottle should be soaked about twice weekly in a solution of vinegar and water to remove sediment, washed with soap and water, and rinsed thoroughly. It is a good idea for the family to have two sets of drainage equipment.

The CHN changes the catheter about once or twice monthly, using a *sterile* technique to lessen chances of a urinary tract infection. It must be stressed that impeccable catheter technique must be used by the CHN and the family, because dying clients are very susceptible to infection. A sterile lubricant such as K-Y jelly should be used on the urethral orifice to decrease tissue damage.

Should the physician choose not to order an indwelling catheter, regular intermittent catheterization or toileting every 2 or 3 hours may alleviate some of the incontinence. In all cases of incontinence, whether bladder or bowel, proper skin care—"clean and dry"—should be emphasized by the CHN.

Both adults and children are very sensitive to the loss of bladder or bowel control; thus, it is important to listen to the concerns of client and family and to offer reassurance and encouragement in this area.

Embarrassment and guilt must particularly be considered when genital care is provided for a parent by his offspring, because it is the epitome of role reversal, involving both intimacy and privacy.

## Bathing

If the client's condition warrants, a daily bed bath, besides being necessary for cleansing, can be a pleasant ritual and a time to observe skin surfaces, change position, and inquire about concerns. It is an excellent time for the CHN or nurse practitioner (NP) to conduct any portion of a physical examination that is deemed necessary. A bath also helps calm the person so that he can rest, if this is indicated.

## Airway maintenance

Airway maintenance should be discussed with all who are involved in the care of the client. It should be discussed as a comfort measure rather than as a life support or resuscitative measure. As indicated previously, proper positioning during and after eating will help prevent possible airway obstruction due to aspiration. If the client experiences nausea, the family should be instructed about the necessity of side or abdominal positioning. If the client is semiconscious or comatose, the nurse should demonstrate how to maintain proper extension of the neck for adequate ventilation. Finally, if the CHN has the assessment skills to check the lungs she should examine the respiratory system for adventitious breath sounds and signs of pneumonia. Oxygen is often administered in a home, so the CHN should teach the family to clean the equipment and to be alert to safety factors. The administration of oxygen is discussed in Chapter 8.

Those who care for the client are most acutely aware of even subtle changes in respiratory quality or pattern. This awareness may be attributed to the proximity of the caregivers as death becomes more imminent. In instances where a nurse is providing weekend or evening on-call availability to a dying client and family, a telephone call to her or the physician indicating that respiratory changes have suddenly occurred (even if the client does not appear distressed) will usually require professional advice or a prompt visit to the home. Whether the change indicates imminent death or gradually declining respiratory effort, the family may desire that a support person be present to assess the changes and discuss the possible significance of these changes.

*Pain control*

Pain is not synonymous with dying; all dying persons do not necessarily experience pain. Yet, when pain occurs, its control is one of the most challenging problems encountered by the client/family unit and the nurse. The perceived pain itself, along with the fear and anxiety that high-level pain can elicit from both client and family, can be almost devastating.

As in all life situations, a sense of control by the dying client over his own life and the immediate environment is essential to mental health. Uncontrolled pain severely threatens such feelings of control. The client's entire store of energy, which may already be depleted by a declining physiological state, is concentrated on the pain, so that he is unable to accomplish other tasks. The CHN has a responsibility to assist the client and family in assessing the pain and the need for analgesics, and to encourage the use of analgesics if necessary.

Personal expressions of pain and fear of pain may be as varied as the types of pain that can occur. Obvious indicators of pain such as crying or facial grimacing are common expressions recognized by even casual observers. Other less obvious expressions that indicate pain include increased irritability, withdrawal from usual activities, more frequent expressions of a need to sleep, and overt demonstrations of anger. If the nurse is aware of these expressions of pain and the possible reasons for the client's use of indirect communication, she will be able to help those caring for the client to recognize and alleviate the pain.

Maintenance of a self-concept as a stoic or uncomplaining person, fear of causing distress to loved ones, and the fear of drug dependence are but a few of the reasons a client may have for not directly expressing pain. The first step in overcoming a client's reluctance to express pain is establishing an atmosphere in which honest communication is welcomed. This may be accomplished through a family discussion of pain in which the expression of thoughts and feelings concerning pain is encouraged. If this kind of sharing is not customary, individual interactions between client and nurse (and family and nurse) may be necessary.

For some individuals, direct communication of pain is more acceptable than any acknowledgment of tension or depression is. There are instances when clients are unable to distinguish pain from depression, and depression may accentuate perceived pain.

There are various aspects of nursing intervention with the use of pharmacological agents for persons dying at home. Family members may need instruction in administering injectable medications. Rotation of injection sites for comfort and maximum absorption should be employed. Because of the frequency of administration, a chart—such as that used by diabetics for the rotation of insulin sites—may be devised (see Figure 8-2). The CHN should instruct the family to record the times of medication administration.

Parenteral medication may not always be necessary. The Brompton Mixture, used for many years in Great Britain, is an oral narcotic mixture that consists of varying amounts of morphine, cocaine, flavoring syrup, and chloroform water, and is available with or without ethyl alcohol. The mixture is given with a potent antiemetic, usually a phenothiazine. Used primarily in treating the chronic pain of advanced malignancies, the Bromptom Mixture is considered extremely effective in eliminating pain while maintaining an unclouded sensorium (Mount, Ajemian, & Scott, 1977). When the Brompton Mixture is utilized, the nurse's responsibility consists primarily of working closely with the client and physician in assessing the effectiveness of each established dose until a pain-free state with minimal sedation is achieved. Thereafter, a recognition of the need for dosage increases or decreases is essential.

Because most neighborhood pharmacies do not stock the quantities of narcotics that may be required for the dying person, the nurse should work with the family to find a convenient pharmacy that will make special arrangements for supplies. Appropriate planning for weekends and holidays when stores may be closed will eliminate the unnecessary stress involved in searching for a supplier while the client waits in fear of uncontrolled pain.

As the nurse discusses pain control with the client and family, at least three points should be discussed: the relief the medication provides; the relative importance and management of drug addiction; and the use of too strong a dosage of medication early in the course of the illness. *The most important reason for the pain medication is relief of pain!* If it does not relieve the pain, the CHN should recommend a change in dosage, an alteration in the duration between administrations, or an alternate drug. The CHN usually does this by telephone or by a note left in the home if the physician's visit is expected. It is the responsibility of the CHN to insure that the telephone order is confirmed with a written medical order.

Drug addition in dying persons is of less consequence than in other clients. Because of general awareness of drugs and addiction, clients and families may fear that their frequent use may compound existing problems. The nurse should listen carefully to these concerns and be aware that hesitancy to take or administer prescribed drugs may be a clue to an unexpressed fear of addiction. Of addiction, Gonda (1970) has said, "It is a trivial side effect of a management that allows the patient to carry on reasonably well and to die in relative comfort" (p. 265). However, if dosages of pain medication are carelessly increased early in the disease process, the client may later require such strong doses for severe pain that it causes depression of the entire nervous system. The nurse needs to educate the client and family about the management of addiction.

Supportive care can greatly enhance the effect of pain medication and/or depression. Other methods of alleviating pain may be selected, such as diversional activities. Because there are fewer restrictions in the home than in the hospital, the creativity of the family can be fully utilized in adapting pleasurable activities to the physical limitation of the client. Simple activities such as listening to music, drawing, and adding to or initiating collections of stamps or coins can have amazing analgesic effects. Maintaining creativity and a sense of usefulness through needlework, simple woodwork, letter writing, use of a two-way radio, or model building may serve as an outlet for expressions of feelings that may otherwise never surface. A well-planned outing, even if no more than a backyard picnic, can bring a sense of relief merely through a change in scenery.

Sharing home movies, slides, or photograph albums might be encouraged. Such activities, while providing diversion, also serve another therapeutic purpose: Some dying persons are aided in their grief process by a review of the meaningful experiences in their lives. Although this task will usually not be completed through the sharing of family movies or pictures in a single evening, a beginning can be made that may be therapeutic for those who participate. An occupational therapist can also be consulted.

Breathing and muscle exercises can also enhance the effect of pain medication. If the client and family are unfamiliar with these techniques, the CHN may demonstrate a few simple exercises and encourage practice as a part of daily routine. Should the methods prove effective, the family can borrow library books that will offer a wider variety of exercises. The family may be surprised to find that they, too, benefit from the exercises and relaxation.

Quite obviously, there is an endless list of activities that can serve as diversion from pain and an outlet for grieving and tension. However, without a supportive and empathetic listener with whom the client can share fears, dreams, concerns, and desires, all efforts to control pain (including massive doses of medication) will prove to be only partially successful.

Meeting the physical needs of a person dying at home can be a monumental task. However, the meaningful time and love that can be shared in both giving and receiving care cannot be replaced. To be a part of these precious weeks, days, or hours is a very special part of being human and a member of the nursing profession.

## Psychological Care during the Terminal Illness

The first days after bringing a dying family member home from the hospital can be overwhelming. Regardless of the preparation and readiness of the family to provide physical care, the psychosocial adjustments can cause severe disequilibrium. Psychosocial nursing intervention for the client and family requires some of the nurse's most creative abilities. Specific interventions are influenced by medical and nursing diagnoses, as well as by the age, cultural background, and religious beliefs of the client. A few conceptual frameworks and the broader areas of concern are discussed in the next section.

### Conceptual frameworks for dying and death

Kübler-Ross (1969) was the first researcher to provide a conceptual framework for the dying process; she depicted a five-stage paradigm through which those facing death proceed. The stages she described include shock, anger, bargaining, depression, and acceptance. While many, particularly those in the health professions, acclaimed the Kübler-Ross framework, it has not been strongly supported by research findings. Now, health professionals are beginning to accept her work for what it is—a theoretical model.

An earlier framework useful in analyzing interactions was that described by Glaser and Strauss (1965). Although originally a description of interactions between dying persons and hospital staff members, it has utility for broader interactions. The categories of interactions are these: closed awareness, suspicion awareness, mutual pretense, and open awareness. Each category carries with it certain assets and liabilities, as well as expected behavioral components. In closed awareness, the interaction proceeds on the basis that the client is unaware of approaching death. In suspicion awareness, the interaction involves means of either allaying or confirming suspicions of the dying state. Mutual pretense involves a mutual understanding of the true situation, but an implicit or explicit agreement not to deal with it openly. Open awareness relies upon a mutual understanding and a willingness to interact openly that is based on that understanding.

The CHN should be familiar with various theoretical frameworks pertinent to dying, and should utilize them insofar as they are appropriate to a particular client and family's situation.

### Contractual agreements as a means of support

The first concern is that of what the client and family expect and need from support persons and what the CHN can realistically offer. The nurse may not initially be able to be specific about which problems can be realistically solved, but may make a contractual agreement to help with any that arise, either through personal intervention or by seeking the services of appropriate others.

Another essential point is the option of returning to hospital care if home care becomes too stressful (Martinson, 1976). Just knowing that the option remains open may reduce panic when difficult situations arise. Severe infections or other complications may make home care impossible and necessitate a return to the hospital. Potential feelings of guilt related to the inability to complete the home care experience may be avoided if an agreement is reached by all concerned before the situation presents itself.

Other topics that might be discussed as part of the contract are the frequency of scheduled visits by the nurse, the actual physical or other nursing care the nurse will participate in, and the issue of responsibility for relaying information to the physician and other health team members, such as an occupational therapist. Certainly the contract may be renegotiated at any time; however, an initial set of agreements will prevent misunderstandings and stress. Contracts are also discussed in Chapter 7.

### Exploration of support systems for the client

Each family will differ in the kind and amount of support it requires. Answers to the following questions will help to examine possible sources of support and enable organization of a system for "on-call" help: Are there other members of the extended family, neighbors, or close friends who have offered time and support? Does the client have a church affiliation from which support persons may be drawn? It is important that the family know, not merely assume, exactly what commitments are offered by others.

A person faced with death usually has at least four important contacts: family, nurse, physician, and clergy. The CHN is probably closely associated with the physician if the client has had care at home from her and the health agency she represents. From the family, physician, and CHN, the client draws physical and psychological support, while the clergyman provides spiritual and psychological strength.

*Role of the physician.* The physician may be in private practice, in a clinic, or in a home care program. The CHN apprises him of the client's condition, and requests medical orders as necessary. For example, as a client becomes sicker, oxygen may be needed and the pain medication may have to be increased. These orders can be taken by telephone, but the CHN should request that the physician also put them in writing, in order to prevent any future misunderstanding or legal problem. It is appropriate for the CHN to request that a physician make a home visit if she considers this essential.

*Role of the clergyman.* The minister, priest, or rabbi is one of the professionals who can give help to the terminally ill. While not all individuals identify themselves with a specific religious group, the majority of clients and families who are faced with terminal illness will want the services of a spiritual advisor as the illness progresses. Counseling is a considerable part of a clergyman's work, and he should be told the client's physical state and the relative imminence of death. The CHN should expect and welcome the visits of the clergy during terminal illnesses; they can and ought to work cooperatively for the welfare of clients and families.

If the nurse perceives that a clergyman has not been notified of the situation, she may ask the client and family if they want one telephoned. The name of the client's clergyman, church affiliation, and telephone number are part of a community health agency's record, as they are of a hospital record. The client may desire that the clergyman, if possible, be present at the time of death. Funeral arrangements are frequently made with the clergy.

The clergy may also be helpful in giving personal support to the CHN who deals extensively with the dying, and should be included in the network of support for professionals who work with the terminally ill (Dumer, 1983).

*Other significant helpers.* Having explored with the client and the family the stability of support persons and their services, the nurse will then be able to help the family plan a system that will effectively provide telephone contact with a helping person every hour of the day and night. Few families will fully use the entirety of the support system, but the knowledge that individuals are available will provide a sense of security.

In assessing the support system, the nurse should be alert to cues that signal a social avoidance of death. As an example, parents of a terminally ill boy were puzzled by and somewhat angry with an elderly neighbor who stopped visiting after their boy became ill. Although the child had not inquired about the neighbor, he frequently positioned himself in bed so that he could look into the man's yard. The CHN asked the parents if it might be that the neighbor felt uncomfortable with the idea of death. The child's father then simply invited the neighbor to visit. Within a few days the neighbor, who obviously had not forgotten the boy, began a series of brief, enjoyable daily visits. This case, like many others of social avoidance of death, was probably caused by fear and lack of knowledge of how to relate to a dying person. The family should be assisted in gaining this type of understanding in order to reduce feelings of rejection.

### Maintenance of the client's autonomy, dignity, and control

Autonomy, dignity, and control are the basis for many of the most cherished human values. To lose our sense of one of these, even for a brief time, causes stress, pain, and sometimes permanent emotional scars. Consider what it might be like to be stripped of all three for as long as life continues—a fairly common phenomenon among persons who become "the dying." Dying persons need to be related to as the living, not as the almost dead (Wentzel, 1976)! The preciousness of living may be lost on the living, who see no end to their days (Paige, 1979).

Home care of the dying client can provide the atmosphere for the maintenance of these rights as no other environment can. The family that has chosen to care for a dying loved one will occasionally usurp some of the client's control, but it is even more likely that persons from outside the intimate unit will unintentionally strip the client of these rights.

If the CHN consciously considers the client's rights in all interactions, these rights can be maintained. First, the CHN should not be guilty of unintentionally challenging or removing these rights; and secondly, the CHN can aid the family in maintaining the client's autonomy, dignity, and control, regardless of others present. Some examples of the unintentional infringement of these rights will serve to illustrate how dying persons may no longer be considered in the same light as living persons.

The dying person may wish to refuse a visit by a relative, friend, health professional, or clergyman, and, like anyone else, may require time alone. Unfortunately, the refusal of the visit may be interpreted as an increase in depression related to the dying process, and further attempts may be made to spend more time in visiting. The person's autonomy is indeed threatened when helping persons assume that the desire to be alone *must* be related to depression.

A simple infringement on dignity is any conversation that takes place in the client's presence as though he were not there. A question such as "How is he today?" spoken to a third person while an alert client sits quietly in the same room can only imply to the client that he is no longer considered able to answer accurately for himself.

Throughout the dying process, clients may be forced to relinquish some control because of declining physical capabilities. It is therefore crucial to provide for personal control and decision making in every possible way. Does the husband of a dying woman force her to relinquish some control when he insists that she nap in the afternoon "for her own good"? Perhaps a nap would be beneficial, but the dying persons needs to be encouraged and assisted in choosing what is personally desirable.

Groenwald and Bermensolo (1978) have summarized the role that all who care for the dying must assume in helping to maintain rights and fulfill needs: "We must let the patient set the stage and direct the play. We are the understudies—available to supply the missing word, the problem solving, the support—when called upon to do so. The most important thing to remember . . . is that it is their life . . . and their death."

### Support for the family

There is one other major concern that should be considered by the CHN. The family members, like the dying client, need to maintain control of their own lives and the situation in which they are participating. Knowledge is essential in the ability to control; the problem identified most often by families is that of coping with the unknown. The nurse can do much to limit the degree of uncertainty for the family.

Questions should be explored and answered, though there are many questions for which there are no certain answers. Families may want to know (but may be afraid to ask) what the actual death will be like. They may be anxious about an increase in pain, the person's appearance, and their own possible reactions to the death. The CHN can offer some general, albeit uncertain, ideas and can allow the family to express concerns. Honest answers, a healthy self-esteem, and a strong support system can significantly reduce the difficulty of coping with the unknown.

*Need for privacy, intimacy, and sexuality
by the client and family*

The proximity of family members within the home environment is one of the advantages of home care of the dying. However, there may be a tendency, most likely related to the uncertainty of time left, to neglect the very important need for privacy. The dying client will need time for private, thoughtful reflection and, as death becomes more imminent, may openly withdraw from loved ones. Families may need help in understanding that time spent alone is important and that withdrawal does not necessarily indicate depression or a decrease in love and affection.

Family members also need privacy and time alone. Signs of increasing irritability, fatigue, and stress may be directly related to the fact that the family member has not allowed adequate time for private reflections or relaxation. Prevention of caregiver "burnout" is essential to maintaining the quality of care. It may be difficult to convince concerned parents involved in the care of their dying child that occasional time away from the child is important. Sometimes a dying child places serious strain on a marriage. Also, the competition among caregivers warrants consideration; for example, a wife can experience tension if she seeks time alone with a dying husband and her husband's parents are present.

An understanding of the effects of stress on the entire family relationship and a choice of alternate activities may make it possible for the family to pursue activities that meet personal needs without feelings of guilt. Sincere praise for efforts made on behalf of the client may provide the family with the encouragement and support necessary for them to permit themselves some private time.

One of the last scenes from the film *Love Story*, a contemporary portrayal of a love relationship through the dying process, depicted a young husband lying next to his dying wife in a hospital bed. This one scene of an intimate embrace said more in a few brief seconds than is found in the scant amount of literature on the intimate and sexual needs of the dying and those they love. The dying person's need to express intimate or sexual feelings does not disappear. Parents do not refrain from holding and soothing their child because the child is dying. Adults, too, need to feel loved and give love, yet the desire and need of a dying person for intimate contact has been all but ignored. There is a strong possibility that, like the elderly in contemporary society, there is a hesitancy on the part of the dying and those who love them to recognize their continuing intimate and sexual needs openly. It is almost as if society has subtly implied that thoughts of intimate and sexual pleasure are inappropriate at such times in life.

A loving touch, an intimate embrace, tender words, and sexual interaction of any kind that is desired between two people can communicate honesty and help to work through feelings. The relaxation and sharing that result from intimate contact can benefit both the dying person and the partner. A sensitive nurse may discover both verbal and nonverbal cues that indicate concerns. If a good rapport has been established, a question such as "Do you ever feel like just holding him quietly?" directed to the spouse of the dying client may open the way for discussion of feelings. The CHN can then share thoughts about intimacy and sex as very special and appropriate forms of communication between loving adults at any time of life. She can also facilitate providing a private environment for the couple to express themselves sexually, if privacy is a problem.

Physical limitations related to medical status and general decline may prevent intimate or sexual contact. A fear of causing further physical discomfort may exist; hormonal and/or psychological shifts can cause fluctuations in sexual drive; or disfigurement may cause embarrassment or revulsion. If the nurse is able to discover the source of the problem, appropriate counseling can then be offered.


At the Time of Death

*Preparations*

The actual event of the death may be a time of anything from intense anxiety for the family to a time of relief and peace. Advance information about the signs of impending death and recognition of the event may reduce anxiety. Families should be prepared for changes in skin color, alterations in respiration (Cheyne Stokes respirations), and variations in level of consciousness.

In the home and other nonacute care settings, the cessation of heartbeat and respiration is generally considered to indicate death. The family should know that it can call upon support people as death nears, and that the physician must be called at the time of death in order to certify and complete the death certificate according to the legal requirements of the state (Creighton, 1979). A client at home is under the care of a physician, who should be the one notified at the time of death.

The family might wish to prepare the body prior to calling the funeral director. Such preparation could include cleansing the skin and removing medical apparatus and jewelry. The family, however, should be encouraged to engage in only those activities with which they feel comfortable, and should understand that funeral directors provide these services as well. A CHN, if present, may suggest that dentures be replaced and that eyelids and the jaw be closed.

The day of death and the following few days are often hectic for the family. Funeral arrangements must be made, relatives and friends must be notified, and most families clean the house and prepare for visitors and socially prescribed mourning rituals. These activities may be carried out in the state of acute grief with its accompanying shock and numbness, or the activities may actually preclude the onset of the grieving process. They are very therapeutic at this time because they allow the loved ones still to do some concrete tasks for the dead person.

### Support of the bereaved

Contemporary nursing literature abounds with concepts of dying and death and theories on grief and bereavement. A sound theoretical base is essential to competent nursing practice, and it is essential that the CHN who participates in home care of the dying client understand these concepts and theories. However, there must be a bridge between theory and practice that spans the wide range of human experience—a process that allows each nurse to offer individualized understanding and care. That bridge involves one basic concept: *Grief is a personal and unique experience for each human being.* With a firm grasp on theory and conscious awareness of the unique experience, the nurse should find it natural to extend reasonable commitment to the bereaved family members.

### The community health nurse's involvement at the time of death

Professional nursing services are usually unwarranted during the days of funeral preparations, although limited participation in the funeral service may be appreciated; a "personal" visit to the funeral home or a telephone call to the family is usually also welcome. Most community health agencies recommend at least one professional nursing visit to the home after the funeral to support the family, help dispose of medical apparatus, and answer remaining questions. The family often asks, "Did I do everything I could have?", to which the CHN responds with assurance. Even if the death has occurred in the hospital, the CHN who has cared for the deceased visits the family afterwards. The visit is also a statement of affirmation of the worth of the deceased and those who survive.

Frequently reported is the need of the bereaved to share thoughts and feelings about the deceased and to relive, through words, the final days and hours spent together. Furthermore, there is a need to be reassured that the waves and pangs of loneliness, fear, panic, anger, and lack of motivation are normal responses to loss. The CHN can offer much as an empathetic listener—one who is willing to hear thoughts on both the good times and the bad, and who understands the purpose of reiterating an incident more than once. The CHN may also aid the bereaved in seeking community support groups, which can serve to meet these and other needs.

The CHN must be specifically alert to the well-being of the bereaved. Loss of appetite, difficulty in sleeping, and weight loss often accompany acute grief. If these become severe or are extended over a long period of time, a referral to the physician for further evaluation is necessary. The survivor might also complain of other physical symptoms, including some that were experienced by the family member who has died. These complaints must never be considered as just part of the grieving process. Numerous studies have indicated an alarming incidence of physical disorders and death within 1 year of the death of a significant other (Lynch, 1977; Parkes, 1972). The CHN can offer assessment, support, and encouragement to seek appropriate medical evaluation if indicated.

## Community Resources and Support Groups

### For Client and Family

The community resources available to support dying persons and their families vary from community to community. In general, urban areas provide the greatest number of agency resources, but informal assistance is often more readily available in small rural communities. In addition to support given by the CHN and the community health agencies, formal agency support may be provided by hospitals and hospices. Services range from complete hospice care programs to telephone hotlines for the general public. Some also provide consultation for the nurse and other caregivers.

Community health agencies keep a directory of various referral services for the CHN to use. Equipment rental places, consultation services, and support groups are provided by such agencies as the American Red Cross, the American Cancer Society, the American Heart Association, and the Kidney Foundation. Local or regional offices are most willing to explain their programs.

Many urban localities have local chapters of the Compassionate Friends—an international organization that promotes mutual group support for persons whose children have died. Some communities offer service programs or support groups for the newly widowed. Most of these groups embrace the philosophy that support can be best provided by other people who have been or are confronted by the same situation. This "people helping people" approach appears to be successful during the normal grieving process and should be seriously considered by the CHN.

Nurses must not overlook the other support resources utilized by families, including voluntary services offered by funeral directors, universities, church groups, clergy, business organizations, unions, fraternal organizations, and social clubs. In those localities where only limited services are available, the CHN may be influential in initiating and organizing these volunteer groups.

## For the Community Health Nurse

While knowledge of community resources for the family is essential for the CHN, she must also be aware of her own personal needs for support. The question of who gives care to the caregiver is a vital one. "Burnout," physical and mental exhaustion, is a critical phenomenon observed among caregivers who deal extensively with the terminally ill and the dying, and support is necessary to prevent this condition. A support network can be established within the employing agency and/or within the local levels of the professional organization to which the CHN belongs.

Furthermore, it is essential that the CHN maintain expertise in the care of the terminally ill and dying. This can be accomplished by reading, attending and giving continuing education workshops, and participating in organizations related to terminal illnesses and care of the dying. Numerous books on the topic of dying, death, and bereavement can be found in public and professional libraries. Professional nursing journals regularly include articles on terminal illness and grief, and thanatological research is reported in at least two journals, *Omega* and *Death Education*. Information on professional care of specific terminal illnesses is available from governmental and voluntary agencies such as the National Cancer Institute and the American Cancer Society, respectively.

Finally, membership is available in organizations that focus on care of the dying, develop standards of care, and disseminate knowledge. One such national organization, the Forum for Death Education and Counseling, is comprised of professionals who practice, teach, or carry out research in all areas of thanatology. Another, the National Hospice Organization, consists of members interested and involved in the various aspects of the hospice movement. At the local level, the nurse may establish study groups within the district nurses' association. Group membership is not only cognitively stimulating, but is also emotionally supportive.

## Summary

The CHN has a very important role in the care of the family faced with death. That role includes the care and support of the dying person and all significant others, both before and after the death. It is a role that embodies much of the essence of nursing—caring. It is a demanding role and one for which nurses must seek additional preparation and support.

Experience with death on any level helps the CHN in subsequent encounters. Each situation reminds us of our own impending death, and that awareness in itself may be problematic. That does not mean, however, that awareness is to be avoided; indeed, it can lead to extensive personal growth, just as care of the dying can lead to great professional reward.

It would be helpful if the CHN could continue to follow the bereaved for a period of months. However, financial arrangements or agency protocol may not allow such follow-up at present. Perhaps the future will bring greater recognition of the importance of bereavement care as essential in community health nursing.

## References

Beeson, P. B., & McDermott, W. *Textbook of medicine*. Philadelphia: W. B. Saunders, 1975.

Benton, R. G. *Death and dying: Principles and practices in patient care*. New York: Van Nostrand Reinhold, 1978.

Cohen, K. P. *Hospice: Prescription for terminal care*. Germantown, Md.: Aspen Systems Corporation, 1979.

Creighton, H. What is death and who determines it? *Supervisor Nurse*, 1979, 9, 74–75.

Dumer, L. H. Unpublished material, March 1983.

Glaser, B., & Strauss, A. *Awareness of dying*. Chicago: Aldine, 1965.

Gonda, T. Pain and addiction in terminal illness. In B. Schoenberg, A. Carr, D. Peretz, & A. Kutscher (Eds.), *Loss and grief: Psychological management in medical practice*. New York: Columbia University Press, 1970.

Groenwald, S., & Bermensolo, P. *Are we death-and-dying our patients to death?* Paper presented at First Annual Conference of the Forum for Death Education and Counseling, Washington, D.C., September 19–22, 1978.

Kübler-Ross, E. *On death and dying*. New York: Macmillan, 1969.

Lynch, J. *The broken heart*. New York: Basic Books, 1977.

Martinson, I. M. *Home care for the dying child*. New York: Appleton-Century-Crofts, 1976.

Milwaukee Hospice. Unpublished material, 1979. (Available from the Hospice at 1022 N. Ninth Street, Milwaukee, Wisc. 53233.)

Mount, B., Ajemian, I., & Scott, J. Use of the Brompton Mixture in treating the chronic pain of malignant disease. *Nursing Digest*, 1977, 1, 49–53.

Paige, R. Living and dying. *American Journal of Nursing*, 1979, 12, 2171–2172.

Parkes, C. *Bereavement: Studies of grief in adult life*. New York: International Universities Press, 1972.

Saunders, C. St. Christopher's Hospice. In E. Schneideman (Ed.), *Death: Current Perspectives*. Palo Alto, Calif.: Mayfield, 1976.

Wentzel, K. The dying are the living. *American Journal of Nursing*, 1976, 6, 956–957.

Whilsmith, G. Father died at home. *The Lutheran*, November 1, 1978, pp. 10–11.

Zorza, V., & Zorza, R. The death of a daughter. *Washington Post*, January 22, 1978, pp. C1 and C4.

# Appendixes

## Appendix A: General Guidelines for a Health History for an Adult or Child*

A. Nature and duration of present health status.
  1. Describe informant (client, spouse, parent) and his reliability.
  2. Describe major concerns about health in the words of the client; if there are chief complaints, describe their onset and history.
B. Past history.
  This section is concerned with the history of wellness and illness in the client and his family.
  1. Childhood illnesses (includes communicable diseases).
  2. Adult illnesses requiring medical attention:
    a. Medications, special regimens prescribed.
    b. Hospitalizations, surgical procedures.
    c. Client/family history:
      1) Genetic illnesses.
      2) Chronic illnesses; tendencies to conditions or diseases. ("Has anyone in your family ever had heart disease, cancer, diabetes, arthritis, hypertension, mental illness, tuberculosis, or alcoholism?") It is sometimes useful to depict the family health history with a family tree or pedigree chart. This should include the index client and at least the two previous generations (parents and grandparents), as well as siblings and offspring.
      3) Allergies: How were these documented (i.e., by reaction to the antigen or skin test)? Describe reactions and effective treatment.
C. Review of body systems as in Appendix C (partial list included here), and assessment of illnesses or symptoms, trauma, and defects. The client will list subjective complaints not detected on a physical examination, such as loss of smell (see 4, below).

*Prepared by Charlene C. Ossler and Dorothy D. Petrowski.

1. Skin—bruises, dermatitis, burns.
2. Eyes—visual loss, glasses, trauma, infections, ocular edema, color blindness, diplopia.
3. Ears—hearing loss, vertigo, tinnitus, earache, discharge from the ear.
4. Senses—loss of smell or taste, nasal obstruction or polyps, epistaxis, rhinitis.
5. Mouth—lesions of the mouth, tongue, gums, dental problems, sore throats, voice changes, hoarseness, tonsillitis, difficulty in swallowing.
6. Neck—stiffness, range of motion, swelling, nodes, glands, goiter.
7. Chest—tuberculosis, pleurisy, bronchitis, pneumonia, asthma, wheezing, pain, cough, sputum (when, amount, color), hemoptysis, night sweats, shortness of breath at rest or upon exertion, previous chest X-rays.
8. Heart—hypertension, enlarged heart, heart attacks, rheumatic fever, precordial and substernal pain or tightness, dyspnea, palpitations, irregular rate or rhythm, previous EKGs, heart murmurs.
9. Gastrointestinal system—indigestion, nausea, vomiting, abdominal pain, stool characteristics (frequency, color, consistency, and changes), use of laxatives, hepatitis, ulcers, colitis, hemorrhoids, rectal problems, diseases of gall bladder or pancreas.
10. Renal system—frequency of urination at day and night, color and clearness of urine, dysuria, hematuria, polyuria, oliguria, incontinence, hesitancy, retention, passed renal calculi.
11. Reproductive system—sexually transmitted disease, vaginal secretion, penile discharge, menstrual cycle, potency, quality of sex, reproductive history (parity, contraception, fertility problems).
12. Skeletal system—fractures, loss of normal range of motion.

D. Mental status assessment.
1. General appearance (calm, agitated).
2. Mood (anxious, cheerful).
3. Thought process (coherent).
4. Cognition (oriented).

E. Immunization status—list date and types of recent immunizations and describe any reaction.
1. Recommended immunization schedules change periodically. The American of Pediatrics and/or the American Medical Association should be consulted for the most recent guidelines. (See the schedule of the American Academy of Pediatrics in Chapter 5, Table 5-2.)
2. Tuberculin skin test: The Mantoux technique with purified protein derivative (PPD) solution is recommended worldwide. Skin tests and chest X-rays as screening techniques are not recommended annually and are done only at the discretion of the practitioner and client. If the client is at risk, this recommendation changes. If the client reacts positively to the skin test, a chest X-ray, sputum smears and/or cultures are usually done.
3. Influenza: Vaccines are available for several strains, and the composition of the vaccine is changed annually. Opinions about the criteria and

need for this immunization differ; it is administered according to the physician's or practitioner's discretion and at a client's request. Clients at risk such as the elderly or those with chronic obstructive pulmonary disease should have this vaccine early each fall.

# Appendix B: Guidelines for Social/Interpersonal Health History or Assessment for an Adult*

A. Marital status and/or presence of significant other person: Describe the client's supportive network upon which he can rely in times of crisis.
B. Religious preference: Describe any implications of client's faith in regard to health intervention (e.g., Jehovah's Witnesses and Christian Scientists do not believe in certain medical practices). It is useful to know how actively the client participates in his religion and the importance of religion to him. It can be helpful to know the location of his church and a clergyman to contact.
C. Occupation, place of employment: Include all work in which the client has ever engaged. Describe the type of business/industry, hazards to which the client may have been exposed, and the frequency, concentration, and duration of exposure. Attempt to elicit information about job satisfaction, occupational stressors, and previous occupation-related injuries or illness.
D. Describe the client's "typical" day in terms of time spent in various activities. This is graphically done with a pie shape, as in Figure B-1. Begin with an empty circle and assist the client in sectioning off a 24-hour period according to his "typical" day's activity. This description will aid the practitioner in understanding the client's life style and time value orientation; it will also provide information about possible stressors and the need to alter some activities. If the time of day for each activity is also listed, the nurse can plan home health care at convenient, acceptable times.
E. Related physiological needs:
   1. Describe sleep patterns (usual amount of nightly sleep, naps, insomnia, need for medication or other devices to encourage sleep, awakening during the night, any interferences with usual sleep pattern (nocturia, environmental noise, dreams). Does the client feel rested upon awakening?
   2. Describe exercise pattern: Does client do a regular exercise program (calisthenics, jogging, running) or regularly participate in any sports? Describe the presence or absence of opportunity to be active at the client's occupational setting. Include those exercise activities that client states he would enjoy doing if he had the time and/or facilities to carry them out.
   3. Degree of physical fitness: Maltz, Zellmer, and Chandler (1973) have identified five specific physiological parameters that are associated with fitness: (1) a slower heart rate during exercise; (2) a more rapid return

*Prepared by Charlene C. Ossler and Dorothy D. Petrowski.

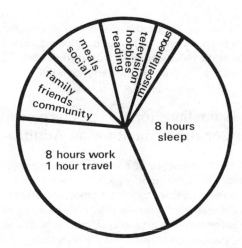

Figure B-1.  Example of a 24-Hour Schedule of Client's Sleep, Work, and Social Activities.

to resting heart rate during exercise; (3) a lower blood pressure before, during, and following exercise; (4) a lower oxygen intake; and (5) less lactic acid in the blood during exercise. Although assessment of some of these parameters requires special equipment, there are simple tests which can be done in any setting. Diekelmann (1977) suggests a specific exercise, which is given in Figure B-2; blood pressure and respiratory rate can also be evaluated during this exercise. Similar experiments for the assessment of physical fitness can be found in Cooper's *The New Aerobics* (1970).

At this point in the assessment, the practitioner may inquire about the client's personal assessment of his state of physical fitness, his desire to increase it, and his need for professional guidance in planning an appropriate exercise program.

4. Relaxation needs:
   a. Describe methods used to induce relaxation (hobbies, recreation, meditation, yoga, music).
   b. Can client induce a state of relaxation upon demand?
   c. If not, the practitioner should discuss the need for relaxation and acquaint the client with the various methods available to teach relaxation response, such as transcendental meditation, biofeedback, and yoga.
5. Driving:
   a. Vehicles used for transportation (motorcycles significantly increase the client's risk of vehicular injury or death).
   b. Miles driven each year.
   c. Exposure to driver education courses.

      d. History of accidents, traffic tickets for violations.

      e. Use of seat belts.

6. Drugs:

      a. Use of alcohol: Frequency, amounts, type (e.g., a six-pack of beer each evening). A response of "social drinking" has no value to the assessor. Ask the client to be more specific. Elicit the pattern of alcohol use for the past 5–10 years. If there seems to be a trend of increasing use of alcohol, evaluate for alcoholism by use of the Alcoholics Anonymous symptoms checklist.

      b. Use of over-the-counter drugs (aspirin, cough syrup).

      c. Use of prescribed medications: Describe the client's positive and adverse reactions to these.

      d. Use of illegal or street drugs.

      e. Caffeine intake (coffee, tea, chocolate, and cola products).

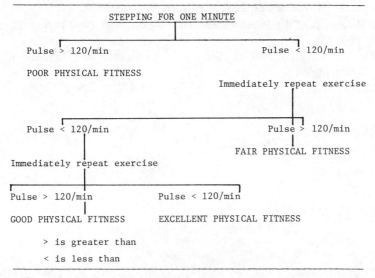

Figure B-2. Assessment of Physical Fitness by Pulse Assessment. The client should select a chair and step up on it for 1 minute in this sequence: Step up with left foot, then the right foot; step down with the left foot, then the right foot. These lifts should be repeated at a pace of 30 steps per minute for a person who weighs 100 to 160 pounds; the pace should be reduced to 20–30 steps per minute for persons exceeding 160 pounds. Immediately after the stepping, the client should sit down and count his pulse. Assessment of physical fitness is based upon the pulse rate, as illustrated in the figure. (Adapted from N. Diekelmann, *Primary Health Care of the Well Adult.* New York: McGraw-Hill, 1977.)

       f. Tobacco.
- 7. Sexual history:
  - a. Need for sexual information.
  - b. Problems with sexual relationships (physical and emotional); ability to achieve orgasm.
  - c. Sexual pattern (frequency, partners).
  - d. Protection from sexually transmitted diseases; knowledge of venereal disease.
  - e. History of venereal disease exposure and treatment.
  - f. History and knowledge of use of contraceptive devices.
  - g. Factors that may influence sexual performance (medical problems, drugs, anxiety or psychological problems, surgical procedures).

## References

Cooper, K. H. *The new aerobics*. New York: Bantam, 1970.

Diekelmann, N. (Ed.). *Primary health care of the well adult*. New York: McGraw-Hill, 1977.

Maltz, S., Zellmer, V., & Chandler, H. *College health science*. Dubuque, Iowa: W. C. Brown, 1973.

# Appendix C: Physical Examination for an Adult*

Height ___    Temperature ___    B.P. lying,    R___ L___

Weight ___    Respirations ___    B.P. sitting    R___ L___

Apical pulse ___    Radial pulse ___    B.P. standing    R___ L___

| | | normal | abnormal | describe and measure |
|---|---|---|---|---|
| SKIN | color | | | |
| | condition | | | |
| | hydration | | | |
| | temperature | | | |
| HEAD and SCALP | shape | | | |
| | condition | | | |
| | hair | | | |
| EYES | vision | | | |
| | cataracts | | | |
| | pupils' reactivity | | | |
| | tonometry | | | |
| EARS | appearance | | | |
| | hearing: acuity, Weber, Rinne | | | |
| | canals | | | |
| | tympanic membranes | | | |
| NOSE and SINUSES | smell | | | |
| | septum | | | |
| | sinus tenderness | | | |
| MOUTH | lips | | | |
| | teeth, dentures | | | |
| | tongue | | | |
| | gums | | | |
| | pharynx | | | |
| NECK | mobility | | | |
| | masses | | | |
| | thyroid | | | |
| | carotids | | | |
| | veins | | | |
| BREASTS | appearance | | | |
| | masses | | | |
| | tenderness | | | |

*Can be adapted for a child.

| CHEST | inspection | | | |
|---|---|---|---|---|
| | expansion | | | |
| | palpation (tactile fremitus) | | | |
| | percussion (resonance) | | | |
| | auscultation (breath sounds) | | | |
| HEART | inspection | | | |
| | palpation (PMI, thrill) | | | |
| | auscultation (S1, S2, S3, S4) | | | |
| | relative intensity (A2 and P2) | | | |
| | murmurs | | | |
| ABDOMEN | inspection | | | |
| | palpation | | | |
| | liver borders | | | |
| | bowel sounds | | | |
| | hernia | | | |
| | kidney tenderness | | | |
| ARTERIES | pulsation in: | | | |
| | brachials | | | |
| | radials | | | |
| | femorals | | | |
| | aorta | | | |
| | popliteals | | | |
| | dorsalis pedis | | | |
| GENITALIA | | | | |
| RECTUS | anus | | | |
| | prostate | | | |
| EXTREMI- TIES | appearance | | | |
| | ROM | | | |
| | joints | | | |
| | varicosities | | | |
| NEURO- LOGICAL | gait | | | |
| | station | | | |
| | Romberg | | | |
| | heel-toe walking | | | |
| | finger-to-nose | | | |
| | heel-to-shin | | | |
| | rapid succession movements | | | |
| | sensory: | | | |
| | pin prick | | | |
| | touch | | | |
| | stereognosis | | | |
| | tendon reflexes: | | | |
| | biceps      R      L | | | |
| | triceps     R      L | | | |
| | radial      R      L | | | |
| | quadriceps R      L | | | |
| | achilles    R      L | | | |

# Index

# Index

Abortion, 160–161, 173
Accident prevention
  preschoolers, 117
  toddlers, 95–96
Adolescents
  acne vulgaris, 155–156
  alcohol and drug abuse, 162–163
  bone and muscle injuries, 167
  clothing, 155
  cuts, bruises, and sprains, 157
  depression, 167–169
  fatigue, 155
  gonorrhea, 164
  headaches, 157
  major health problems of early,
    159–163
  major health problems of late,
    164–170
  menstrual irregularities, 156
  minor health problems, 155–156
  minor illnesses, 157
  mononucleosis, infectious, 166–
    167
  needs assessment for (form), 175–
    178
  nutrition, 157
  personal hygiene, 154–155
  physical examination, guidelines
    for (tab.), 149
  poor posture, 155
  pregnancy among, 23–25, 159–162
  relationship with opposite sex,
    159–162

relationship with others, 158–159
self-esteem, 157–158
sexually transmitted diseases,
  164–165
suicide, 169–170
syphilis, 164–165
trichomoniasis, 165–166
wellness promotion, 157–159
Alcohol abuse
  among adolescents, 162–163
  among young adults, 172, 174
  sources of information on, 178–
    179
Anal cancer, see Colostomy

Blood pressure
  of grade school children, 146–147
  high, see Hypertension
Breast cancer
  chronicity, 253–255
  morbidity and mortality, 247
  nursing care in clinic, 255
  occupational health, 255–256
  postoperative care at home, 249–
    251
  presentation and diagnosis, 248
  psychological counseling, postop-
    erative, 251–253
  radical mastectomy, 249
  risk factors, 247
  statistics on, 247–248
  survival rates, 247–248
  total mastectomy, 249–256